Molecular Mechanism of Congenital Heart Disease and Pulmonary Hypertension

Toshio Nakanishi · H. Scott Baldwin
Jeffrey R. Fineman · Hiroyuki Yamagishi
Editors

Molecular Mechanism of Congenital Heart Disease and Pulmonary Hypertension

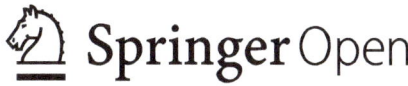

Springer Open

Editors
Toshio Nakanishi
Department of Pediatric Cardiology
Tokyo Women's Medical University
Tokyo
Japan

Jeffrey R. Fineman
UCSF Benioff Children's Hospital
University of California
San Francisco, CA
USA

H. Scott Baldwin
Department of Pediatrics and Cell and
Developmental Biology
Vanderbilt University Medical Center
Nashville, TN
USA

Hiroyuki Yamagishi
Division of Pediatric Cardiology
Department of Pediatrics
Keio University School of Medicine
Tokyo
Japan

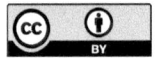

This book is an open access publication.
ISBN 978-981-15-1184-4   ISBN 978-981-15-1185-1   (eBook)
https://doi.org/10.1007/978-981-15-1185-1

This Springer imprint is published by the registered company Springer Nature Singapore Pte Ltd.
The registered company address is: 152 Beach Road, #21-01/04 Gateway East, Singapore 189721,
Singapore

Preface

How does the advance in science happen? Is it a sudden phenomenon like an unexpected illumination or a result of collective addition of many small facts?

This book is based on the 8th Takao International Symposium on Molecular Mechanism of Cardiopulmonary Disease—New Insight into the Development of Pulmonary Circulation and Ductus Arteriosus—in October 2017 in Matsue, Japan.

The Takao International Symposium was first held in 1978 by Dr. Atsuyoshi Takao who was a professor and the chief of Pediatric Cardiology at the Heart Institute of Japan in Tokyo Women's Medical University from 1972 to 1990 (passed away on August 8, 2006, at the age of 81). In the 1970s, Dr. Takao wanted to facilitate basic science in pediatric cardiology by holding international conferences, putting researchers together in a small place, and letting them discuss the etiology of congenital heart diseases (CHD). Since the success of the first symposium, it has been held every 4–5 years and after he passed away, twice in recent 5 years. The proceeding books were published after each symposium in 1980, 1984, 1990, 1995, 2000, 2005, 2015, and this time in 2020. It is amazing that so much advance in science has been accomplished since the first Takao symposium, with path-breaking changes occurring in fields ranging from experimental teratology to molecular biology.

At this time of the 8th Takao symposium, we, organizers, thought that it might be a good time to change the field of discussion somewhat from cardiac morphogenesis to lung development. Pulmonary circulation consists of airway, lung parenchyma, and pulmonary vessels, and each component can have diseases closely related with CHD. Development of the lung in the embryonic stage may have a common pathway of heart development. Researchers in the field of cardiac morphogenesis may be interested to talk with researchers in the field of pulmonary circulation. Also, between the heart and lung, there is a ductus arteriosus, which has unique characteristics, although it is so close to the pulmonary artery. Thus, the 8th Takao symposium focused on new insights into the development of pulmonary circulation as well as basic science of pulmonary hypertension (PH) and ductus arteriosus. The aim of the meeting was to mix old friends studying cardiac morphogenesis with new friends studying pulmonary circulation and ductus arteriosus.

Although PH in the field of pediatric cardiology shares common features of adult PH, it is associated with diverse diseases with onset at any age. The etiology of pediatric PH is quite different to that of adults, including idiopathic pulmonary arterial hypertension, PH associated with CHD, and/or developmental lung diseases.

Recently, medical and surgical treatment of CHD has been well established, and the associated PH and/or pulmonary arterial disorders have become important causes of morbidity and mortality in children. The management of such children remains challenging as treatments are basically dependent on evidence-based studies in adult and/or the clinical expertise of pediatric cardiologists. Moreover, there is still a lack of data on treatment strategies, effectiveness, pharmacokinetics as well as basic science of pulmonary vascular development and disorders.

The ductus arteriosus is an essential fetal structure, which provides a fetal arterial shunt between the main pulmonary artery and the descending aorta. Normally, the ductus arteriosus begins to close immediately after birth, but in some cases, it remains patent after birth and results in severe complications including PH, right ventricular dysfunction, and respiratory failure. On the other hand, patent ductus arteriosus after birth is required for patients with some complex CHD in which the systemic or pulmonary circulation is dependent on the blood flow through the ductus arteriosus. Understanding of the precise molecular mechanism underlying ductus closure is, therefore, important in the field of pediatric cardiology. The final step of ductus closure is as a result of vascular remodeling events driven by the cascade of signaling pathways that have not been fully elucidated.

In this proceedings book, many interesting results in the field of "Basic Science of Lungs and Pulmonary Circulation," "Clinical/Translational Science of Pulmonary Hypertension," "Basic and Clinical Science of Ductus Arteriosus and Vessels," as well as "Development and Regeneration of Cardiovascular System" are presented. These interactive chapters must contribute to an enthusiastic and exciting advance in science. We hope to shed light on the basic mechanisms of PH by studying basic science in the development of the lung, pulmonary vessels, ductus arteriosus, and heart.

Finally, we would like to note that the Takao symposium and its publications have been supported by the Akemi-chan Fund from The Sankei press since its inception. The Akemi-chan Fund was set up over 50 years ago to save the life of Akemi-chan who was a Japanese girl with ventricular septal defect. Since that time, the fund has been supported by the donation from many persons from all over Japan. Also, we would like to appreciate the support from the Japanese Society of Pediatric Cardiology and Cardiac Surgery, Japan Research Promotion Society for Cardiovascular Diseases, and the Cardiovascular Development Forum in Japan. The purpose of this Forum is to study the etiology and management of CHD, from both basic and clinical aspects, as well as to exchange the results among the members in order to contribute to the development of medicine which totally overlaps with the concept propounded by Dr. Takao. We do hope that this book would shed light on the direction in which we should proceed in the research field in the next 5 years, to ultimately save the lives of those who suffer from congenital and acquired heart and lung diseases.

Tokyo, Japan   Toshio Nakanishi
Tokyo, Japan   Hiroyuki Yamagishi

Contents

Part IV   Development and Regeneration of the Cardiovascular System

Part I

Basic Science of Pulmonary Development and Pulmonary Arterial Disease

Perspective for Part I

Hiroyuki Yamagishi

The lungs are the primary organs of the respiratory system in vertebrates, other than fish, that function as an efficient gas exchanger. This respiratory system is physically and physiologically connected to the cardiovascular system to extract oxygen from the atmosphere and transfer it into the bloodstream and to release carbon dioxide from the bloodstream into the atmosphere. The normal pulmonary circulation, in contrast to the systemic circulation, has low pressure because of a low-resistant vascular bed that enables highly efficient gas exchange between the millions of alveoli and capillaries. Pulmonary hypertension (PH) is a rare pulmonary arterial disease with a high mortality and morbidity although treatment options have improved in the last decades. PH is defined by a mean pulmonary artery pressure (mPAP) greater than or equal to 20 mmHg at rest and is classified into five main subgroups based on the etiology and hemodynamic criteria. Because PH is heterogeneous at the genetic and molecular levels, a deeper understanding is required for the development of more effective therapies.

In Part I, the basic science for the development of the lungs and the pathogenesis of PH is discussed towards a better understanding of the etiology and pathophysiology of PH. Drs. Hogan and Morimoto overview the morphogenesis and epithelial development of the lung. Each alveolus in lungs is composed of epithelial and mesenchymal populations. Dr. Hogan (Chap. 2) focuses on the interesting function of Type 2 epithelial cells, as epithelial stem cells for the alveoli, capable of long-term self-renewal and differentiation into Type 1 epithelial cells that are extremely large and thin to be specialized for gas exchange. The relative contribution of the WNT, FGF, EGF, and BMP signaling pathways as well as cytokines produced by immune

H. Yamagishi (✉)
Division of Pediatric Cardiology, Department of Pediatrics,
Keio University School of Medicine, Tokyo, Japan
e-mail: hyamag@keio.jp

© The Editor(s) (if applicable) and The Author(s) 2020
T. Nakanishi et al. (eds.), *Molecular Mechanism of Congenital Heart Disease and Pulmonary Hypertension*, https://doi.org/10.1007/978-981-15-1185-1_1

cells to alveolar homeostasis, repair and regrowth is discussed. Dr. Morimoto (Chap. 3) focuses on Notch signaling as a reciprocal mesenchymal-epithelial interaction that controls the development of the airway branching structure. Notch-mediated cell fate selection is utilized to organize three epithelial cell types during the bronchial tree is extending. As for the mesenchymal population that gives rise to endothelial cells, pericytes, several different fibroblast subpopulations, and immune cells, Dr. Uchida et al. (Chap. 8) suggest that the expression of a transcription factor Tbx4 in the lung mesenchyme may be involved in the formation of both airways and vessels in the lungs using animal experiments. It is also known that mutations of the TBX4 gene lead to PH in human. Dr. Ishizaki et al. (Chap. 9) demonstrate that pulmonary arterial smooth muscle layers, probably derived from mesenchyme of the mesodermal origin, may elongate gradually from the proximal pulmonary arterial trunk to bilateral peripheral pulmonary arteries by using a transgenic mouse line harboring the LacZ reporter gene in the specific locus. This observation supports the "distal angiogenesis" model for pulmonary arterial development.

PH is also known as a progressive pulmonary vascular remodeling disease. Histopathological changes in PH include an increase in smooth muscle cells in the pulmonary vasculature with muscularization of normally non-muscularized distal pulmonary arterioles. Dr. Greif's team (Chap. 4) identified novel smooth muscle cell progenitors located at the muscular-unmuscular arteriole border that have a unique molecular signature and are the source of the vast majority of pathological distal arteriole smooth muscle cells in PH. Molecular mechanisms underlying induction, proliferation, migration, and differentiation of these specialized progenitor cells are discussed. In addition to the above-described fashions to increase smooth muscle cells in the pulmonary vasculature of PH, recent studies have demonstrated that a part of smooth muscle cells from intimal and plexiform lesions has an endothelial origin through the process of endothelial-mesenchymal transition (EMT). Dr. Ranchoux et al. (Chap. 6) describe how EMT appears to play a crucial role in PH progression including the underlying molecular mechanisms. As another advanced understanding for pathogenesis of PH, Drs. Chen and Raj (Chap. 7) focus on extracellular vesicles. Subsets of extracellular vesicles are microvesicles, exosomes, and apoptotic bodies. They are released from a variety of cell types and carry cargo such as proteins and microRNAs that may play an important role in the pathogenesis of PH.

Utilizing animal models, three important findings about the pathogenesis of PH are also discussed in Part I. Dr. Nakanishi et al. (Chap. 11) show morphological changes of pulmonary microvasculature in the mouse model of bronchopulmonary dysplasia (BPD). As BPD is often associated with PH, their study may provide insights into secondary PH due to pulmonary diseases. Dr. Zhang et al. (Chap. 12) identify significant increased expression of chemokine receptor type 4 (CXCR4) and some stem cell markers in PH model rats as putative mediators of pulmonary vascular remodeling. Dr. Shibata et al. (Chap. 13) demonstrate that Ca^{2+} signal through the inositol trisphosphate receptor (IP_3R) may be involved in the pathophysiology of PH using IP_3R knockout mice. CXCR4 or IP_3R might be a potential candidate for new therapeutic targets of PH.

Finally, Dr. Clapp's group (Chap. 5) discuss about basic science for the treatment of PH. Although there were no treatments available for PH 20 years ago, current therapies come from four drug classes, namely, prostanoid analogs, endothelin receptor antagonists, phosphodiesterase type 5 inhibitors, and soluble guanylate cyclase stimulators, and through focused research, there are more in development. Intravenous prostacyclin, as a prostanoid analog, remains the most efficacious treatment for PH, and several prostacyclin analogs are approved for use via different administration routes. They act as vasodilators but potently inhibit platelet aggregation, cell proliferation, and inflammation. Dr. Clapp et al. discuss how prostacyclins might rescue BMPR2 and TASK-1 dysfunction and the importance of prostanoid EP2 receptors as negative modulators of vascular tone, proliferation, and fibrosis. BMPR2 is known as the most important genetic cause of PH, and TASK-1 is a TWIK-related acid-sensitive potassium channel that, they believe, is likely to be a key target for prostacyclins. As basic research for future stem cell therapy of PH, Dr. Maeda et al. (Chap. 10) suggest that stem cell antigen-1 in the pulmonary endothelium may potentially make progenitor cell populations stay resident in adult murine lungs.

The field of pulmonary vascular biology continues to capitalize on advances in basic science. Part I includes a number of exciting advances in basic science and how these advances are impacting the patient with PH. This knowledge should be required for physicians and scientists to be translated into future clinical practice.

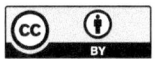

The Alveolar Stem Cell Niche of the Mammalian Lung

2

Brigid L. M. Hogan

Abstract

The alveolar region of the mammalian lung evolved to enable highly efficient gas exchange between the millions of air-filled sacs known as alveoli and blood circulating through the pulmonary vessels. Each alveolus is composed of epithelial and mesenchymal populations; Type 1 (AT1) and Type 2 (AT2) epithelial cells line the sacs while the mesenchymal compartment is composed of endothelial cells, pericytes, several different fibroblast subpopulations, and immune cells. Compared with organs such as the intestine and skin, there is normally little cell turnover in the adult lung. However, if the alveolar epithelium is damaged, for example, by toxic agents or viral infections, or if a lung lobe is removed, there is extensive repair or compensatory regrowth (neoalveolarization) of the tissue. It is now well accepted that AT2s function as epithelial stem cells for the alveoli, capable of long-term self-renewal and differentiation into AT1s. However, many important questions remain, in particular, about the functional heterogeneity of AT2s and how the different components of their local environment or niche interact to regulate their proliferation and differentiation. Known signaling factors include ligands and antagonists of the WNT, FGF, EGF and bone morphogenetic (BMP) signaling pathways as well as cytokines produced by immune cells. The relative contribution of these factors to alveolar homeostasis, repair and regrowth is discussed.

Keywords

Lung · Alveolar stem cell niche · Compensatory regrowth · Signaling pathways

B. L. M. Hogan (✉)
Department of Cell Biology, Duke University Medical School, Durham, NC, USA
e-mail: brigid.hogan@duke.edu

© The Editor(s) (if applicable) and The Author(s) 2020
T. Nakanishi et al. (eds.), *Molecular Mechanism of Congenital Heart Disease and Pulmonary Hypertension*, https://doi.org/10.1007/978-981-15-1185-1_2

7

2.1   Introduction: The Alveolar Type 2 Epithelial Stem Cell Niche

Our current understanding of the alveolar stem cell niche of the mammalian lung is schematized in Fig. 2.1 [1–4]. Each alveolus contains two kinds of epithelial cells: Type 2 cells (AT2s), specialized for producing, secreting and recycling surfactant lipids and proteins, and Type 1 cells (AT1s) that are extremely large and thin and specialized for gas exchange [5]. It is now well accepted AT2s that express surfactant protein C (Sftpc) can function as stem cells during homeostasis and repair by self-renewing and giving rise to AT1s. However, the rate at which AT2s proliferate and differentiate depends on local "demand." At steady state the rate is very low. If lungs are experimentally depleted of only AT2s then their proliferation increases but differentiation is still minimal [6]. However, if AT1s are also damaged or if whole new alveoli need to be generated in response to partial (left lobe) pneumonectomy (PPnx), then AT2s both self-renew and show robust AT1 differentiation [7–9]. How AT2s detect the absence of AT1s is unclear; perhaps they sense denuded basal lamina or a reduction in cellular contacts with AT1s or, in the case of PPnx, an increase in mechanical tension [10].

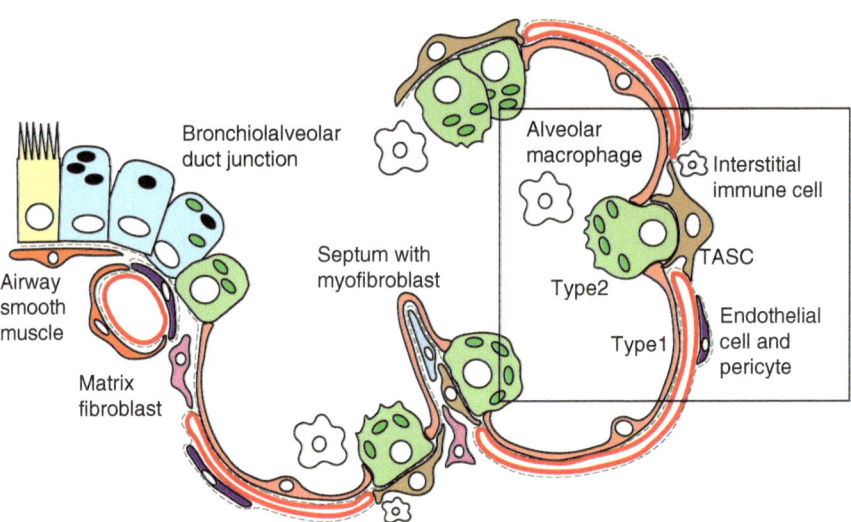

Fig. 2.1 Schematic representation of the alveolar region of the mouse lung. The Type 2 stem cell niche (boxed) includes fibroblasts known as TASCs that have long cytoplasmic extensions, AT1 cells, capillary endothelial cells and pericytes as well as alveolar macrophages and interstitial immune cells. Alveolar septae contain myofibroblasts, and other fibroblast cell types (matrix fibroblasts) are present in the stroma

2.2   Evidence for Heterogeneity in the AT2 Population

An important unanswered question is whether *all* AT2s have the same stem cell potential or whether this is a property of a privileged few. Significantly, two groups have recently shown that at steady state a minority of AT2s express a reporter for *Axin2*, a downstream target of canonical Wnt signaling. One group [11] found that only 1% of the AT2s were positive although more cells became active in response to injury. By contrast, a second group [12] reported that 20–30% of AT2s were positive at steady state and constituted a stable subpopulation which they termed alveolar epithelial progenitors (AEPs). In both cases evidence was presented that the Wnt ligand responsible for upregulating *Axin2* and promoting AT2 proliferation is produced by niche fibroblasts in close proximity to AT2s, termed MANCs (mesenchymal alveolar niche cells). These cells can also produce Wnt antagonists, which reduce AT2 proliferation and promote differentiation, and may, therefore, fine tune the dynamic response of the stem cells during repair [13].

In the light of these studies, one may ask whether AT2 subpopulations have been detected by single-cell transcriptomic analysis. One recent study does show a minor AT2 subpopulation in the steady state lung, defined as "alveolar bipotential progenitors" [14]. However, these cells are distinguished by co-expressing markers of AT2s and AT1s but not by *Axin2* levels. In support of the single-cell RNA-seq data, a recent report [8] identified by immunohistochemistry a small subpopulation (less than 1%) of AT2s co-expressing Sftpc and Ager (advanced glycosylation and end product-specific receptor, a marker for AT1s). The proportion of these dual-positive cells increases to 20% by 7 days after PPnx when compensatory cell proliferation is active. In addition, when isolated AT2 cells are placed in 3D organoid culture under conditions in which single cells give rise to structures known as "alveolospheres" containing both AT2s and AT1s, all of the cells initially and transiently become dual positive for Sftpc and Ager [8]. This behavior may indicate a reversion of mature AT2s to a more plastic, bipotential state under conditions promoting repair. New genetic tools are clearly needed to test the in vivo significance of the dual-positive cells and their relation, if any, to Axin2+ epithelial cells [11, 12].

2.3   Signaling Pathways in the Stem Cell Niche

Besides WNTs and their antagonists, a number of other signaling factors have been identified as playing a role in the mouse lung alveolar stem cell niche. Pathways include those regulated by Fgfs (largely produced by fibroblast populations), Vegf (secreted by AT2s), Bmps and Egfs. Egf signaling is thought to be mediated both by the ligand itself and by peptides released from the extracellular matrix after injury. This latter mechanism has been proposed for the proliferation of AT2s after PPnx [15]. Specifically, it appears that in response to PPnx pulmonary capillary endothelial cells (PCECs) activate the expression of the matrix metalloproteinase MMP14. This degrades laminin and releases peptides with a cryptic Egf domain that can bind to Egf receptors in the AT2 cells. Changes in PCECs and perivascular macrophages have also been implicated in the response of the alveolar region to damage by bleo-mycin or HCL [16]. In this case, it is argued that the notch ligand Jagged1 is upregu-lated in the damaged PCECs, affecting the behavior of adjacent fibroblasts. Given the recent finding that lung microvasculature is a major site of platelet biogenesis and a reservoir for hematopoietic progenitors [17] there are likely many other ways in which cytokines and angiocrine factors produced by the vascular compartment influence the stem cell niche.

BMP signaling in the alveolar niche has not received much attention until recently since most research has focused on the pathway in the etiology of pulmo-nary hypertension. However, immunohistochemistry with antibodies to phosphoS-mad1/5/8 shows that BMP signaling is active in both epithelial and stromal cells of the alveolar region. Signaling is transiently downregulated after PPnx when AT2s are proliferating and preparing to differentiate into AT1s. This transient downregu-lation is likely brought about by the upregulation of BMP antagonists, including follistatin and follistatin-like 1 by stromal cells rather than downregulation of BMP ligands [8].

2.4   The Role of Immune Cells and Stromal Cells in Alveolar Repair and Regeneration

One of the major roadblocks to our understanding of the alveolar stem cell niche is the precise identification of the different mesenchymal/mesoderm-derived cell types in the region. This population includes lipofibroblasts (cells with varying numbers of lipid inclusion), myofibroblasts (cells rich in smooth muscle actin) and "matrix fibroblasts" and their progenitors [13, 14, 18]. The lung also contains a rich and varied population of resident immune cells with multiple subclasses of dendritic cells and innate lymphoid cells, and interstitial and alveolar macrophages. Immune cells are recruited to the alveolar niche after injury and can play important roles in repair and regrowth. Recent studies have shown a role for bone marrow–derived macrophages in compensatory regrowth after PPnx [9]. Genetic deletion of the bone marrow-derived macrophages, or the innate immune cells thought to activate them, results in reduced AT2 proliferation and regrowth. In the future, it will be important to determine the precise mechanism by which the macrophages promote repair, for example, whether they produce cytokines acting directly on AT2s or function indi-rectly through other components of the niche.

Progress in defining the precise physiological function of the different stromal populations in the alveolar region has been hampered by the relative paucity of tools for genetically manipulating and lineage tracing specific cell types. We, therefore, generated a new *Pdgfra-CreEr* knock-in allele (Jackson Lab stock number 032770) to test the function of genes expressed in fibroblasts expressing the Pdgf receptor alpha. This is a heterogeneous population but includes cells intimately associated with AT2s that we have called Type 2 associated stromal cells, or TASCs [8]. These cells have a very distinct morphology with long cellular extensions and may be the same as the MANCs described by others [13]. They likely represent the mouse equivalent of cells described in the human lung that make contact with AT2, AT1 and endothelial cells [19] and are, therefore, well positioned to integrate signaling pathways within the niche.

2.5   Future Directions and Clinical Implications

This review highlights recent advances in our understanding of the cells and signaling pathways that regulate AT2 proliferation and differentiation in the alveolar niche of the mouse lung. In the long term, this information may inspire new clinical strategies for promoting alveolar repair from remaining endogenous stem cells in damaged human lungs. A major challenge is to translate techniques used with mouse cells to primary cells isolated from the human lung. For example, the "alveolosphere" organoid culture system that has been used so successfully to screen for factors that regulate AT2 stem cell behavior is much less efficient with human AT2 cells for reasons that are currently unclear [20]. Nevertheless, progress is being made and we should expect to see important advances in the near future.

Acknowledgment   Work from the authors' laboratory was funded by the USA National Heart, Lung and Blood Institute.

References

1. Leach JP, Morrisey EE. Repairing the lungs one breath at a time: how dedicated or facultative are you? Genes Dev. 2018;32(23-24):1461–71.
2. Hogan BL, et al. Repair and regeneration of the respiratory system: complexity, plasticity, and mechanisms of lung stem cell function. Cell Stem Cell. 2014;15(2):123–38.
3. Tata PR, Rajagopal J. Plasticity in the lung: making and breaking cell identity. Development. 2017;144(5):755–66.
4. Borok Z, et al. Cell plasticity in lung injury and repair: report from an NHLBI workshop, April 19-20, 2010. Proc Am Thorac Soc. 2011;8(3):215–22.
5. Weibel ER. On the tricks alveolar epithelial cells play to make a good lung. Am J Respir Crit Care Med. 2015;191(5):504–13.
6. Barkauskas CE, et al. Type 2 alveolar cells are stem cells in adult lung. J Clin Invest. 2013;123(7):3025–36.
7. Desai TJ, Brownfield DG, Krasnow MA. Alveolar progenitor and stem cells in lung development, renewal and cancer. Nature. 2014;507(7491):190–4.
8. Chung MI, et al. Niche-mediated BMP/SMAD signaling regulates lung alveolar stem cell proliferation and differentiation. Development. 2018;145(9)
9. Lechner AJ, et al. Recruited monocytes and Type 2 immunity promote lung regeneration following pneumonectomy. Cell Stem Cell. 2017;21(1):120–134.e7.
10. Liu Z, et al. MAPK-mediated YAP activation controls mechanical-tension-induced pulmonary alveolar regeneration. Cell Rep. 2016;16(7):1810–9.
11. Nabhan AN, et al. Single-cell Wnt signaling niches maintain stemness of alveolar type 2 cells. Science. 2018;359(6380):1118–23.
12. Zacharias WJ, et al. Regeneration of the lung alveolus by an evolutionarily conserved epithelial progenitor. Nature. 2018;555(7695):251–5.

13. Zepp JA, et al. Distinct mesenchymal lineages and niches promote epithelial self-renewal and myofibrogenesis in the lung. Cell. 2017;170(6):1134–1148.e10.
14. Han X, et al. Mapping the mouse cell atlas by Microwell-Seq. Cell. 2018;172(5):1091–1107. e17.
15. Ding BS, et al. Endothelial-derived angiocrine signals induce and sustain regenerative lung alveolarization. Cell. 2011;147(3):539–53.
16. Cao Z, et al. Targeting of the pulmonary capillary vascular niche promotes lung alveolar repair and ameliorates fibrosis. Nat Med. 2016;22(2):154–62.
17. Lefrancais E, et al. The lung is a site of platelet biogenesis and a reservoir for haematopoietic progenitors. Nature. 2017;544(7648):105–9.
18. Tabula Muris C, et al. Single-cell transcriptomics of 20 mouse organs creates a Tabula Muris. Nature. 2018;562(7727):367–72.
19. Sirianni FE, Chu FS, Walker DC. Human alveolar wall fibroblasts directly link epithelial type 2 cells to capillary endothelium. Am J Respir Crit Care Med. 2003;168(12):1532–7.
20. Barkauskas CE, et al. Lung organoids: current uses and future promise. Development. 2017;144(6):986–97.

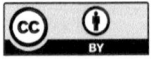

Lung Development and Notch Signaling

3

Mitsuru Morimoto

Abstract

The respiratory system is connected to the cardiovascular system physically and physiologically. This chapter overviews the morphogenesis and epithelial development of the lung. The airway branching structure is formed as development progresses and is controlled by reciprocal mesenchymal-epithelial interactions. During the branching process, the distal terminal buds are thought to contain a population of multipotent epithelial progenitors that are more proliferative than proximal cells. This predominant proliferation in the distal tip leads to the lung bud extension toward the distal end. As the bronchial tree extends further, descendants of these multipotent cells give rise to lineage-restricted progenitors in the conducting airways. Notch signaling is used repeatedly to organize three epithelial cell types: Club, ciliated, and neuroendocrine (NE) cells. The Notch-mediated fate selection of Club/ciliated cells and of the size of NE cell clusters is regulated by different mechanisms. The Club/ciliated cell fate decision is mediated exclusively by Notch2 in response to Jag1. In contrast, all three Notch receptors contribute to robustly regulate the NE cell-cluster size. High-resolution whole-mount imaging of the developing lung revealed that the NE cell cluster appears at the stereotypic positions at the bifurcating area of the branching airways. Moreover, the 4D imaging, 3D plus live-imaging, method for developing lung epithelial cells discovered dynamics of NE cell clustering in which NE cells appear at inter-bifurcation area as solitary cells and migrate toward the branching points to form clusters. Further analyses determined that Notch signaling regulates the number of solitary NE cells in a lateral-inhibition fashion.

M. Morimoto (✉)
RIKEN Center for Biosystems Dynamics Research, Laboratory for Lung Development and Regeneration, Kobe, Japan
e-mail: mitsuru.morimoto@riken.jp

© The Editor(s) (if applicable) and The Author(s) 2020
T. Nakanishi et al. (eds.), *Molecular Mechanism of Congenital Heart Disease and Pulmonary Hypertension*, https://doi.org/10.1007/978-981-15-1185-1_3

13

Keywords

Lung · Notch signaling · Cell fate selection · Live imaging · Directional cell migration

3.1   Introduction

The lung facilitates gas exchange by maximizing ventilation efficiency and the surface area of interface to the capillaries. The developing lung forms an intricate, but stereotypic, branching airway structure and arrayed epithelial cells (Fig. 3.1). Air from the external environment includes viruses, bacteria, and toxic chemical compounds, which means that the airways may become damaged and need to be repaired rapidly. For these reasons, the lung is a useful model organ for studying cellular events that are conserved between organogenesis in the embryo and tissue regeneration in the adult.

3.2   Morphogenesis and Epithelial Progenitors

For the last two decades, extensive studies using mouse models have revealed biological processes and genes that regulate lung development. Although there are significant differences in tissue size, the lungs in human and mouse display similar

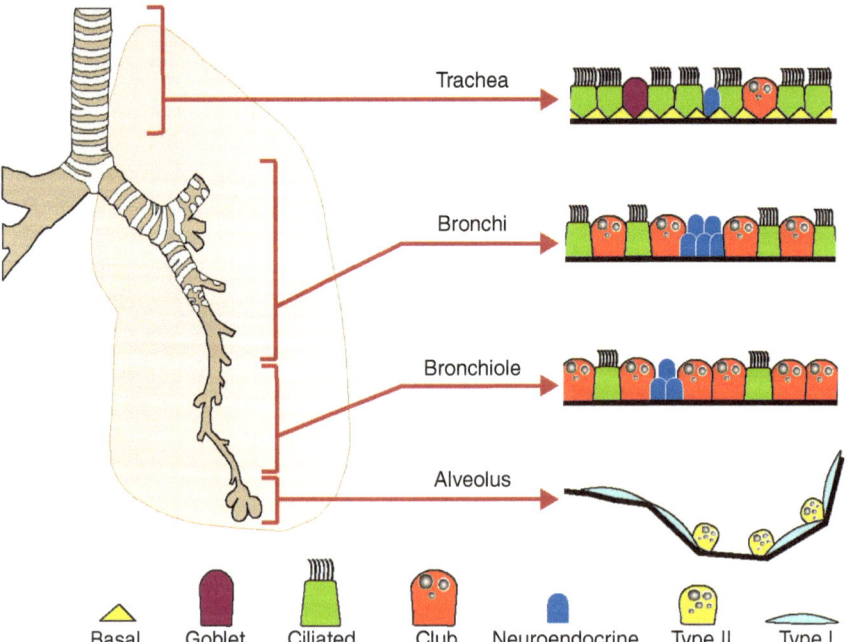

Fig. 3.1 The structure of the lung airways and their epithelial components

Fig. 3.2 The distal tip stem cells and proximal differentiated cells in developing airways during pseudoglandular stage

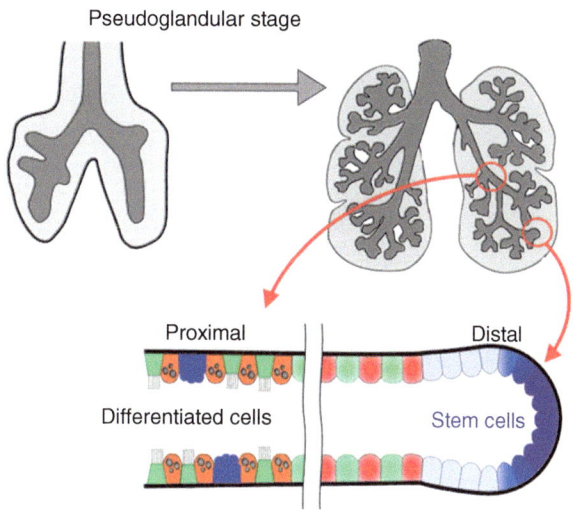

histology and pathology [1], suggesting that the mouse lung may be a useful model system for investigating organ biology and human disease. Lung development relies on reciprocal mesenchymal-epithelial interactions orchestrated by temporal and spatial expression waves of multiple secreted factors and their downstream effectors [2]. Airway branching morphogenesis takes place at E11.5–16.5 in the mouse and at 5–17 weeks in human embryo (known as pseudoglandular stage, during which most of airway branching morphogenesis takes place); it is thought that the terminal buds contain a population of multipotent epithelial progenitors (Fig. 3.2) [3]. While the buds extend and branch in a genetically coordinated stereotypic pattern [4], the progenitors give rise to lineage-restricted descendants that produce at least seven major cell types in the 'stalk' region [3, 5]. Thus, the early stalks form the proximal airway, then the distal airways, and finally the alveoli [6]. In the proximal airway, the tracheal epithelium consists of the basal, goblet, Club (secretory), and ciliated cells. Smaller bronchi contain the latter two cell types and pulmonary neuroendocrine (NE) cells. The distal-most airway, the alveolus, is lined with thin layers of flat Type I cells and cuboidal Type II cells (Fig. 3.1).

3.3 Notch Signaling Controls Both Epithelial Cell Fates and Distributions

One of the outstanding questions in the field is how epithelial cells interact and exchange information to generate and maintain the appropriate balance in their respective cell numbers and distributions. Using genetic engineering methods, we have performed stepwise removal of the components of Notch signaling, a key signaling in cell fate decisions in developing lung epithelium, and revealed that Notch signaling is used reiteratively to organize three major epithelial cell types: Club,

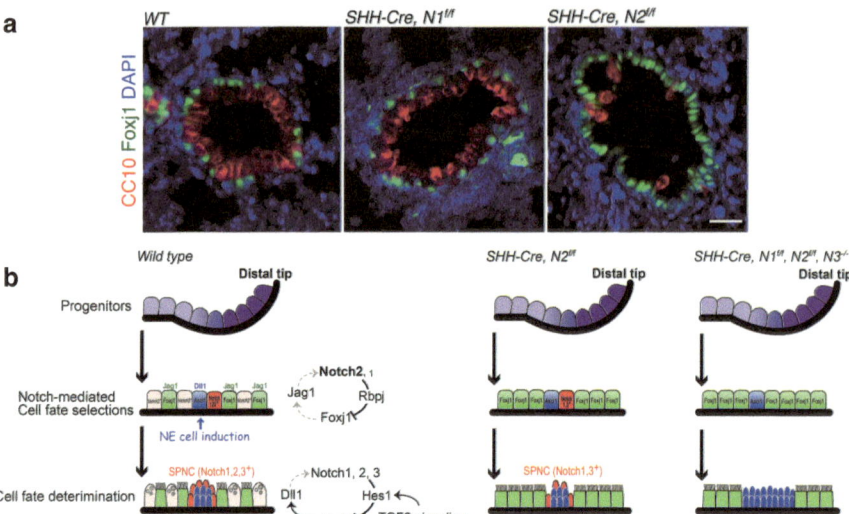

Fig. 3.3 Loss of Notch signaling phenotypes within airway epithelium. (**a**) Immunostainings for Club (CC10, Red) and ciliated (Foxj1, Green) cells of epithelial Notch1 or 2 conditional KO lung. (**b**) Schematic diagrams of the proposed regulatory mechanisms involved in Notch-mediated cell fate determination during bronchial epithelial development. In the pseudoglandular stage, epithelial progenitors (purple) located at the distal tip produce descendants that differentiate into Club (pink), ciliated (green), SPNC (red) and NE (blue) cells

ciliated, and NE cells [7, 8]. We also identified significant differences between the selection of Club/ciliated cells and the size regulation of NE cell clusters. The Club/ciliated cell fate decision is mediated exclusively by Notch2 in response to Jag1 with negligible contributions from Notch1 and 3 (Fig. 3.3a). In contrast, all three Notch receptors respond to Dll1 and contribute in an additive manner to regulate NE cell cluster numbers and size (Fig. 3.3b). These results indicate that two distinct Notch signaling pathways, involving Jag1-Notch2 and Dll1-Notch123 signaling, respectively, coordinate the number and distribution of the major epithelial cell types of the conducting airway in lung organogenesis. However, at the time we were unable to clarify the Notch-mediated mechanism by which the NE cell number and cluster size are regulated.

3.4 Development of NE Cell Clusters on Bifurcating Area of Branching Airways

The pulmonary NE cells are thought to function as chemoreceptors and as a component of the stem cell niche and are also the cells of origin in small-cell lung cancer. NE cells often localize at bifurcation points of airway tubes, forming small clusters called neuroepithelial bodies (NEBs). These are referred to as "nodal" NEBs [9] whereas NEBs in inter-bifurcation regions are called "internodal" (Fig. 3.4). Despite

Fig. 3.4 Immunohistochemistry of the NE cell marker CGRP (brown) for E18.5 mouse lung. The arrowheads indicate the NEBs on bifurcation points (black) or inter-bifurcation region (gray)

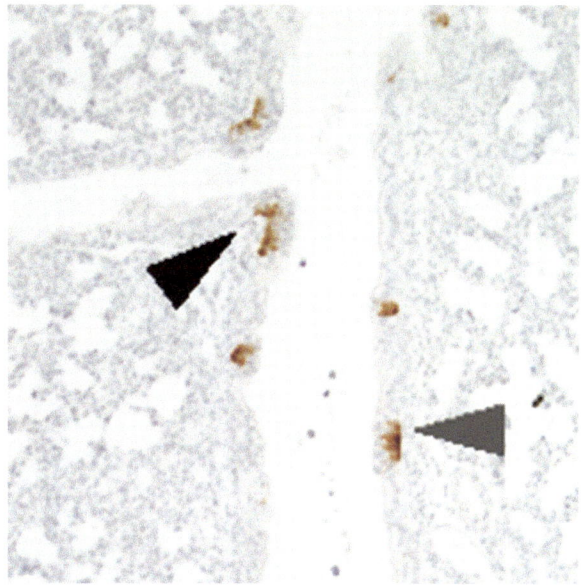

the functional importance of NE cells and NEBs, their developmental course remains unclear in part because of technical limitations in obtaining high-resolution images and quantitative analysis of the behavior of epithelial cells in the context of a 3D branching morphology. We have established methods for 3D mapping of lung epithelial cells and ex vivo 4D imaging of the developing lung [10].

To accurately map the positions of all NEBs throughout the entire respiratory tree, we used two-photon microscopy to image whole-mount lungs in a transgenic mouse strain, $Ret^{EGFP/+}$; $SHH^{Cre/+}$; $R26R^{H2B-mCherry}$ mice visualizing NE cells in the epithelium (EGFP+; mCherry+) and neuronal cells in the mesenchyme (EGFP+; mCherry−). Lungs were collected at E14.5, E15.5, and E16.5 and cleared using clear, unobstructed brain imaging cocktail (CUBIC) solution [11]. The 3D architecture of mCherry+ lung epithelium was extracted computationally from 3D image stacks by removal of mesenchymal signals, and data on the positions of all epithelial and NE cells were recorded (Fig. 3.5a). These 3D imaging and quantitative analyses revealed that nodal NEBs are significantly larger than internodal NEBs at each stage. We redefined the localization of nodal NEBs by close examination of their positions within the entire geometric architecture of the airway tubes (Fig. 3.5b). These geometric analyses revealed that nodal NEBs are located at stereotypic positions in airway branching structures.

3.5 Notch-Hes1 Signaling Is Required for Restricted Differentiation of Solitary NE Cells

To determine the mechanisms of Notch-mediated NEB development, we genetically ablated *Hes1* gene, which is the target of Notch signaling and a regulator of NE cell development [12], from endodermal epithelium by generating $SHH^{Cre/+}$;

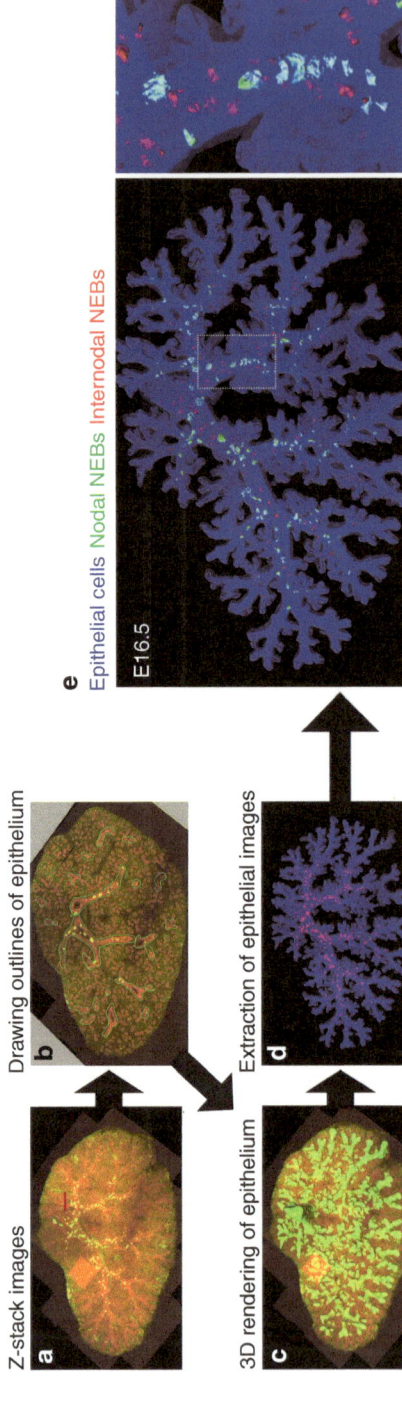

Fig. 3.5 Processes of 3D image analysis. Z-stack images of *SHH^Cre/+*, *R26R^H2B-mCherry*, *RET^eGFP/+* lungs were collected (**a**). The outlines of the epithelium are labeled on each 2D image using IMARIS drawing mode (**b**). The enclosed regions of the raw images were processed with 3D rendering (**c**). Epithelium was colored in blue and the NEB signals were regionalized (**d**). Finally, the NEBs were classified as nodal (green) or internodal (red) NEBs by their positions on the bifurcating tissue structure (**e**)

Hes1$^{f/f}$ mice. Ascl1-positive primordial NE cells were examined at E13.5. Compared with normal epithelium, the Hes1-deficient epithelium showed abundant NE cells that tended to adjoin each other at the proximal region in Hes1-deficient epithelium (Fig. 3.6a). The punctate distribution of NE cells in the normal E13.5 lung and the disruption of this pattern in Hes1 mutants suggest that Notch-Hes1 signaling suppresses NE cell fate in a classical lateral inhibition fashion (Fig. 3.6b). To analyze the effect of Hes1 depletion in NEB formation, we performed NEB 3D mapping by generating *SHH*$^{Cre/+}$; *R26R*$^{H2B-mCherry}$; *Ret*$^{EGFP/+}$; *Hes1*$^{f/f}$ embryos and imaged the cranial lobes at E16.5. In contrast to the wide distribution of NE cells at E13.5, we noted markedly enlarged NEBs throughout the proximal to distal airways (Fig. 3.6c).

3.6   Directional Migration of NE Cells Toward Bifurcation Points Creates Nodal NEBs

We hypothesized that NE cells emerge as solitary cells and, subsequently, migrate toward a bifurcation point to form NEBs. To test this hypothesis, we established a 4D imaging method for the developing lung, involving 3D plus time-lapse imaging of living tissue. We cultured E13.5 cranial lobes at the air-liquid interface on a membrane filter that becomes transparent in liquid (Fig. 3.7a). In these 4D images, NE cells initially appear as individual cells, in line with our expectations. These cells subsequently migrated toward a bifurcation point located in a more distal region and accumulated there to form an NEB (Fig. 3.7b). Some NE cells also clustered at inter-bifurcation areas. These observations support the idea that NE cells emerge as solitary cells via Notch-mediated cell fate selection and, subsequently, migrate toward bifurcation points on the basement membrane to form nodal NEBs (Fig. 3.8). Internodal NEBs may be generated by a population of cells that are arrested during this migration. In this study, we described a spatial relationship between 3D branching morphology and nodal NEB localization. We also provided direct evidence showing that cell-autonomous Notch-Hes1 signaling inhibits NE cell differentiation in a classical lateral inhibition fashion, giving rise to a limited number of NE cells. Our results suggest the presence of at least three factors (or combinations of factors) that control NE cell clustering, working to attract them to the distal trap at bifurcation points and induce their aggregation [10]. We are now investigating molecular mechanisms explaining directional migration and clustering at the bifurcating area of the developing airways.

Given that NE cells are thought to be the cells of origin in highly malignant small-cell lung cancers, investigating the molecular mechanisms of NE cell migration may provide important clues toward the development of new therapeutic approaches to mitigate this malignancy.

Acknowledgments Research in the Morimoto lab is supported by Grants-in-Aid for Scientific Research (B) and Young Scientists (A) 26713029 and 23689044 of the Ministry of Education, Culture, Sports, Science and Technology, Japan, and The Takeda Science Foundation for the Life Science (M.M.).

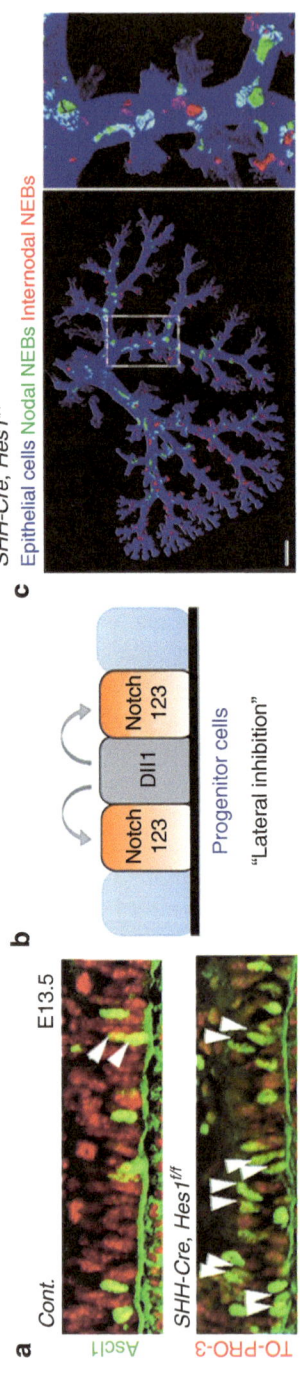

Fig. 3.6 The center lines (red lines) of airway epithelium (blue) and intersection points (white spots) were defined. Right panel shows the magnified view of the dotted square in the left panel. Redefining stereotypic pattern of nodal NEB distributions with 3D information of NE cells and epithelial tube. The NEBs all were ranked by distance from a correlated the centroid of triangle (Red X shows the centroid), and the angle bisector (Red line shows the angle bisector). Rank 1 means the selected nodal NEB is the closest to the point or line among the all NEBs

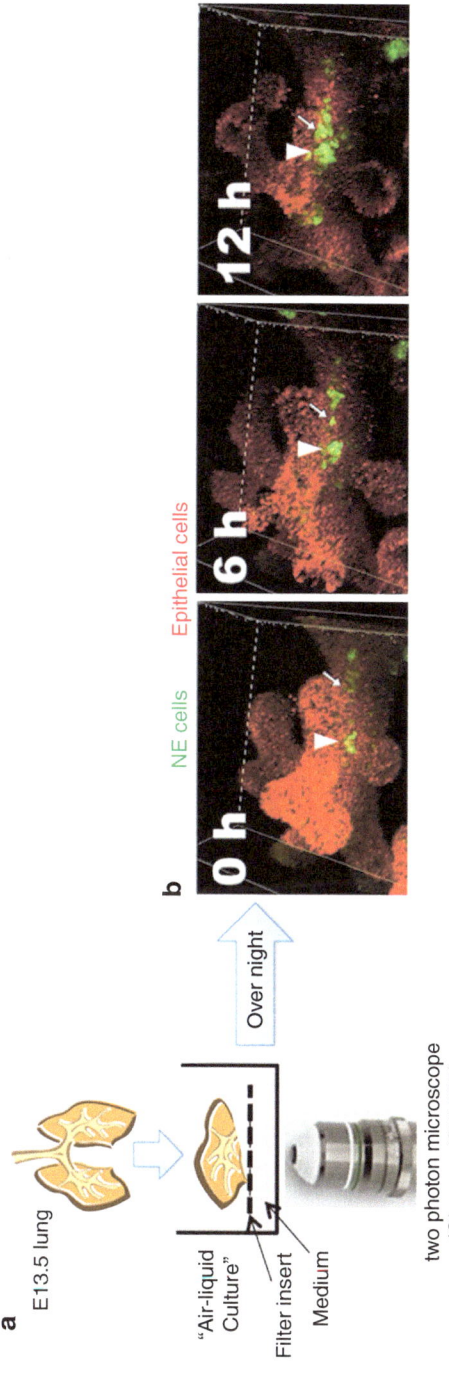

Fig. 3.7 (**a**) Schematic images of lung organ culture for 4D imaging. (**b**) Snapshot images of supplementary movie 5 at 0, 6, and 12 h. Arrowheads indicate NE cell clusters at bifurcation point. Arrows show migrating solitary NE cells

Fig. 3.8 Conclusion

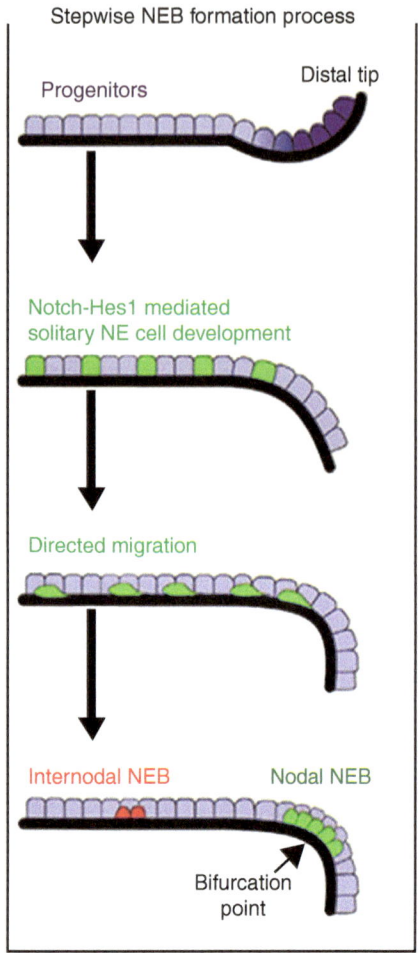

Stepwise NEB formation process

Progenitors

Distal tip

Notch-Hes1 mediated
solitary NE cell development

Directed migration

Internodal NEB   Nodal NEB

Bifurcation
point

References

1. Hogan BL, Barkauskas CE, Chapman HA, et al. Repair and regeneration of the respiratory system: complexity, plasticity, and mechanisms of lung stem cell function. Cell Stem Cell. 2014;15(2):123–38.
2. Morrisey EE, Hogan BL. Preparing for the first breath: genetic and cellular mechanisms in lung development. Dev Cell. 2010;18(1):8–23.
3. Perl AK, Wert SE, Nagy A, et al. Early restriction of peripheral and proximal cell lineages during formation of the lung. Proc Natl Acad Sci U S A. 2002;99(16):10482–7.
4. Metzger RJ, Klein OD, Martin GR, et al. The branching programme of mouse lung development. Nature. 2008;453(7196):745–50.
5. Rawlins EL, Clark CP, Xue Y, et al. The Id2+ distal tip lung epithelium contains individual multipotent embryonic progenitor cells. Development. 2009;136(22):3741–5.
6. Cardoso WV, Lu J. Regulation of early lung morphogenesis: questions, facts and controversies. Development. 2006;133(9):1611–24.

7. Morimoto M, Liu Z, Cheng HT, et al. Canonical notch signaling in the developing lung is required for determination of arterial smooth muscle cells and selection of Clara versus ciliated cell fate. J Cell Sci. 2010;123(Pt 2):213–24.
8. Morimoto M, Nishinakamura R, Saga Y, et al. Different assemblies of notch receptors coordinate the distribution of the major bronchial Clara, ciliated and neuroendocrine cells. Development. 2012;139(23):4365–73.
9. Cutz E, Chan W, Sonstegard KS. Identification of neuro-epithelial bodies in rabbit fetal lungs by scanning electron microscopy: a correlative light, transmission and scanning electron microscopic study. Anat Rec. 1978;192(3):459–66.
10. Noguchi M, Sumiyama K, Morimoto M. Directed migration of pulmonary neuroendocrine cells toward airway branches organizes the stereotypic location of neuroepithelial bodies. Cell Rep. 2015;13(12):2679–86.
11. Susaki EA, Tainaka K, Perrin D, et al. Whole-brain imaging with single-cell resolution using chemical cocktails and computational analysis. Cell. 2014;157(3):726–39.
12. Ito T, Udaka N, Yazawa T, et al. Basic helix-loop-helix transcription factors regulate the neuroendocrine differentiation of fetal mouse pulmonary epithelium. Development. 2000;127(18):3913–21.

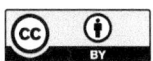

Specialized Smooth Muscle Cell Progenitors in Pulmonary Hypertension

4

Fatima Zahra Saddouk, Aglaia Ntokou, and Daniel M. Greif

Abstract

The accumulation of excessive and ectopic smooth muscle cells (SMCs) is integral to the pathogenesis of diverse cardiovascular diseases, including atherosclerosis, restenosis and pulmonary hypertension. Unfortunately, underlying mechanisms are poorly understood which markedly limits therapeutic options. In the idiopathic form of pulmonary hypertension, reduced pulmonary artery compliance is a strong independent predictor of mortality (Mahapatra et al. J Am Coll Cardiol 47(4):799–803, 2006). Distal arteriole endothelial tubes in the normal lung lack a SMC coating, and pathological distal arteriole muscularization contributes to the reduced compliance. Recently, we identified specialized progenitors that are located at the muscular-unmuscular border of each arteriole in the normal lung and express markers of SMCs and the undifferentiated mesenchyme marker platelet-derived growth factor receptor-β (Sheikh et al. Cell Rep 6(5):809–17, 2014; Sci Transl Med 7(308):308ra159, 2015). Upon exposing mice to hypoxia, these "primed" SMC progenitors are induced to express the pluripotency factor Kruppel-like factor 4 (Sheikh et al. Sci Transl Med 7(308):308ra159, 2015). Subsequently, one of these primed cells migrates distally and in a cell autonomous hypoxia-inducible factor (HIF)1-α-dependent manner and clonally expands, giving rise to distal arteriole SMCs (Sheikh et al. Sci Transl Med 7(308):308ra159, 2015; Cell Rep 23(4):1152–65, 2018). Additionally, endothelial cell HIF1-α-dependent signaling contributes in a non-cell autonomous manner, regulating induction, proliferation and differentiation of primed cells (Sheikh et al. Cell Rep 23(4):1152–65, 2018).

F. Z. Saddouk · A. Ntokou · D. M. Greif (✉)
Section of Cardiovascular Medicine, Department of Internal Medicine, Yale Cardiovascular Research Center, Yale University School of Medicine, New Haven, CT, USA

Department of Genetics, Yale University School of Medicine, New Haven, CT, USA
e-mail: daniel.greif@yale.edu

© The Editor(s) (if applicable) and The Author(s) 2020
T. Nakanishi et al. (eds.), *Molecular Mechanism of Congenital Heart Disease and Pulmonary Hypertension*, https://doi.org/10.1007/978-981-15-1185-1_4

25

Keywords
Smooth muscle cells · Pulmonary hypertension · Progenitors · Clonality · Vascular

4.1   Introduction

Physiologically, pulmonary hypertension (PH) is defined by a mean pulmonary artery pressure greater than or equal to 25 mm Hg at rest. PH encompasses heterogeneous entities that the World Health Organization has classified into five groups by etiology as follows: Group 1—pulmonary arterial hypertension (PAH); Group 2—PH due to left heart disease; Group 3—PH due to lung disease and/or chronic hypoxia; Group 4—PH due to chronic thromboembolism; and Group 5—PH with unclear multi-factorial mechanisms [1]. Overall, PH is a grave complication of other pathologies as well as a devastating disease in its own right: indeed, within seven years of initial diagnosis of PAH, one-half of patients have died [2].

Histopathological changes in PH include an increased SMC burden in the pulmonary vasculature with muscularization of normally non-muscularized distal pulmonary arterioles. Reduced compliance of the pulmonary arterial vasculature is an independent predictor of mortality in idiopathic PAH [3], and the distal extension of SMC coverage to normally unmuscularized distal arterioles contributes to this reduced arterial compliance. Treatments for PAH are largely limited to therapies that primarily induce vascular dilation, but these approaches do not ameliorate the hypermuscularization. The lack of therapeutic options that combat hypermuscularization is striking but perhaps not surprising given our limited understanding of the molecular and cellular processes underlying distal arteriole muscularization. To begin to delineate these mechanisms, our group utilized a reductionist approach and investigated in-depth, the process of hypoxia-induced distal muscularization of select arteriole beds in the murine lung. We identified novel SMC progenitors located at the muscular-unmuscular arteriole border that have a unique molecular signature and are the source of the vast majority of pathological distal arteriole SMCs in PH. During the muscularization process, these progenitors and their daughter cells undergo a stereotyped program of gene expression, migration and proliferation, which is subjected to intricate cell autonomous and non-cell autonomous regulation.

4.2   Hypoxia-Induced Distal Pulmonary Arteriole SMCs Derive from Specialized SMC Progenitors

Chronic hypoxia is a common cause of PH in humans and is widely used in a rodent model of PH, resulting in muscularization of distal pulmonary arterioles [4, 5]. At each arteriole muscular-unmuscular transition zone in the normal lung, we identified a pool of cells that express SMC markers (α-smooth muscle actin [SMA], smooth muscle myosin heavy chain [SMMHC]) and the undifferentiated mesenchyme marker platelet-derived growth factor receptor (PDGFR-β) [6, 7]. Because of their gene expression and position, we assessed if these cells give rise to distal pulmonary arteriole SMCs during PH through fate mapping in mice carrying the ROSA26R-mTmG Cre reporter and either *Acta2-CreER*^*T2* to induce recombination in SMCs (*Acta2* is the gene encoding SMA) or *Pdgfrb-CreER*^*T2* [6–9]. Treatment of these mice with hypoxia revealed that more than 80% of the distal pulmonary arteriole SMCs derive from primed SMCs [6, 7]. Thus, we termed these PDGFR-β⁺SMA⁺SMMHC⁺ progenitors as "primed" cells by virtue of their head start on other SMCs with regard to muscularizing the distal arteriole due to their location and PDGFR-β expression.

4.3 Stereotyped Program of Distal Muscularization

During the distal muscularization process, the primed SMC-derived lineage undergoes stereotyped steps of dedifferentiation (downregulation of SMMHC and maintenance of PDGFR-β expression) and migration beyond the muscularized-unmuscularized arteriole border and finally differentiation (upregulation of SMMHC and downregulation of PDGFR-β) [6]. In addition, analysis of bromodeoxyuridine (BrdU) incorporation indicates that proliferation of distal arteriole SMCs peaks at day 7 of hypoxia with remarkably ~2/3 of distal arteriole SMCs staining for BrdU, four hours after a single BrdU injection (100 mg/kg) [6].

4.4 Monoclonal Expansion of SMCs in PH

Furthermore, we analyzed the clonal relationship of hypoxia-induced distal arteriole SMCs. For these studies we used *Acta2-CreER*^*T2* mice also carrying the multicolor Rainbow (Rb) Cre reporter; a *ROSA26R(Rb/+)* cell that has undergone Cre-induced recombination will randomly and permanently express a specific fluorophore—Cerulean, mCherry or mOrange—and all of the cell's progeny will express this same fluorophore [10, 11]. Remarkably, for each distal arteriole, almost all of the pathological distal SMCs are marked by a single color (Fig. 4.1) and thus derive from clonal expansion of a single SMA⁺ cell and based on the fate mapping studies described above, from a single primed SMC [6, 7].

4.5 Signaling Pathways Regulating Primed Cells

The expression of the pluripotency factor Kruppel-like factor 4 (KLF4) in primed cells is essential for their initial migration in response to hypoxia, but KLF4 is dispensable for subsequent steps of SMC proliferation [7]. Interestingly, the hypermuscularized arterioles of human PH patients have a marked upregulation of KLF4 [7]. Platelet-derived growth factor (PDGF)-B is integral in primed cell KLF4 expression and distal muscularization as *Pdgfb*(+/−) mice are protected against these hypoxia-induced changes and do not develop PH [7].

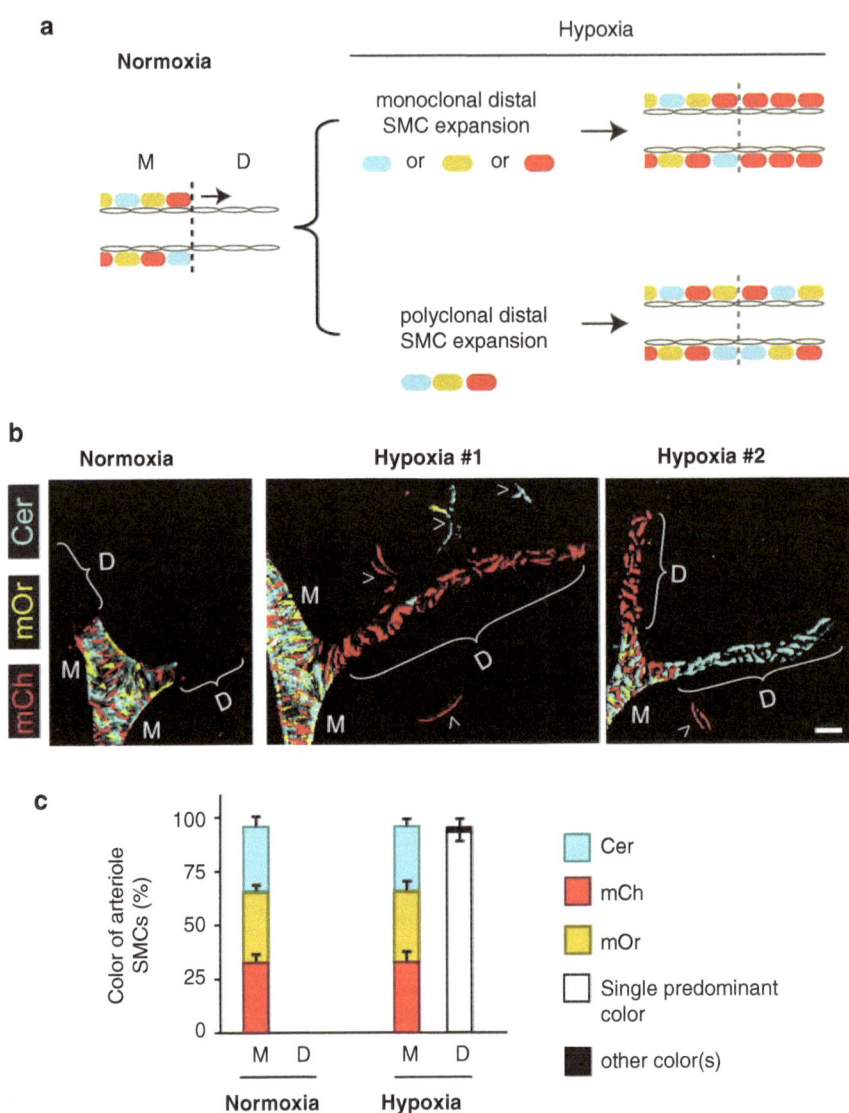

Fig. 4.1 The vast majority of hypoxia-induced SMCs in each pulmonary arteriole derive from a single pre-existing SMC. *Acta2-CreER* mice also carrying the multi-color Rainbow (Rb) Cre reporter *ROSA26R(Rb/+)* were induced with tamoxifen, rested and then exposed to normoxia or hypoxia (FiO₂ 10%) for 21 days. (**a**) Potential patterns of Rb colors in pulmonary arteriole SMCs. Middle (*M*) arteriole SMCs are present in normoxia and marked by different Rb colors [i.e., Cerulean (blue), mOrange (yellow) or mCherry (red)]. Hypoxia-induced distal (*D*) arteriole SMCs will be a single color if they derive from a single pre-existing SMC. Instead, distal arteriole SMCs will be of multiple colors if they derive from multiple SMCs. (**b**), Lung sections from a normoxic mouse and two hypoxic mice and imaged for Rb colors. Middle arteriole SMCs are polyclonal whereas distal arterioles are almost entirely monoclonal. Alveolar myofibroblasts are also marked (arrowheads). (**c**) Quantification of arteriole SMCs by size (*M, D*) and color. *n* = 4 lungs, 2–3 arterioles per lung (Adapted from reference [7])

Hypoxia-inducible factors (HIFs) are key transcription factors in PH. Deletion of *Hif1a* in SMMHC⁺ cells attenuates hypoxia-induced pulmonary vascular remodeling [12]. In contrast to KLF4, our studies suggest that HIF1-α in PDGFR-β^+ cells is not required for initial primed cell migration but is needed for the subsequent clonal expansion. In ECs, HIF1-α is upstream of PDGF-B, and EC deletion of either of these genes non-cell autonomously attenuates hypoxia-induced primed cell KLF4 expression, distal muscularization and PH [7, 13].

4.6 Future Direction and Clinical Implications

A number of questions are raised by these findings. From a developmental perspective, it is interesting to consider what is the role of primed cells in morphogenesis of the pulmonary vasculature and when do primed cells form. It remains to be determined whether the primed SMCs clonally expand in models of PH other than the hypoxia model and whether primed cells are present in the pulmonary arterioles of other animals beyond mice and in humans. Yet, the clonal expansion of SMC marker⁺ progenitors in pathological settings is not limited to hypoxia-induced PH as a series of recent studies demonstrate marked expansion of rare SMCs during atherogenesis in mice [14–16]. The need for effective and safe treatments for PH is dire, and further studies that investigate the role of primed cells and underlying signaling pathways in pathogenesis are critical and likely to provide key steps in the development of novel therapeutic approaches.

Acknowledgments F.Z.S was supported by Yale University (Brown-Coxe fellowship). This work was funded by the March of Dimes (Basil O'Connor Award, 5-FY13-208 and Gene Discovery & Translational Grant, 6-FY15-223 to D.M.G.), American Lung Association (Biomedical Research Grant, RG-310716 to D.M.G.), American Heart Association (National Innovative Research Grant, 15IRG23150002 to D.M.G.) and National Institutes of Health (R01HL125815, R01HL133016 and R01HL142674 to D.M.G. and CTSA 5UL1RR024139-08, National Center for Research Resources).

References

1. Simonneau G, Gatzoulis MA, Adatia I, Celermajer D, Denton C, Ghofrani A, et al. Updated clinical classification of pulmonary hypertension. J Am Coll Cardiol. 2013;62(25 Suppl):D34–41.
2. Benza RL, Miller DP, Barst RJ, Badesch DB, Frost AE, McGoon MD. An evaluation of long-term survival from time of diagnosis in pulmonary arterial hypertension from the REVEAL Registry. Chest. 2012;142(2):448–56.
3. Mahapatra S, Nishimura RA, Sorajja P, Cha S, McGoon MD. Relationship of pulmonary arterial capacitance and mortality in idiopathic pulmonary arterial hypertension. J Am Coll Cardiol. 2006;47(4):799–803.
4. Stenmark KR, Fagan KA, Frid MG. Hypoxia-induced pulmonary vascular remodeling: cellular and molecular mechanisms. Circ Res. 2006;99(7):675–91.
5. Stenmark KR, Meyrick B, Galie N, Mooi WJ, McMurtry IF. Animal models of pulmonary arterial hypertension: the hope for etiological discovery and pharmacological cure. Am J Physiol Lung Cell Mol Physiol. 2009;297(6):L1013–32.

6. Sheikh AQ, Lighthouse JK, Greif DM. Recapitulation of developing artery muscularization in pulmonary hypertension. Cell Rep. 2014;6(5):809–17.
7. Sheikh AQ, Misra A, Rosas IO, Adams RH, Greif DM. Smooth muscle cell progenitors are primed to muscularize in pulmonary hypertension. Sci Transl Med. 2015;7(308):308ra159.
8. Muzumdar MD, Tasic B, Miyamichi K, Li L, Luo L. A global double-fluorescent Cre reporter mouse. Genesis. 2007;45(9):593–605.
9. Wendling O, Bornert JM, Chambon P, Metzger D. Efficient temporally-controlled targeted mutagenesis in smooth muscle cells of the adult mouse. Genesis. 2009;47(1):14–8.
10. Greif DM, Kumar M, Lighthouse JK, Hum J, An A, Ding L, et al. Radial construction of an arterial wall. Dev Cell. 2012;23(3):482–93.
11. Rinkevich Y, Lindau P, Ueno H, Longaker MT, Weissman IL. Germ-layer and lineage-restricted stem/progenitors regenerate the mouse digit tip. Nature. 2011;476(7361):409–13.
12. Ball MK, Waypa GB, Mungai PT, Nielsen JM, Czech L, Dudley VJ, et al. Regulation of hypoxia-induced pulmonary hypertension by vascular smooth muscle hypoxia-inducible factor-1alpha. Am J Respir Crit Care Med. 2014;189(3):314–24.
13. Sheikh AQ, Saddouk FZ, Ntokou A, Mazurek R, Greif DM. Cell autonomous and non-cell autonomous regulation of SMC progenitors in pulmonary hypertension. Cell Rep. 2018;23(4):1152–65.
14. Chappell J, Harman JL, Narasimhan VM, Yu H, Foote K, Simons BD, et al. Extensive proliferation of a subset of differentiated, yet plastic, medial vascular smooth muscle cells contributes to neointimal formation in mouse injury and atherosclerosis models. Circ Res. 2016;119(12):1313–23.
15. Jacobsen K, Lund MB, Shim J, Gunnersen S, Fuchtbauer EM, Kjolby M, et al. Diverse cellular architecture of atherosclerotic plaque derives from clonal expansion of a few medial SMCs. JCI Insight. 2017;2(19)
16. Misra A, Feng Z, Chandran RR, Kabir I, Rotllan N, Aryal B, et al. Integrin beta3 regulates clonality and fate of smooth muscle-derived atherosclerotic plaque cells. Nat Commun. 2073;9(1):2018.

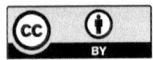

Diverse Pharmacology of Prostacyclin Mimetics: Implications for Pulmonary Hypertension

5

Lucie H. Clapp, Jeries H. J. Abu-Hanna, and Jigisha A. Patel

Abstract

Pulmonary arterial hypertension (PAH) is a progressive vascular remodelling disease where patients ultimately die from heart failure. Increased production of vasoconstrictors (endothelin-1 and thromboxane A_2) accompanied by loss of prostacyclin, nitric oxide (NO), bone morphogenetic protein receptor type 2 (BMPR2) and TASK-1 combine to cause endothelial apoptosis, smooth muscle hyperactivity and thickening of the blood vessel wall. Prostacyclin remains the most efficacious treatment for PAH, and several prostacyclin analogues are approved for use via different administration routes. They act as vasodilators but potently inhibit platelet aggregation, cell proliferation and inflammation. The pharmacology of each prostacyclin (IP) receptor agonist is distinct, with other targets contributing to their therapeutic and side-effect profile, including prostanoid EP_1, EP_3, EP_2 and DP_1 receptors, alongside peroxisome proliferator-activated receptors (PPARs), to which prostacyclin and some analogues directly bind. To improve selectivity, selexipag, a non-prostanoid was developed, whose only significant biological target is the IP receptor, but is a partial agonist in cyclic AMP assays and has no anti-aggregatory properties in vivo. Prostanoid receptor expression profiles in the normal and diseased lung demonstrate loss of the IP receptor and upregulation of EP_2 and EP_3 receptors in PAH, affecting the action of prostacyclin mimetics in different ways. We discuss how prostacyclins

L. H. Clapp (✉) · J. A. Patel
Centre for Cardiovascular Physiology and Pharmacology, Institute of Cardiovascular Science, University College London, London, UK
e-mail: l.clapp@ucl.ac.uk

J. H. J. Abu-Hanna
Centre for Cardiovascular Physiology and Pharmacology, Institute of Cardiovascular Science, University College London, London, UK

Centre for Rheumatology and Connective Tissue Disease, Division of Medicine, University College London, London, UK

© The Editor(s) (if applicable) and The Author(s) 2020
T. Nakanishi et al. (eds.), *Molecular Mechanism of Congenital Heart Disease and Pulmonary Hypertension*, https://doi.org/10.1007/978-981-15-1185-1_5

31

might rescue BMPR2 and TASK-1 dysfunction and the importance of EP_2 receptors as negative modulators of vascular tone, proliferation and fibrosis. Alongside DP_1 and EP_4 receptors, they have specific roles in veins and airways. Whether drugs selective for the IP receptor confer a superior or reduced therapeutic benefit remains an important clinical question as do the role of platelets in PAH.

Keywords
Prostanoid receptors · Prostacyclin mimetics · Vascular smooth muscle · Pulmonary hypertension · Cell proliferation

5.1 Introduction

Pulmonary arterial hypertension (PAH) is a progressive and fatal disease. Patients suffer from elevated pulmonary artery pressure (PAP) and right ventricular (RV) heart failure [1]. Without treatment, adults have a median life expectancy of 2.8 years from diagnosis, while children have less than 10 months [2, 3]. Narrowing of the small pulmonary arteries involves proliferation of endothelial cells, smooth muscle cells and fibroblasts and is associated with inflammatory cell infiltration and the formation of thrombotic lesions [4, 5]. The highly proliferative phenotype is driven by elevated levels of mitogens (endothelin-1, thromboxane A_2 and 5-HT) and growth factors (platelet-derived growth factor, transforming growth factor $\beta1$ and fibroblast growth factor) concomitant with a reduction in the endogenous levels of nitric oxide (NO) and prostacyclin, agents which have potent anti-proliferative and anti-inflammatory properties in many different cell types [6].

Pulmonary hypertension (PH) is classified by the World Health Organization (WHO) into five clinical groups, with patients diagnosed as having PAH belonging to Group I [5, 7]. PAH is further classified as being idiopathic (of no known cause), heritable (genetic component) or secondary to other lung or systemic diseases, including connective tissue disease (CTD), congenital heart disease (CHD) and HIV [5, 7]. It is estimated that around 10% of all patients are described as having heritable PAH (HPAH). From this, a significant proportion of patients (~70–80%) have a mutation in the bone morphogenetic protein receptor type 2 (BMPR2), a member of the transforming growth factor beta (TGF-β) receptor family [7, 8]. The consequence of such mutations is to lead to a pro-proliferative phenotype in pulmonary arterial smooth muscle cells (PASMCs) and a high vascular permeability in endothelial cells leading to apoptosis [9, 10]. It is also important to note that downregulation of the BMPR2 protein occurs in around 25% of patients with idiopathic PAH (IPAH) [8, 11].

Additional and rarer heterozygous germline mutations in the TGF-β pathway have also been implicated, with studies confirming activin-like kinase-type (ALK-1), endoglin and various members of the SMAD (SMAD 9, 4, 5, 1) family contributing to the pathogenesis of HPAH [8]. ALK is a type-1 receptor phosphorylated when BMPR2 is activated by a BMP ligand and endoglin encodes a type III or accessory receptor to BMPR2, while phosphorylation of SMAD 1,5 and 8(9) leads to their association with the nuclear chaperone SMAD4, resulting in translocation of the SMAD complex to the cell nucleus to regulate transcription [8]. Furthermore, loss of function mutations in the potassium channel KCNK3 (TASK-1) have been described in patients with either HPAH or IPAH, representing a mechanistically novel cause of PAH [12]. This parallels the downregulation of Kv channels that has been implicated to underlie hypoxic-induced vasoconstriction and abnormal proliferation of smooth muscle cells from patients with IPAH [12].

5.2 Development of Prostacyclin Mimetics and Their Diverse Pharmacology

Prostacyclin, a prostanoid produced in endothelial and smooth muscle cells by the cyclooxygenase (COX) pathway, was discovered in 1976 by a group of scientists led by John Vane as a potent vasodilator and anti-thrombotic agent of the vasculature [13, 14]. It was the first treatment to routinely be used in PAH, with the primary clinical benefit resulting from a reduction in PAP and resistance thereby improving cardiac output [15]. Shortly thereafter, chemically stable analogues of prostacyclin with a longer half-life in the blood were synthesised, including beraprost, iloprost, treprostinil and cicaprost. Apart from cicaprost, these analogues have been in use for PAH since the early to mid-1990s, with iloprost and treprostinil receiving FDA approval in 2002 and 2004, respectively, whereas beraprost is currently only licensed in Asia. Initial work presumed prostacyclin drugs produced their effects via binding to the Gs-coupled prostacyclin (IP) receptor leading to the activation of adenylate cyclase and the cellular accumulation of intracellular cyclic-3′,5′-adenosine monophosphate (cAMP) [16]. Consistent with this notion, the blood pressure–lowering, vasodilatory and anti-aggregatory properties of cicaprost were abolished in IP receptor null mice [17]. Indeed the IP receptor appears to largely account for the pharmacological properties of prostacyclins in humans, including vasodilator [18, 19] and anti-proliferative effects [20–22] in normal pulmonary smooth muscle as well as inhibition of platelet function in healthy individuals [23, 24]. However, early on in their development, prostacyclin and its analogues were found to regulate gene transcription via peroxisome proliferator-activated receptors (PPARs), which would concur with the strong perinuclear expression of prostacyclin synthase [13] with cyclooxygenase enzymes [25], both the enzymes required for prostacyclin synthesis. Some analogues (but not cicaprost) were shown to bind and activate PPARα and PPARβ, an effect reported to be independent of the IP receptor and cAMP generation [26, 27]. Such a mechanism might help to explain the enigmatic observation (at the time) that abolition of the iloprost-induced elevation in cAMP by adenylate cyclase inhibition had no significant effect on vascular relaxation by this agent in guinea-pig aorta [28]. However, it was not until a decade later did evidence emerge for the explicit role of PPARs in mediating some of the functional effects of prostacyclin analogues on vascular tone, cell proliferation and endothelial cell integrity (reviewed in [6]). Indeed, studies in genetically modified mice show that distinct phenotypes are generated when the IP receptor and the prostacyclin synthase gene are deleted; the former are normotensive but do show an increased susceptibility to thrombosis, while the latter are hypertensive and show fibrosis and vascular remodelling in the kidney [6]. This strongly suggests that PPARs are involved in regulating blood pressure and is consistent with the known vasodilatory effects of ligands activating all three PPAR (α, β, γ) isoforms [29, 30].

At the same time as the discovery of signalling through PPARs, prostacyclin and its analogues were found to activate multiple prostanoid receptors, including EP$_1$, EP$_3$, EP$_4$, TP and FP [16, 31]. Given that all (bar EP$_4$) are contractile receptors linked to either calcium elevation or inhibition of cAMP generation (Fig. 5.1), and thus their activation might promote unwanted side effects or physiologically oppose IP receptor signalling, prompted the search for more selective IP receptor agonists. Based on this rationale, selexipag, a novel non-prostanoid moiety with a high selectivity for the IP receptor was developed [32, 33] and subsequently approved in 2015 for the treatment of PAH [34]. Selexipag, which is structurally different from prostacyclin, is broken down in the liver to form MRE-269 (known also as ACT 333679), a metabolite with a significantly increased affinity for the IP receptor but with essentially weak or no activity at other prostanoid receptors [32]. Along the same lines, a new series of potent, non-prostanoid and relatively

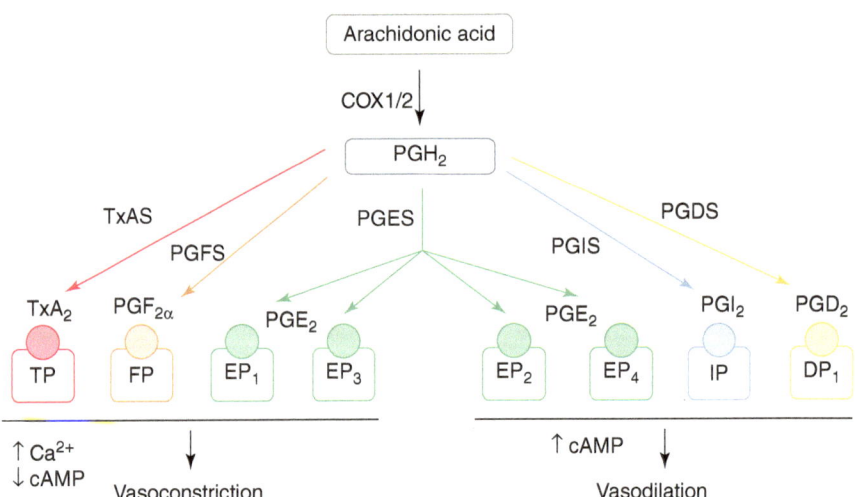

Fig. 5.1 Synthesis of prostanoids and their downstream receptors. Oxidation of arachidonic acid by cyclooxygenase (COX-1 and COX-2) enzymes converts it to an unstable intermediate, prostaglandin H$_2$, the common precursor for five principal bioactive derivatives. Thromboxane A$_2$ (TXA$_2$), prostaglandin F$_{2\alpha}$, (PGF$_{2\alpha}$), prostaglandin E$_2$ (PGE$_2$), prostacyclin and prostaglandin D$_2$ (PGD$_2$) are then generated by the action of individual prostaglandin synthase enzymes (TxAS, PGFS, PGES, PGIS and PGDS). Once generated, the different prostanoids exert their biological effects by binding to and activating specific membrane bound G-protein-coupled receptors. TP, FP, EP$_1$ and EP$_3$ receptors are contractile receptors coupled to Gq and Gi that either elevate intracellular Ca^{2+}and/or reduce cAMP, respectively. EP$_2$, EP$_4$, IP and DP$_1$ receptors are vasorelaxant receptors coupled to Gs that will activate adenylate cyclase and elevate intracellular cAMP

selective IP receptor agonists were recently synthesised, with ralinepag (APD811) in clinical development as a next generation, once a day oral for the treatment of PAH [35]. Other novel approaches are being taken, including the development of ONO-1301, a non-prostanoid with a dual function of activating the IP receptor and inhibiting TXA_2 synthase [24]. The latter property of the molecule appears to protect the IP receptor from undergoing desensitisation, which is often observed with repeated prostacyclin or analogue administration. This suggests a major role for the TP receptor in promoting IP receptor desensitisation.

All prostacyclin mimetics used clinically display high affinity binding to the human IP receptor. Potency varies, with those having a Ki of 2–4 nM (prostacyclin, iloprost and ralinepag) and those having a tenfold lower affinity with a Ki of 20–38 nM (MRE-269, treprostinil and beraprost), or lower still, with selexipag having a Ki of 250 nM [6, 35]. Esuberaprost (beraprost-314*d*), a reformulated single isomer of beraprost, may be the most potent IP agonist developed so far for therapeutic use [36] and is now in a phase III clinical trial as an oral with inhaled treprostinil. It remains to be determined whether high selectivity towards the IP receptor, which typifies the two non-prostanoid IP receptor agonists, will give rise to therapeutically superior effects and/or a better side-effect profile compared to prostacyclin mimetics that can act at other membrane and nuclear receptors.

Mechanistic and functional differences between prostanoid and non-prostanoid IP agonists are now beginning to emerge that need to be carefully considered in a clinical context. Both ralinepag and MRE-269 behave as partial agonists in cAMP assays in CHO cells stably expressing the human IP receptor and in human PASMCs from PAH patients [35, 37, 38]. Partial agonism may in part explain why MRE-269 was about 65-fold less potent than iloprost at inhibiting contractions in human pulmonary arteries [19] and why selexipag has little overall effect on platelet aggregation in vivo [39]. The latter might suggest the inability of the active metabolite to raise cAMP levels sufficiently to oppose platelet aggregation by endogenous mediators like thromboxane A_2 (TXA_2), which in itself can lower cAMP levels through IP receptor desensitisation, Gi coupling to adenylate cyclase or Ca^{2+} activation of cAMP-dependent phosphodiesterases [6, 24]. High EP_3 receptor activity is also likely to have a similar effect as this receptor is negatively coupled to adenylate cyclase.

The role of platelets as a disease-modifying process in PAH is neither well understood nor the nature of the benefit derived from anti-coagulant therapy [40, 41]. This is an issue that needs to be further investigated as activated platelets produce and release vasoactive substances such as TXA_2, 5-HT and platelet-derived growth factor [41, 42], which may cause harmful vasoconstriction and vascular remodelling in PAH. However, as internal bleeding is a potential risk factor for all prostacyclin analogues [41], and thrombocytopenia a complication of long-term use with epoprostenol (synthetic prostacyclin) in some PAH patients [43], the ability to switch to an IP agonist devoid of anticoagulation properties might be considered beneficial in some patients.

There are also key mechanistic differences in how prostacyclin analogues and non-prostanoid IP agonists inhibit pulmonary arterial smooth muscle proliferation in cells derived from PAH patients. The anti-proliferative responses to treprostinil and iloprost show weak effects of IP receptor inhibition with RO1138452 [22, 44] whereas the same antagonist completely reversed the effects to both MRE-269 and ralinepag, suggesting inhibition of cell proliferation was fully IP receptor-dependent [37, 44]. These results suggest that non-IP receptor targets play a significant role in mediating the effects of some prostacyclin analogues in PAH whereas the IP receptor is likely to be the only significant biological target for MRE-269 and ralinepag. In the search for an explanation to the original 2010 observation, radioligand-binding assays against human prostanoid receptors demonstrated unexpectedly that treprostinil had a tenfold higher affinity for the DP_1 and EP_2 receptor (Ki 4.4 and 3.6 nM, respectively) than the IP receptor [45]. On the other hand, iloprost had a $\geq$240-fold lower affinity for DP_1 and EP_2 but was equipotent at the IP and EP_1 receptor [45]. A similar potency pattern was observed in functional assays (cAMP and calcium) in the same study, confirming the unique pharmacology of treprostinil [6], which was subsequently independently verified [46]. It is known that receptor affinities can differ significantly between species for natural ligands as well as for their agonists [6] and antagonists [47] so future experiments should be directed towards obtaining the binding affinity profile of treprostinil at mouse and rat prostanoid receptors (and for that matter some prostacyclin drugs) and how different models of PAH affects receptor expression in relevant tissues and cells.

The receptor selectivity of prostacyclin and its mimetics could greatly impact on their control of pulmonary haemodynamics and vascular remodelling in PAH as well influence their side-effect profile. It is presumed that the IP receptor-selective agonists will have fewer adverse events than those agents which activate multiple receptors although this remains to be determined clinically. For the remainder of this chapter, the physiological and pathophysiological context of these distinct membrane receptor profiles for the different prostacyclin mimetics will be evaluated. Comparative prostanoid receptor expression profiles in normal and diseased lung will be described and how this has the propensity to affect the mode of action of prostacyclin mimetics in arteries and veins and other cell types in PAH. We will also focus on the importance of EP_2 and EP_4 receptors as negative modulators of pulmonary artery smooth muscle tone, cell proliferation and fibrosis, and how these receptors alongside DP_1 receptors may have a specific role in the veins and the airways. Other data suggests that limiting EP_3 receptor activation will be beneficial in PAH as this receptor is upregulated by hypoxia and activates TGF-β signalling and may thus oppose signalling through BMPR2 receptors.

5.3 Prostanoid Synthesis and Receptor Expression

Prostanoids are derived from cyclooxygenase isoenzymes (COX-1 and COX-2), which convert arachidonic acid to an unstable intermediate, prostaglandin H_2, the common precursor for five principal bioactive derivatives. TXA_2, prostaglandin $F_{2\alpha}$, prostaglandin E_2 (PGE_2), prostacyclin and prostaglandin D_2 (PGD_2) are then generated by the action of individual prostaglandin synthase enzymes. Once generated, the different prostanoids exert their pharmacological and biological effects by binding to and activating specific membrane bound G-protein-coupled receptors (Fig. 5.1). EP_1, EP_3, FP and TP receptors are contractile receptors coupled to Gq and Gi that either elevate intracellular $Ca^{2+}$and/or reduce cAMP, respectively. EP_2, EP_4, IP and DP_1 receptors are vasorelaxant receptors coupled to Gs that will activate adenylate cyclase and elevate intracellular cAMP (Fig. 5.1). The DP_2 (CRTH2) receptor, which has no significant homology to other prostanoid receptors, recognises PGD_2 as its endogenous ligand and is involved in allergic or T-helper 2 cell inflammation, with antagonists currently being trialled as a novel therapy for asthma. As the receptor is not activated to any significant extent by prostacyclin mimetics [48], for this reason it will not be further discussed.

As mentioned already, prostacyclin analogues have diverse effects on prostanoid receptors, with different IP receptor agonists likely to activate EP_1 (iloprost), EP_3 (prostacyclin) and EP_2 or DP_1 (treprostinil) receptors within their therapeutic dose range [6]. TP receptor activation by prostacyclin might come into play if either the plasma concentration is in excess of 50 nM (twice the reported plasma concentration in patients [49]), the receptor becomes primed by other vasoconstrictor agents (cross-sensitization), and/or its activity increases because the receptor becomes uncoupled from IP receptors, dimerization of which normally limits the deleterious effects of thromboxane [6]. Thus in order to understand the mode of action of these drugs in the therapeutic setting, it is important to assess the relative expression, function and impact of PAH on prostanoid receptors in small arteries and veins, the major sites of vessel disease. We have, therefore, sought to assess their expression in lung sections from control and PAH patients with end-stage disease using methods previously described [44]. For comparison, bronchial sections were examined and acted as a positive control since the staining for IP, EP_{1-4} and DP_1 was strong to moderately strong for all of these receptors in the respiratory epithelium (Fig. 5.2).

5.3.1 Bronchial Smooth Muscle

IP, EP_2 and EP_3 receptor staining was strong in the bronchial smooth muscle, with EP_2 being the strongest (Fig. 5.2a). DP_1 staining was moderately strong, and EP_4 staining less uniform, but nonetheless the smooth muscle stained positively, while overall EP_1 receptor expression was weak. In studies conducted nearly 20 years ago, IP, EP_2 and to a lesser extent DP_1 receptors, but not the EP_4 receptor, were reported to be associated with human bronchus relaxation as assessed by prostacyclin analogues, PGE_2 and PGD_2 [50]. Furthermore, PGE_2 did not induce relaxation in tracheal smooth muscle preparations from EP_2 receptor knockout mice [51], consistent with these earlier observations of a dominant role for EP_2 receptors in regulating airway smooth muscle tone. However, more recent studies using highly specific receptor agonists and antagonists suggest that the EP_4 receptor is the main receptor subtype to promote relaxation to PGE_2 in human small airways [52]. However, in

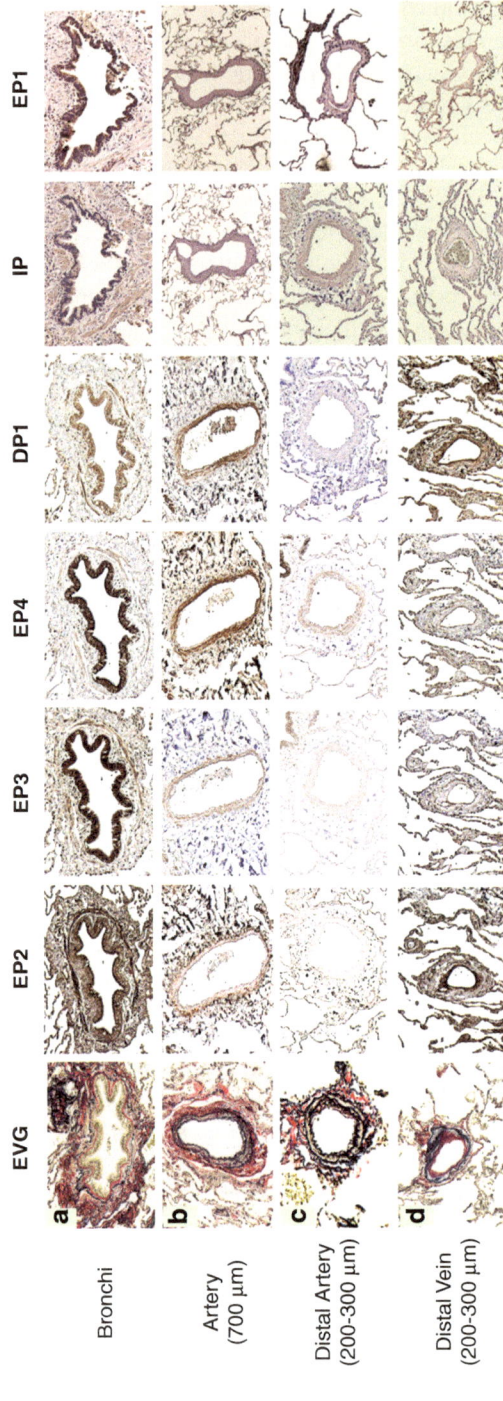

Fig. 5.2 Prostanoid EP_{1-4}, DP_1 and IP receptor expression in a human lung section from a control patient. Immunohistochemical staining was carried out in 10 µm sections of human lung tissue from a control patient. Each row from A to D represents sections of pulmonary bronchi, large artery (700 µm), distal artery (200–300 µm) and distal veins (200–300 µm), respectively. Far left panel, Van Gieson stain (EVG) shows collagen in red and elastic fibres in black. This was followed by antibody staining for different prostaglandin receptors: EP_2, EP_3, EP_4, DP_1, IP and EP_1 (from left to right columns) visualised by diaminobenzidine (brown) in sections counterstained with haematoxylin. All receptors are heavily expressed in the respiratory epithelium and act as a control for antibody staining in the arteries and veins

the same study, EP_2 receptors were reported to inhibit mast cell-mediated broncho-constriction, highlighting a novel and potentially important function of EP_2 receptors. Inhibition of mast cell function might be considered beneficial in the context of PAH. Increasingly mast cells are thought to promote vascular remodelling in lung disease, including in PAH, releasing a number of mediators like histamine, PGD_2, leukotrienes, pro-inflammatory cytokines and growth factors like TGF-β [53].

With respect to contractile prostanoid receptors in the bronchus, TP receptors are the predominant functional contractile prostanoid receptor and appear to mediate contractions induced by high concentrations of PGE_2 [52, 54]. The latter would fit in with the relatively weak expression of EP_1 receptors that we observed in the human bronchus muscle (Fig. 5.2a). Based on this pharmacology, and that neither treprostinil nor iloprost has significant activity at TP receptors, it is suggested that these agents will be effective bronchial dilators through the IP receptor. EP_4 receptors may contribute to iloprost-induced relaxation, though given iloprost has a Ki of 212 nM at this receptor [45], the inhaled drug would have to reach concentrations in excess of 100 nM in order to do so. This is highly unlikely given the upper plasma concentrations of iloprost in patients is ~1 nM [6]. DP_1 receptors are, however, likely to contribute to treprostinil-induced bronchial relaxation. As EP_2 receptors were the most highly expressed prostanoid receptor in the bronchus smooth muscle, this might indicate a significant role for these receptors although further work is required to understand their function in small bronchi.

5.3.2 Pulmonary Blood Vessels

5.3.2.1 Endothelium

There was moderate to strong expression of all prostanoid receptors in the endothelium of large and small pulmonary arteries (Fig. 5.2b, c) although the strongest expression was observed in small veins (Fig. 5.2d), suggesting the endothelium may be particularly important for maintaining the patency of blood vessels in the venous circulation. Few studies have investigated the involvement of human prostanoid receptors expressed on the endothelium and none in small pulmonary vessels. Moreover, studies have often assessed prostanoid effects on vascular tone in the presence of inhibitors of nitric oxide (NO) synthase and COX to prevent the release of endogenous prostanoids and NO (e.g. [55, 56]), thus masking the potential effect/role of the endothelium. Nonetheless, NO synthase inhibition was reported to augment the contractile function of PGE_2 in rat pulmonary arteries [57]. Furthermore, a significant dependency on endothelial-derived NO for relaxation induced by beraprost and treprostinil in rat and human pulmonary arteries has been reported [58, 59], which is likely to be associated in part by activation of the IP receptor. Curiously, both MRE-269 and iloprost show no endothelial dependence to their vasorelaxant actions in pulmonary arteries [58, 59], demonstrating a differential mechanism of these two prostacyclin mimetics compared to beraprost and treprostinil. The clinical significance of these findings is unclear but may suggest differences in the clinical efficacy of combination therapies based around potentiation of NO signalling (e.g. phosphodiesterase type 5 inhibitors).

5.3.2.2 Pulmonary Artery

There was expression of all prostanoid receptors in the medial layer of large arteries, though EP_1 receptor expression was moderate to weak, as was EP_2 receptor staining which was mainly confined to the outer medial layer (Fig. 5.2b). Our immunostaining data broadly support many of the previously published findings investigating receptor expression and contractile function in large (control) pulmonary blood vessels from humans. In arterial preparations, the IP receptor was found to be the predominant receptor involved in relaxation [55], while EP_3 and TP receptors were the main contractile receptors to counteract this [60]. In other studies, EP_4 and DP_1 receptors were found to be expressed in human pulmonary arteries whereas EP_2 and EP_1 receptors were not [19, 56]. This would generally fit with the moderate to strong IP, EP_3, EP_4 and DP_1 receptor staining, the generally weaker staining of the EP_1 receptor we observed in larger arteries coupled with the overall weak staining of EP_2 receptors that was recently reported in large and small pulmonary arteries [44].

5.3.2.3 Differential Prostanoid Expression in Distal Pulmonary Artery and Veins

There were some distinctive features of prostanoid receptor expression in small arteries (Fig. 5.2c) and veins (Fig. 5.2d) in control sections of lung tissue that are worth noting. Staining for EP_2 receptors was weak in the medial layer of arteries, but strong in veins, with a broadly similar picture for DP_1 receptors. By contrast, EP_3 staining was observed throughout the media in arteries but was generally confined to the outer layer of the vein juxtaposed with the adventitia although the endothelium was, however, strongly stained. Likewise, the EP_4 receptor antibody stained the medial layer of the distal artery, and greater staining was observed in the vein compared to EP_3. With respect to the IP receptor, staining appeared stronger in the artery compared to the vein, while the EP_1 receptor antibody moderately stained both small artery and vein.

5.3.2.4 Distal Pulmonary Veins

Previous experiments in human proximal veins have provided clear evidence that prostanoid IP, DP_1 and EP_4 receptors mediate relaxation to prostanoids whereas TP and EP_1 receptors mediate constriction [55, 56, 61]. The particularly strong expression of EP_2 and DP_1 receptors in the endothelium and medial layer of small veins suggest a functional role of these two prostanoid receptors in regulating venous tone. Such an observation may explain why PGE_2 and PGD_2 are strong relaxants of human proximal pulmonary veins constricted with phenylephrine whereas they fail to cause relaxation in pulmonary arteries under similar experimental conditions [55, 56]. DP_1 receptors are expressed at the protein level in veins and reported to underlie in part the venorelaxation to treprostinil [19]. This is consistent with the observation of only a partial dependence of the IP receptor in mediating relaxation to treprostinil in both human [19] and rat pulmonary veins [62]. Furthermore, 40% of relaxation to treprostinil in human vessels still remained in the presence of both a DP_1 and IP receptor antagonist, suggesting an additional mechanism contributing to relaxation [19], possibly via EP_2 receptors. Indeed, functional EP_2 receptors have been reported in large human pulmonary veins, with the EP_2 agonist, ONO-AE1-259, causing relaxation, albeit at relatively high concentrations [56]. The prediction is that EP_2 receptors will play a greater role in small pulmonary veins, given its strong expression both in the endothelium and in the medial layers. To our knowledge, there have been no reports investigating the role of EP_2 receptors in small pulmonary vessels, so the functional consequence of these receptors requires investigation. Elsewhere in the vasculature, the main vasodilator response to PGE_2 appears to be driven by the EP_2 receptor as PGE_2 produces hypotension in wild-type mice compared to substantial hypertension in EP_2 null mice [63]. This suggests a major role for EP_2 receptors in regulating vascular tone, at least in mice.

In terms of the function of other prostanoid receptors, EP_4 receptor agonists (e.g. ONO-AE1–329) strongly relax human pulmonary veins, and these were partially inhibited by an EP_4 antagonist as were PGE_2-induced relaxations [56]. Surprisingly, iloprost relaxations in pulmonary veins (and also arteries) were insensitive to EP_4 receptor antagonists [19]. Thus the EP_4 receptor as a proposed target for iloprost-mediated vasodilation during therapeutic use in human PAH [64] is so far not supported experimentally. Whether this relates to iloprost acting at various receptor targets (IP, EP_4 and PPARs) to cause relaxation, thus requiring the simultaneous treatment with multiple antagonists to inhibit functional responses is unclear, but supported by experimental observation in other vascular tissues [65]. EP_4 activation may be thwarted by the potent actions of iloprost at EP_1 receptors. Indeed EP_1 antagonists enhance iloprost and PGE_2 relaxation in human pulmonary veins and also underlie contractions seen by these two agents in the same tissue [55, 56, 61]. Likewise, the presence of an EP_1 antagonist was required before the relaxant effect of prostacyclin in pulmonary veins approached that in pulmonary arteries [66]. Furthermore, beraprost strongly relaxed human pulmonary arteries but not veins [19] whereas treprostinil was a stronger venorelaxant than an arterial relaxant in rat distal pulmonary blood vessels [62], presumably through its combined action at IP, DP_1 and EP_2 receptors. Such findings might provide a rationale for investigating the effects of treprostinil in pulmonary hypertension (PH) associated with post-capillary disease, of which PH due to left heart dysfunction is characterised predominantly by venoconstriction and remodelling (see later).

5.3.3 Prostanoid Receptor Expression in PAH

In lung sections derived from a patient with PAH, prostanoid receptor expression in the bronchi remained largely unchanged, the exception being the DP_1 receptor, expression of which went up in the bronchial smooth muscle (Fig. 5.3a). In contrast, there were marked changes to expression in pulmonary blood vessels (Fig. 5.3b–d). There was a reduction in the expression of all prostanoid receptor subtypes in the endothelium of arteries and veins, with IP and EP_1 receptor staining barely evident in small arteries, while EP_3 receptor expression appeared particularly reduced in the vein. Some loss of staining is undoubtedly due to endothelial damage which was apparent in many blood vessels. The pattern of prostanoid receptor expression

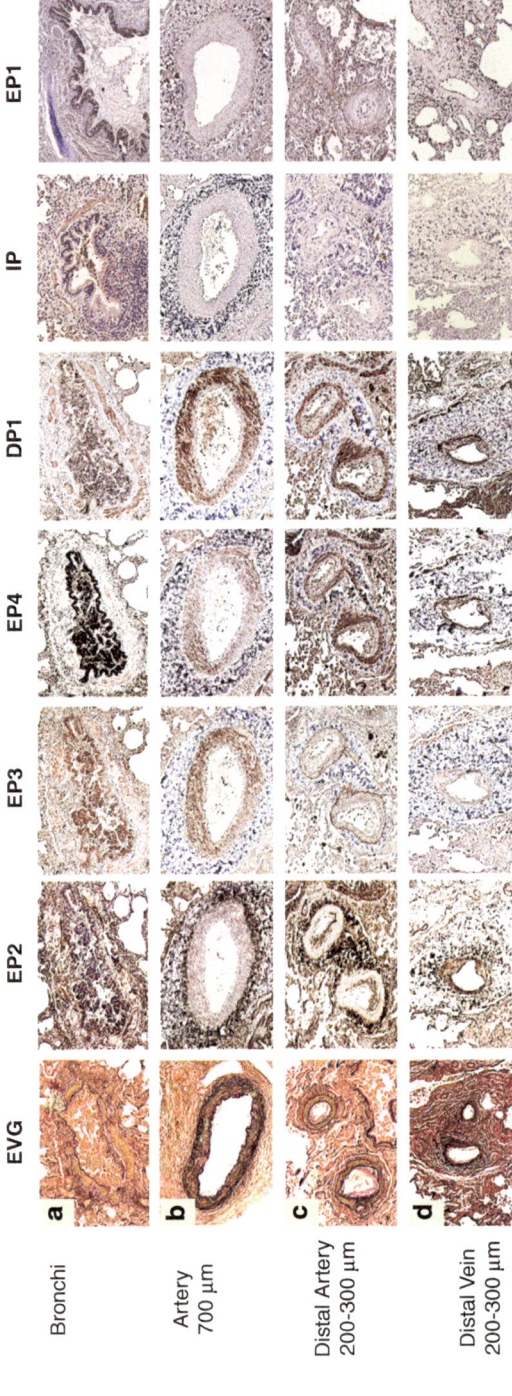

Fig. 5.3 EP_{1-4}, DP_1 and IP receptor expression in a human lung section from a PAH patient. Immunohistochemical staining was carried out in 10 μm serial sections of human lung tissue from patient with pulmonary arterial hypertension (PAH). Each row from **a** to **d** represents a sections of pulmonary bronchi; large artery (700 μm), distal artery (200–300 μm) and distal vein (200–300 μm) respectively. Far left panel, Van Gieson stain (EVG) shows collagen in red and elastic fibres in black. This was followed by antibody staining for different prostanoid receptors: EP_2, EP_3, EP_4, DP_1 IP and EP_1 (from left to right columns) visualised by diaminobenzidine (brown) in sections counterstained with haematoxylin

was somewhat different in smooth muscle. Prostanoid EP_3 receptor staining was increased in the medial layer of large and small arteries and in the vein compared to control, while EP_4 and EP_2 receptor antibody staining was increased in small arteries and veins. Similar to EP_2 and EP_4 receptors, DP_1 receptors were found to be strongly expressed in the small artery and vein. In contrast, IP receptor expression was weak in arteries and veins. Finally, the expression of EP_2 receptors in the adventitial layer of both large and small arteries and veins was marked, being particularly strong in PAH lung sections as was the case for the EP_4 receptor in small arteries (Fig. 5.3c). Staining in the adventitial layer is likely to come from fibroblasts, which preside predominately in this layer, undergoing proliferation in PAH and producing significant amounts of collagen to increase adventitial thickness [67, 68]. This was evidenced by the Van Gieson (EVG) stain which showed extensive collagen deposition (red staining). We cannot rule out the possibility that EP_2 and EP_4 receptor staining comes from inflammatory cell types, particularly monocytes and dendritic cells, which can be found in the adventitia of remodelled arteries in PAH [4, 67] and which express functional EP_2 and EP_4 receptors [60, 69]. Whether EP_4 receptors can account for any of the IP receptor-independent effects of iloprost on cell growth in PASMCs from PAH patients, where EP_4 function may be upregulated, requires investigation.

5.3.3.1 Downregulation of IP Receptors in PAH

It was not unexpected to find that IP receptor expression was downregulated in the arteries and veins in PAH, as previous studies have shown that mRNA and protein levels are substantially reduced both in the lungs and in PASMCs derived from PAH patients compared to controls [22, 64]. Furthermore, in a rat monocrotaline model of PAH, IP receptor mRNA levels were decreased while EP_4 and EP_2 receptor expressions were preserved [64], although in another study using the same model, no decrease in the IP receptor expression was found [33]. In a sugen/hypoxia model of severe PAH, the IP receptor was minimally expressed in whole lungs, and iloprost did not reduce mean PAP despite improving cardiac output [70]. This might suggest that in severe disease IP receptor function in the pulmonary circulation may be limited or be curtailed by the activation of prostanoid vasoconstrictor pathways opposing signalling through this receptor. That IP receptors were still functional in cultured PASMCs from PAH patients and significantly contributed to the anti-proliferative effects of non-prostanoid IP agonists may, however, be counterintuitive. It might be expected that due to the substantive drop in IP receptor expression found even in cell culture, combined with cells having been exposed to long-term prostacyclin therapy (epoprostenol or iloprost) for several months prior to isolation [22, 44], this would lead to substantive receptor desensitisation. Because this did not happen, it might suggest either a large IP receptor reserve (redundancy) in the system and/or that IP function recovers sufficiently well in culture before agonist treatment. Other studies have suggested that partial agonism leads to limited β-arrestin recruitment and less IP receptor internalisation, and hence a lower likelihood of receptor desensitisation with MRE-269 compared to other analogues [38]. Against this notion, MRE269 still remains the weakest anti-proliferative agent when compared to other prostacyclin analogues in the same assay [37].

5.3.3.2 Robust Expression of EP$_2$ and EP$_4$ Receptors in PAH: Key Anti-Fibrotic Targets

A striking difference in the pattern of prostanoid receptor mRNA expression was recently reported in human PASMCs derived from control versus PAH patients [44]. While prostanoid IP, EP$_2$ and EP$_4$ receptor mRNA levels were similarly expressed in control cells, the relative expression of EP$_2$ or EP$_4$ over the IP receptor was enhanced 84- and 15-fold, respectively, in PAH cells, suggesting that signalling through these receptors may be well-maintained or even upregulated in PAH [44]. Indeed, EP$_2$ and EP$_4$ receptors, as evidenced by the use of butaprost (selective EP$_2$ agonist) and iloprost, respectively, were functionally coupled to cAMP generation in PASMCs cells derived from either patients or rats with PAH [44, 64]. Moreover, using the selective EP$_2$ receptor antagonist, PF-04418948 [71] as well as EP$_2$ receptor siRNAs, the anti-proliferative effects of treprostinil were found to be mediated by this receptor over a wide concentration range (0.1–1000 nM) in human PASMCs from PAH patients [44]. This corroborates with an earlier observation that an IP receptor- and adenylate cyclase-independent mechanism was largely responsible for the anti-proliferative effects of treprostinil in the same diseased cell type, and appeared also to be the case for iloprost [22]. With respect to treprostinil, PPARγ plays a significant role in mediating the anti-proliferative effects of treprostinil in human PASMCs isolated from PAH patients [22] and by inference involves the EP$_2$ receptor in its activation although this remains to be established. Other PPARs may contribute to the anti-proliferative effects of beraprost [72] though this has not been investigated in PASMCs.

From a pharmacological perspective, this switch towards signalling via the EP$_2$ receptor with treprostinil may with hindsight not be surprising. Based on the high relative EP$_2$/IP receptor expression (84-fold) and that treprostinil has a tenfold greater affinity at the EP$_2$ receptor compared to the IP receptor [45], it suggests that it is >800× more likely to activate the EP$_2$ over the IP receptor in PAH cells. This does not necessarily mean that the IP receptor would not be activated by treprostinil at therapeutic doses as IP receptor activation could be observed under conditions of substantial EP$_2$ antagonism [44]. The situation is in stark contrast to the mode of action of the non-prostanoid IP agonists, MRE-269 and ralinepag, where the IP receptor appears to be entirely responsible for their anti-proliferative properties in cells from PAH patients assessed under similar experimental conditions [37, 44]. At this stage it is unknown whether non-prostanoid IP agonists can bind to PPARs and act in concert with the IP receptor [73] to promote their biological effects, but this is key information to ascertain.

The observation that EP$_2$ receptor expression was abundant relative to other prostanoid receptors may imply that it is upregulated as a consequence of disease. In this respect, EP$_2$ receptor expression can be enhanced in response to platelet-derived growth factor [74, 75] and transforming growth factor β [76], key drivers of smooth muscle proliferation in PAH [4]. Moreover, significantly more EP$_2$ receptors per cell (but not EP$_4$) were detected in asthmatic airway smooth muscle cells compared with non-asthmatic cells, and were found to be associated with enhanced sensitivity to the anti-proliferative effects of both PGE$_2$ and butaprost but not to either prostacyclin or forskolin [74]. Likewise, EP_2 (and EP_4) receptor expression was enhanced in lung fibroblasts derived from patients with chronic obstructive pulmonary disease [77, 78]. Such observations are consistent with enhanced EP_2 receptor function/activity in airway remodelling as well as in PAH. While the role of the EP_2 receptor in the context of remodelling in PAH is unknown, it should be noted that the activation of EP_2 receptors has a range of inhibitory effects on fibroblast function that could have beneficial effects in PAH. Treatment of human lung fibroblasts with either PGE_2 or butaprost inhibits migration [79]. In addition, PGE_2 inhibits the transition of fibroblasts to myofibroblasts [80] and is capable of suppressing fibroblast proliferation and collagen synthesis through EP_2 receptor-mediated pathways [81]. Indeed, anti-fibrotic properties of treprostinil have been reported both *in vivo* (bleomycin-induced pulmonary fibrotic model) and *in vitro* (inhibition of TGF-β-stimulated collagen production), though the receptor involved was not defined in these studies [82, 83]. It should also be mentioned that some of the above effects can be replicated by EP_4 receptors [47, 84], suggesting some overlapping function of EP_2 and EP_4 receptors in regulating fibroblast function. Iloprost appears to ameliorate established cardiac fibrosis by preventing collagen synthesis and increasing collagen turnover, and though the receptor mechanism was not specifically established in this study, evidence was presented that the IP receptor was probably not involved [70]. It is worth noting that in a high-throughput screen to assess the therapeutic potential of novel drugs in pulmonary fibrosis, drugs acting at either the EP_2 or EP_4 receptor were identified as amongst the most effective agents at inhibiting TGF-β-induced myofibroblast differentiation via the SMAD2/3 pathway [85].

5.3.3.3 EP_3 Receptors May Contribute to Disease Pathology in PAH

It is important to understand the role of contractile prostanoid receptors as these could limit the doses of prostacyclin mimetics given therapeutically or potentially give rise to unwanted side effects. Of note, EP_3 expression went up in small arteries from PAH patients, as has been reported in the airway smooth muscle cells derived from asthmatic patients compared to controls [74]. Likewise, enhanced EP_3 expression was observed in rodent models of PAH [33, 86] and was associated with increased sensitivity to the EP_3 agonist, sulprostone, suggesting a gain of function at this receptor [33]. Elevated EP_3 receptor expression would be predicted to dampen cAMP signalling in cells and hence potentially reduce prostanoid-induced relaxation in pulmonary blood vessels as well as relaxation to non-prostanoid IP agonists. Prostacyclin action may be curtailed since it potently binds to the EP_3 receptor (Ki of ~10–40 nM) and the plasma concentration in patients (~25 nM) would be in the range for receptor activation [6, 49]. Many studies have provided evidence that the contractile effects of prostacyclin analogues are mediated through EP_3 receptors [33, 58, 65, 87] and that their inhibition can enhance vasorelaxation induced by these agents [33, 65]. However, based on binding affinities, EP_3 receptors are unlikely to be activated by prostacyclin analogues in the clinical setting; the upper plasma concentration achieved in humans is ~1 nM for iloprost and ~50 nM for treprostinil which is 50× the Ki for both drugs [6]. Consistent with this interpretation, the contractile effects of prostacyclin analogues are only observed at high concentrations (≥1000 nM) in distal rat pulmonary arteries although priming of the tissue with phenylephrine was required before contractions to treprostinil were even observed [87]. Thus any counteracting effect of EP_3 is likely to arise from basal activity of the receptor and not from direct activation by prostacyclin analogues. EP_3-TP-induced vasoconstrictive synergism has been described in blood vessels where priming with a TXA_2 mimetic markedly increases both the potency and size of contraction to EP_3 agonists (see [87]). Enhanced synergy between EP_3 and TP receptors could occur in PAH because of increased TXA_2 levels [88] and because of enhanced activity of EP_3 receptors. Such an interaction might provide an explanation of why iloprost showed far less relaxation and sensitivity in human pulmonary arteries when contracted with the TXA_2 mimetic (U46619) as opposed to phenylephrine [87]. This might suggest that the vasodilatory responses of prostacyclin and iloprost in the lung may be more adversely affected in patients with high TXA_2 levels compared to other IP receptors agonists which either have less sensitivity towards the EP_3 receptors or do not activate them.

EP_3 receptors may contribute to disease pathology in PAH as inhibition of EP_3 receptors either pharmacologically or through deletion of smooth muscle EP_3 receptors attenuated right ventricular systolic pressure (RVSP) and vascular wall thickness in rats with mild (chronic hypoxia), moderate (monocrotaline) or severe (sugen/hypoxia) PAH [86]. Interestingly, the mechanism appeared related to hypoxia-induced TGF-β activation via Rho-associated kinase, with the downstream activation of SMAD2/3 leading to extracellular matrix remodelling via upregulation of collagen 1, fibronectin and tenascin-C genes. Effects were, however, independent of cell proliferation [86], so this suggests that the main role for the EP_3 receptor is to module vascular tone and stiffness in PAH through TGF-β-induced changes in extracellular matrix remodelling.

5.3.3.4 Role of the Veins in PAH and Other Classified Groups of PH

The extent to which venous remodelling contributes to the pathology in PAH is currently a subject of much debate [89] and is thwarted by the lack of good venous biomarkers and the difficulty in identifying veins that might masquerade as a remodelled artery. We can functionally distinguish distal arteries from veins on the basis of their differential response to PGD_2 and PGE_2 in blood vessels pre-contracted with U46619 (thromboxane mimetic). The former relaxes veins while having little effect on tone in arteries, contrasting with PGE_2, which has potent contractile effect in arteries but is minimally contractile in veins under similar experimental conditions (unpublished observations). Whether this will be observed in remodelled veins and arteries is unknown but should be investigated. Strong expression of DP_1 and EP_2 and EP_4 receptors in veins suggests this pattern of response may be preserved.

Elucidating the role of venous remodelling in PH and what might be an effective treatment strategy is complicated by their being a spectrum of disease. This might be seen as a continuum from pure pre-capillary disease (perhaps defined as IPAH) to secondary causes giving rise to a mixed pre- and post-capillary disease (e.g. CTD) through to a predominantly post-capillary phenotype, epitomised by PH due pulmonary venocclusive disease or left heart disease. Interestingly, increased pulmonary venous remodelling has recently been demonstrated in PAH patients harbouring

BMPR2 mutations compared to those without, showing a somewhat similar histological presentation to inoperable chronic thromboembolic pulmonary hypertension (CTEPH) with persistent PH, i.e. fibrotic lesions associated with bronchial to pulmonary shunting [90, 91]. In the context of PH, targeting the veins is important as remodelled veins will significantly contribute to PVR, and mismatching (dilation in arterial but not venous side) will cause higher sheer stress in veins and increase PAP. Enhanced collagen deposition, which makes veins less distensible, would also contribute to the elevated pressure. In primary PH (IPAH), intimal and adventitial thickening of pulmonary veins <250 µm was estimated to be observed in ~50% of cases [92]. Given this study predates the discovery of BMPR2 mutations in the IPAH population [8, 11], and that the current definition of IPAH has a more stringent hemodynamic definition (lower mean PAP and pulmonary artery wedge pressure), suggests that this figure might be overestimated and should thus be re-evaluated [93].

In humans, pulmonary veins have a greater vasoconstrictor sensitivity towards ET-1, TXA_2, leukotrienes and platelet activating factor (PAF) than in arteries, a finding reported in many animal species as well [94]. In addition, numerous studies have shown intense constriction of pulmonary veins in response to hypoxia in a variety of species which may involve the release of ET-1 and TXA_2 [94]. The consequence of venous constriction will be to increase pulmonary capillary pressure and thus promote pulmonary oedema. ET-1 is known to increase capillary permeability via post-capillary vasoconstriction, which is also dependent on the presence of inflammatory cells [95]. Experiments in EP_3 receptor null mice suggest that the EP_3 receptor is responsible in part for oedema triggered by PAF in rat lungs [96] and, as discussed above, is also linked to enhanced collagen production [86]. It also suggests that hypoxia in the veins may be an underlying trigger for oedema via this prostanoid receptor.

The potential for the deleterious effects of prostacyclin (epoprostenol) in patients with severe congestive heart failure and POVD, and the failure of agents that increase cGMP (riociguat and sildenafil) to show significant improvement in the context of PH with left heart disease, has led to the belief that vasodilatory therapy is not appropriate or at least controversial in this setting [89, 97, 98]. Several factors may account for the problems faced with epoprostenol use in patients with diagnosed venous disease. Not only is this agent predicted to be a poor venodilator in humans [19], due in part to its actions on the EP_1 receptor in veins [66], but also the activation of the EP_3 receptor is likely to cause oedema and perpetuate vasoconstriction [94]. The latter may help to explain why pulmonary oedema is commonly reported in POVD patients on epoprostenol therapy [98], particularly in those patients on higher doses of the drug, which would give rise to significant activation of the EP_3 receptor. In severe venous disease, the hypoxic environment coupled with high TXA_2 levels and low IP receptor function might actually be predicted to convert prostacyclin into a venoconstrictor, which would have detrimental consequences (c.f. [97]). For similar reasons, the use of iloprost and beraprost may also be contraindicated in PH-related venous disease. Both, particularly beraprost, are better arterial dilators than venodilators in human pulmonary blood vessels. Iloprost has potent actions on the contractile EP_1 receptor [45] which is functionally expressed in veins, while repeated administration with beraprost in mice has been reported to increase circulatory TXA_2 levels [24]. Whether such an effect occurs in humans remains to be determined, but this might explain why beraprost is a particularly poor venodilator and why effects may not be sustained in PAH patients [1]. In contrast, MRE-269, which is devoid of significant EP_3 receptor activity, is surprisingly a slightly better veno than an arterial vasorelaxant, the significance of which remains unclear but might suggest some usefulness in treating venous disease.

The pharmacological profile of treprostinil suggests it should be seriously considered as a treatment option in PH associated with venous remodelling. Its ability to activate IP, DP_1 EP_2 receptors coupled to the robust expression of the latter two receptors in PAH suggests that its use could provide a beneficial response both as a venodilator and as an anti-fibrotic agent even in the absence of the IP receptor. As such, the efficacy of oral treprostinil, in a multi-centre randomised double blinded trial, is currently being investigated in patients with PH in heart failure with preserved ejection fraction (TDE-HF-301). On a cautionary note, in a retrospective analysis of a PAH cohort (1996–2006) with high rate of contamination from post-capillary disease (of different aetiologies), patients with a mean pulmonary artery wedge pressure (PAWP) >12 did not show meaningful changes in PVR or PAP whereas those classified as having 'pure' pre-capillary disease did [93]. This occurred despite patients having a significant increase in cardiac output and a placebo-corrected improvement in 6-min walk test of 35 m compared to 23 m in the IPAH group. Interestingly, in another randomised study of non-operable CTEPH or persistent PH pulmonary hypertension, patients did respond to treprostinil with significant hemodynamic improvement, including in PVR and mean PAP [99]. The extent to which these patients had venous disease was not reported, but it is possible that venous improvement may have occurred.

5.4 BMPR2 and TGF-β Signalling in PAH and Impact of Prostacyclin Analogues

Since the original discovery of a loss-of-function mutation in the gene encoding for BMPR2 being associated with PAH, more than 300 disease-causing mutations have been described throughout the BMPR2 gene, including critical regions such as the kinase domain [8, 11]. BMPR2 is a transmembrane serine-threonine kinase, which serves as a receptor for bone morphogenetic proteins (BMPs). In association with a co-receptor, usually BMPR1A, BMPR2 can signal through multiple pathways, including the canonical Smad1/5/8-dependent pathway (Fig. 5.4) [5, 6, 8]. The impact of prostacyclin analogues on BMPR2 signalling was investigated by Yang and colleagues in 2010 [9]. They found that iloprost and treprostinil enhanced BMP-induced phosphorylation of Smad1/5 and caused induction of the inhibitor of DNA-binding protein 1 (Id1), both of which are downstream effectors of BMPR2 in normal PASMCs (Fig. 5.4). The growth-suppressive effects of BMPs were re-established in PASMCs derived from patients harbouring BMPR2 mutations without restoring BMPR2 protein levels, consistent with a mechanism that

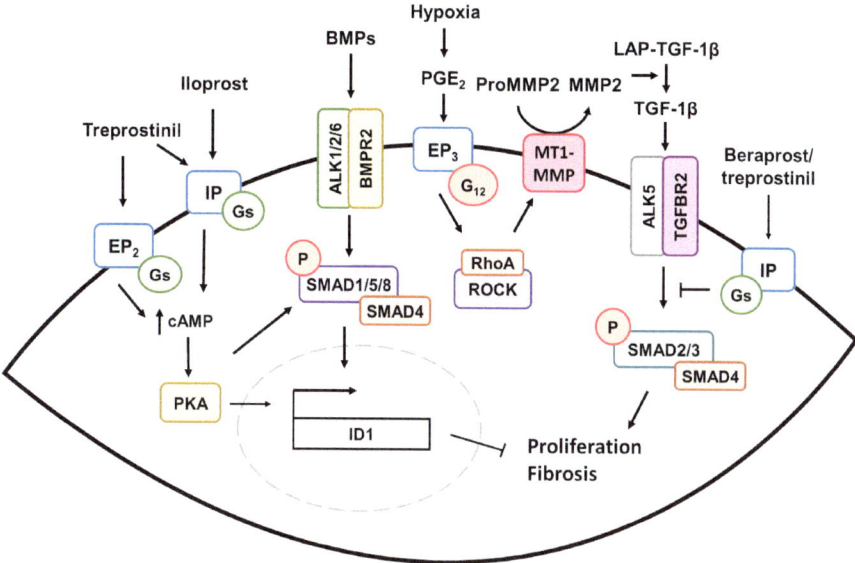

Fig. 5.4 Prostacyclin analogues can enhance bone morphogenic protein receptor type 2 (BMPR2) signalling and oppose cell growth induced via the transforming growth factor beta 1 (TGF-1β) receptor pathway. Upon ligand binding, the BMPR2 receptor phosphorylates a type I receptor (ALK1, ALK2, or ALK6) leading to the phosphorylation of SMAD 1/5/8. The subsequent phosphorylation of SMAD 4 causes translocation of the phosphorylated SMADs to the nucleus to modulate the expression of target genes that inhibit pulmonary artery smooth muscle cell (PASMC) growth and promote apoptosis. Iloprost and treprostinil enhance BMPR2-mediated SMAD 1/5/8 phosphorylation and inhibitory DNA binding protein 1 (ID1) transcription by recruiting IP and EP₂ receptors and activating cAMP-dependent protein kinase A (PKA); induction of ID1 expression can also occur independently of SMADs. Activation of EP₃ receptors by hypoxia in PASMCs pulmonary leads to Rho-dependent activation of metalloproteinase type 2 (MMP2), with the release of active TGF-1 β and the downstream activation of SMAD2/3 via TGF-1β type II receptor (TGFBR2), which phosphorylates a type I receptor, ALK5. The consequence will lead to enhanced proliferation and collagen deposition

bypasses the defective receptor. The prostanoid receptor involved remains undetermined although prostacyclin analogue effects on BMPR2 signalling were shown to be cAMP/PKA-dependent. Likewise, the phosphodiesterase type 5 inhibitor, sildenafil, another PAH therapy, was able to enhance BMPR2 signalling either in normal or mutant cell PASMCs by acting through cyclic GMP-dependent protein kinase I [100]. Thus, prostacyclin drugs known to act by increasing NO (beraprost, epoprostenol and treprostinil) might be predicted to promote a more robust activation of this pathway, with or without sildenafil.

In addition to a deficit in Smad1/5 phosphorylation, heightened Smad2/3 phosphorylation and transcriptional activity have been demonstrated in BMPR2-mutant PASMCs, indicative of increased pro-proliferative TGF-β signalling unopposed by growth-suppressive BMPR2 signalling [101]. Moreover, in contrast to normal PASMCs, upon which TGF-β has growth-suppressive effects, TGF-β promotes the proliferation of BMPR2-mutant PASMCs. The prostacyclin analogue beraprost inhibited TGF-β-induced Smad2/3-dependent signalling (Fig. 5.4) and was more effective at inhibiting the proliferation of BMPR2 mutant PASMCs than that of their wild-type equivalent. Beraprost, like iloprost and treprostinil, could, therefore, be rescuing the diminished BMRP2 signalling while inhibiting the augmented TGF-β signalling to reduce the proliferative capacity of BMPR2-mutant PASMCs. Such a mechanism may also be important in the heart where beraprost was shown to inhibit rat cardiac fibroblast proliferation by activating IP receptors and suppressing the TGF-β/Smad signalling pathway [102].

5.5   Regulation of TASK-1 By Prostacyclin Mimetics: Implications in PAH

Two-pore domain potassium channels of the KCNK gene subfamily, designated K_{2P} channels, mediate leak or background potassium currents (I_{KN}) and underlie the high-membrane permeability to K^+ at physiological resting membrane potentials [103]. KCNK3 encodes a TWIK-related acid-sensitive potassium channel, also known as TASK-1, and is the only TASK subunit to be expressed in either normal or PAH patient lungs [104]. In many cell types, including PASMCs, extracellular acidosis strongly and reversibly inhibits TASK-1 currents and causes membrane depolarisation whereas extracellular alkalosis enhances the currents mediated by TASK-1 to hyperpolarise the membrane. Several lines of evidence suggest a key role for TASK-1 in regulating pulmonary vessel diameter and, hence, vascular tone through its sensitivity to vasoactive mediators, pH, membrane stretch and hypoxia [105, 106]. TASK-1 currents are switched off by hypoxia in PASMCs and are proposed to contribute to standard terminology in the field [106].

In 2013, using whole-exome sequencing, novel heterozygous mutations in the KCNK3 gene were identified in patients with IPAH and HPAH [107]. Subsequently, homozygous KCNK3 mutations were later reported in patients with very aggressive and early-onset forms of PAH [108]. All KCNK3 mutations have severely reduced whole-cell TASK-1 currents recorded from COS-7 as well as from PASMCs expressing both wild-type and mutant TASK-1 subunits to reproduce the heterozygosity observed in carriers of the mutations [104, 107]. Moreover, TASK-1 expression levels were found to be markedly reduced in the explanted lungs of patients with IPAH but lacking disease-causing KCNK3 mutations [109], suggesting more widespread dysfunction of TASK-1 in PAH. Consistent with this notion, rats chronically treated with A293, a selective blocker of TASK-1 channels, were shown to develop early manifestations of PAH, including muscularisation of distal pulmonary arteries (normally non-muscular) and elevated RVSP [109]. Histological analysis of pulmonary arteries from these A293-treated rats revealed marked proliferation of pulmonary arterial endothelial cells (PAECs), PASMCs and pulmonary adventitial fibroblasts [109]. Moreover, TASK-1 currents were also shown to be attenuated in PAECs and PASMCs derived from the lungs of patients with HPAH due to BMPR2 mutations, suggesting that TASK-1 channel downregulation might represent a second hit required for PAH to manifest in carriers with BMPR2 mutations [109].

Activation of different potassium channel types represents an important mechanism underlying the vasorelaxing properties of prostacyclin analogues, including large-conductance calcium-activated, ATP-sensitive and TASK-1 potassium channels [6, 110]. TASK-1 appears to be a downstream target of the IP receptor where iloprost and treprostinil have both been shown to equipotently (EC_{50} 1 nM) enhance I_{KN} currents through TASK-1 channels in normal human PASMCs [110]. The effects of iloprost and treprostinil on TASK-1 currents were mimicked by 8-br-cAMP, a membrane-permeant form of the second messenger cAMP, and blocked by the protein kinase A (PKA) inhibitor, KT5720 and the IP receptor antagonist, RO1138452, suggesting that in healthy human PASMCs prostacyclin analogues signal primarily via the IP/cAMP/PKA pathway to increase TASK-1 currents (Fig. 5.5) [106, 110]. Consensus PKA phosphorylation motifs were also identified within TASK-1 and treprostinil was shown to promote the phosphorylation of these sites [106]. Interestingly, cAMP-dependent PKA was reported to promote

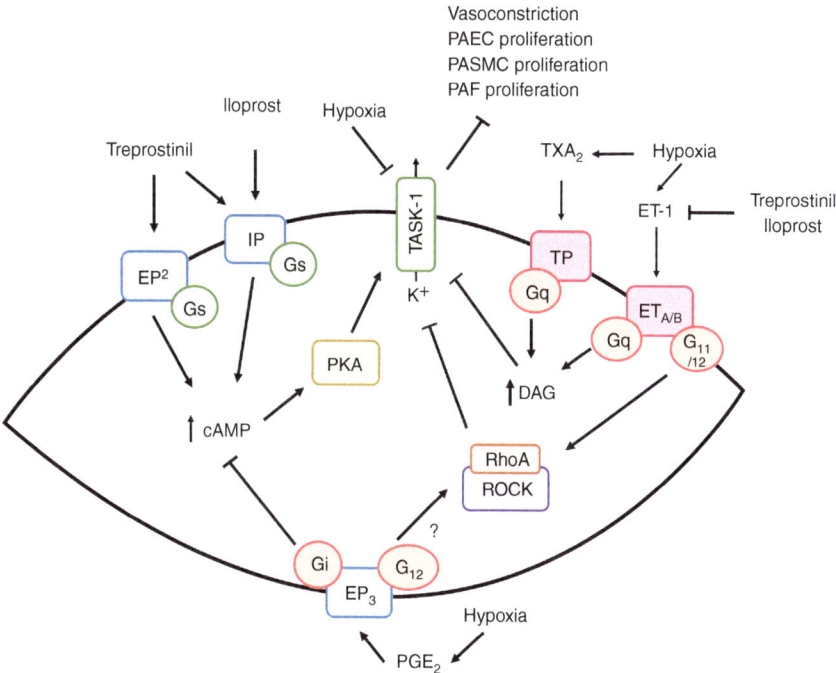

Fig. 5.5 Opposing regulation of TASK-1 by prostacyclin analogues and by hypoxia. TASK-1 in pulmonary arterial smooth muscle cells (PASMCs) is activated by prostacyclin analogues via the IP or EP_2 receptor, while EP_3 receptors oppose this action either through lowering cyclic AMP (cAMP) or via activation of the Rho pathway. Hypoxia-induced synthesis of thromboxane A_2 (TXA_2) or endothelin-1 (ET-1) will inhibit TASK-1 though activation of Gq or $G_{11/12}$. *DAG* diacylglycerol, *PKA* protein kinase A, *ROCK* Rho-associated protein kinase

the forward trafficking of TASK-1 channel subunits from the ER (where they are synthesised) to the plasma membrane where they assemble to form functional, current-conducting channels [111, 112]. Thus, treprostinil or iloprost could be increasing TASK-1 currents in human PASMCs by promoting the forward trafficking of TASK-1 channel subunits from the ER to the sarcolemma. Whether iloprost and treprostinil can rescue the depressed TASK-1 currents in PASMCs from patients with PAH, and whether these channels contribute to the anti-proliferative effects of prostacyclin analogues, remain to be established. Downregulation of the IP receptor in PAH could mean that iloprost becomes less effective at enhancing TASK-1 currents than treprostinil, which is also able to recruit the EP_2 receptor to enhance TASK-1 currents [113].

Several mechanisms may account for the depressed function of TASK-1 in PAH. Gq-coupled receptors, including those activated by ET-1, 5-HT and TXA_2, suppress current through TASK-1 channels (Fig. 5.5) [103]. Given that all these mediators would be elevated in PAH [5, 88, 114], this may lead to a generalised inhibition of the channel. Prostacyclin analogues are potent inhibitors of ET-1 synthesis, both in pulmonary endothelial and smooth muscle cells [6], so these agents could negate the inhibitory effects of ET-1 on TASK-1. The mechanisms by which hypoxia inhibits TASK-1 currents are unclear but may involve increased ET-1 production, given that ET-1 expression and secretion have been shown to be induced by hypoxia in pulmonary endothelial, smooth muscle cells and fibroblasts [94, 114]. ET-1 has been shown to reduce TASK-1 currents in PASMCs by recruiting the RhoA/Rho kinase pathway [115, 116]. EP_3 receptors have been shown to be upregulated in PASMCs in response to hypoxia and are directly linked to activation of the RhoA/Rho kinase pathway [86], so may, like ET-1, inhibit TASK-1 currents through this pathway (Fig. 5.5). EP_3 receptors also couple to $G_{i/o}$ to inhibit cAMP production and so could counteract the effect of prostacyclin analogues on TASK-1 currents, particularly under hypoxic conditions.

5.6   Prostacyclin Effects on Vascular Remodelling In Vivo: Outstanding Issues

The key question is whether prostanoid drugs used to treat PAH patients have positive effects on vascular remodelling associated with the abnormal proliferation of different cell types within the blood vessel wall. In vitro studies reported from a number of laboratories using vascular cells isolated from the lungs of patients with end-stage disease suggest that they should do so *in vivo* [9, 22, 83, 101]. Our own studies directly comparing the anti-proliferative properties of several clinically approved therapies in PASMCs from PAH patients showed hugely variable responses with the lowest dose to significantly inhibit cell proliferation varying some 10,000-fold from 0.1 nM for treprostinil up to 1 μM for the ET-1 receptor antagonist bosentan [117]. By inference, therapies are, therefore, likely to have vastly different effects on the remodelling process *in vivo* and pose challenges when designing protocols. Nonetheless, translation into positive effects on vascular remodelling has been consistently reported in a monocrotaline model of PAH where treprostinil, beraprost and iloprost all significantly improved pulmonary haemodynamics as well as reducing muscularisation and the cell proliferation index of small blood vessels [9, 118–120]. This may in part be due to the analogue effects on inflammatory cell types like macrophages, dendritic cells and mast cells [6], which play a pivotal role in regulating pulmonary vascular remodelling in the monocrotaline model [121] and also in humans [53, 67, 89]. Dysfunctional BMPR2 signalling can also be rescued by prostacyclin analogues through their downstream enhancement of phosph-Smad1/5 and Id1 gene expression in monocrotaline-induced PAH in rats [9], which may act in concert with analogue effects on inflammatory cell types, particularly dendritic cells [6].

With respect to the Sugen 5416/hypoxia model of severe PH, which is a mixed model of group 1 (PAH) and group 3 (due to lung disease and/or hypoxia) PH, all analogues improved cardiac function either by reducing RVSP and RV hypertrophy (beraprost and treprostinil), by increasing exercise capacity and reducing cardiac fibrosis (iloprost) or by improving the ultrastructure of the heart [70, 119, 122]. This would fit with data suggesting that prostacyclins have positive effects on RV function in the heart [123]. Beraprost, given at a high dose as an inhaled bolus in nanoparticles (150 µg/kg), was the only analogue to reduce the muscularisation of arteries, possibly suggesting under dosing may have occurred in the other two studies [70, 119, 122]. The interpretation and significance of the above results would be greatly enhanced if the impact of Sugen 5416/hypoxia on prostanoid receptor and PPAR expression was known, and if hypoxia is a confounding factor in limiting the ability of prostacyclin drugs to activate any of their downstream targets. This could occur, for example, through the excessive production of TXA_2 and ET-1 within the blood vessel wall by hypoxia. This would lead to activation of TP receptors which may cause substantial IP receptor desensitisation and/or enhance EP_3 receptor activation and may thus affect some analogues (iloprost and prostacyclin) more than others. Rats have the peculiar property in that prostacyclin analogues do not relax pulmonary arteries constricted with ET-1 at all whereas they strongly relax human arteries [47]. Whether this means that these agents are not, therefore, able to reverse the mitogenic effects of ET-1 in rats should be considered. Dysfunctional BMPR2 signalling with depressed phospho-Smad1/5 and Id expression is a key feature of the monocrotaline-induced PAH model [9, 10] whereas surprisingly it does not appear to be a feature of the sugen/hypoxia model of PAH as reported in a recent study [122]. This represents a potentially key difference between how PAH is generated in these two classic models. Likewise, many drugs, including potent anti-cancer or anti-angiogenic drugs, do not reverse remodelling in sugen/hypoxia either [124], possibly suggesting that enhanced drug resistance is occurring in this experimental setting, for example, from the inactivation of regulators of the tumour suppressor gene, p53. The use of simvastatin in PAH is not supported by clinical trial data in patients [125] but is one of the very few drugs shown to reduce the number of obliterated lung vessels in the Sugen 5416/hypoxia model. This demonstrates the unpredictability of translating results from animal models into the clinical area.

Another reason why it may be difficult to translate prostanoid receptor function in rodents directly into humans is that, depending on the species, IP and EP_2 receptors can have pro- or anti-inflammatory actions in rat/mouse [126] and human [127] macrophages, respectively. This may confound the interpretation of prostacyclin action in animal models of PAH. The significance of the curious absence of perivascular infiltration of inflammatory cell types in the sugen/hypoxia model [128] needs to be addressed. Moreover, the rat expresses an atypical IP receptor which has a relatively low affinity for the selexipag metabolite compared to the human receptor [32], making it difficult to assess the properties of MRE-269 with other prostacyclin analogues. The same may be true in mice, the other species regularly used to model PAH disease. In this respect, there is no published data on prostanoid receptor affinities in the rat and mouse for treprostinil or much knowledge about prostanoid expression in the lung of these species and whether/how this differs to the pattern of expression in the human lung.

5.7   Future Work and Clinical Implications

Studies suggest that TASK-1 is likely to be a key target for prostacyclins either through the IP or EP_2 receptor. It will be important to understand the role of this channel in experimental PAH models, dysfunction of which is known to promote vasoconstriction, cell proliferation and resistance to apoptosis in cells [12]. Whether prostacyclins can rescue such dysfunction, and thus become a treatment strategy for those patients harbouring TASK-1 mutations, remains to be determined. Along the same lines, upfront prostacyclin therapy should be considered for patients with dysfunctional TGF-β1 and BMPR2 signalling, and those with venoconstriction or remodelling the use of treprostinil considered. Interestingly, in a small scale study in children, only epoprostenol appeared to provide significant improvement out of all the standard PAH therapies in patients habouring BMPR2 and ALK-1 mutations [129]. Furthermore, a number of patients were found to respond to oxygen therapy. It is tempting to speculate here that switching off of the hypoxic-sensitive EP_3 receptor, which is linked to TGF-β receptor activation, may provide some clinical benefit as might activating the hypoxia-sensitive TASK-1 channel. This remains an interesting area for further research.

We have little knowledge about prostacyclin signalling in human distal pulmonary vessels, and to our knowledge no studies have specially investigated vascular reactivity and remodelling processes in small veins in PAH. Clearly future experiments should focus on bridging these gaps. The diverse pharmacology of prostacyclin, its analogues and the newly developed non-prostanoid selective IP agonists potentially give each one of them advantages and disadvantages in different clinical scenarios that should be exploited by patient stratification of PAH and PH subtypes as well as from a personalised medicine approach. These agents are not just vasodilators; they are potent anti-proliferative agents in smooth muscle, and increasing evidence suggests that they act to dampen down fibrosis through their actions on the pro-fibrotic TGF- β signalling pathway, and some of this may also translate into long-term improvements of heart function. The inhibitory action of prostacyclins on platelet function should not be underestimated in PAH, and having a selective IP agonist like selexipag, which is seemingly devoid of *in vivo* action on platelets, may help to tease out their role. From a clinical standpoint, treprostinil through its potent action on EP_2 and DP_1 receptors may provide another treatment option in those patients seen not to be responding well to IP receptor-selective agonists, who are subsequently identified with having low IP receptor expression or limited functional capacity of the receptor. Its pharmacological profile suggests it should also be a good venodilator and strong anti-fibrotic agent through its action on the EP_2 receptor.

Acknowledgements Some of the research described in this article was funded by United Therapeutics (529389) and UCL and supported by the National Institute for Health Research University College London Hospitals (UCLH) Biomedical Research Centre. Jeries Abu-Hanna is funded by a UCL overseas PhD scholarship and Dr. Jigisha Patel is funded in part by a grant from the Biomedical Research Centre (BRC499/CM/LC/101320).

Declaration of Interest Statement L.H.C. has acted as a consultant for United Therapeutics Corp, Arena Pharmaceuticals and Bayer but has received no personal remuneration from these activities. She has also received educational grants from United Therapeutics and Lung Biotechnology PBC which supported part of the work described in this article. The funders had no input into the writing of this manuscript.

References

1. Humbert M, Ghofrani HA. The molecular targets of approved treatments for pulmonary arterial hypertension. Thorax. 2016;71:73–83.
2. D'Alonzo GE, Barst RJ, Ayres SM, et al. Survival in patients with primary pulmonary hypertension. Results from a national prospective registry. Ann Intern Med. 1991;115:343–9.
3. Sandoval J, Bauerle O, Gomez A, et al. Primary pulmonary hypertension in children: clinical characterization and survival. J Am Coll Cardiol. 1995;25:466–74.
4. Hassoun PM, Mouthon L, Barbera JA, et al. Inflammation, growth factors, and pulmonary vascular remodeling. J Am Coll Cardiol. 2009;54:S10–9.
5. Rabinovitch M. Molecular pathogenesis of pulmonary arterial hypertension. J Clin Invest. 2012;122:4306–13.
6. Clapp LH, Gurung R. The mechanistic basis of prostacyclin and its stable analogues in pulmonary arterial hypertension: Role of membrane versus nuclear receptors. Prostaglandins Other Lipid Mediat. 2015;120:56–71.
7. Simonneau G, Gatzoulis MA, Adatia I, et al. Updated clinical classification of pulmonary hypertension. J Am Coll Cardiol. 2013;62:D34–41.
8. Liu D, Morrell NW. Genetics and the molecular pathogenesis of pulmonary arterial hypertension. Curr Hypertens Rep. 2013;15:632–7.
9. Yang J, Li X, Al-Lamki RS, et al. Smad-dependent and Smad-independent induction of Id1 by prostacyclin analogues inhibits proliferation of pulmonary artery smooth muscle cells in vitro and in vivo. Circ Res. 2010;107:252–62.
10. Long L, Ormiston ML, Yang X, et al. Selective enhancement of endothelial BMPR-II with BMP9 reverses pulmonary arterial hypertension. Nat Med. 2015;21:777–85.
11. Thomson JR, Machado RD, Pauciulo MW, et al. Sporadic primary pulmonary hypertension is associated with germline mutations of the gene encoding BMPR-II, a receptor member of the TGF-beta family. J Med Genet. 2000;37:741–5.

12. Boucherat O, Chabot S, Antigny F, et al. Potassium channels in pulmonary arterial hypertension. Eur Respir J. 2015;46:1167–77.
13. Smith WL, DeWitt DL, Allen ML. Bimodal distribution of the prostaglandin I2 synthase antigen in smooth muscle cells. J Biol Chem. 1983;258:5922–6.
14. Gryglewski RJ. Prostacyclin among prostanoids. Pharmacol Rep. 2008;60:3–11.
15. Rubin LJ, Groves BM, Reeves JT, et al. Prostacyclin-induced acute pulmonary vasodilation in primary pulmonary hypertension. Circulation. 1982;66:334–8.
16. Narumiya S, Sugimoto Y, Ushikubi F. Prostanoid receptors: structures, properties, and functions. Physiol Rev. 1999;79:1193–226.
17. Murata T, Ushikubi F, Matsuoka T, et al. Altered pain perception and inflammatory response in mice lacking prostacyclin receptor. Nature. 1997;388:678–82.
18. McLaughlin VV, McGoon MD. Pulmonary arterial hypertension. Circulation. 2006;114:1417–31.
19. Benyahia C, Boukais K, Gomez I, et al. A comparative study of PGI$_2$ mimetics used clinically on the vasorelaxation of human pulmonary arteries and veins, role of the DP-receptor. Prostaglandins Other Lipid Mediat. 2013;107:48–55.
20. Wharton J, Davie N, Upton PD, et al. Prostacyclin analogues differentially inhibit growth of distal and proximal human pulmonary artery smooth muscle cells. Circulation. 2000;102:3130–6.
21. Clapp LH, Finney PA, Turcato S, et al. Differential effects of stable prostacyclin analogues on smooth muscle proliferation and cyclic AMP generation in human pulmonary artery. Am J Respir Cell Mol Biol. 2002;26:194–201.
22. Falcetti E, Hall SM, Phillips PG, et al. Smooth muscle proliferation and role of the prostacyclin (IP) receptor in idiopathic pulmonary arterial hypertension. Am J Respir Crit Care Med. 2010;182:1161–70.
23. Jones RL, Wise H, Clark R, et al. Investigation of the prostacyclin (IP) receptor antagonist RO1138452 on isolated blood vessel and platelet preparations. Br J Pharmacol. 2006;149:110–20.
24. Kashiwagi H, Yuhki K, Kojima F, et al. The novel prostaglandin I2 mimetic ONO-1301 escapes desensitization in an antiplatelet effect due to its inhibitory action on thromboxane A2 synthesis in mice. J Pharmacol Exp Ther. 2015;353:269–78.
25. Parfenova H, Parfenov VN, Shlopov BV, et al. Dynamics of nuclear localization sites for COX-2 in vascular endothelial cells. Am J Physiol Cell Physiol. 2001;281:C166–78.
26. Hertz R, Berman I, Keppler D, et al. Activation of gene transcription by prostacyclin analogues is mediated by the peroxisome-proliferators-activated receptor (PPAR). Eur J Biochem. 1996;235:242–7.
27. Forman BM, Chen J, Evans RM. Hypolipidemic drugs, polyunsaturated fatty acids, and eicosanoids are ligands for peroxisome proliferator-activated receptors alpha and delta. Proc Natl Acad Sci U S A. 1997;94:4312–7.
28. Turcato S, Clapp LH. The effects of the adenylyl cyclase inhibitor SQ22536 on iloprost-induced vasorelaxation and cAMP elevation in isolated guinea-pig aorta. Br J Pharmacol. 1999;126:845–7.
29. Linz W, Wohlfart P, Baader M, et al. The peroxisome proliferator-activated receptor-α (PPAR-α) agonist, AVE8134, attenuates the progression of heart failure and increases survival in rats. Acta Pharmacol Sin. 2009;30:935–46.
30. Jimenez R, Sanchez M, Zarzuelo MJ, et al. Endothelium-dependent vasodilator effects of peroxisome proliferator-activated receptor beta agonists via the phosphatidyl-inositol-3 kinase-Akt pathway. J Pharmacol Exp Ther. 2010;332:554–61.
31. Abramovitz M, Adam M, Boie Y, et al. The utilization of recombinant prostanoid receptors to determine the affinities and selectivities of prostaglandins and related analogs. Biochim Biophys Acta. 2000;1483:285–93.
32. Kuwano K, Hashino A, Asaki T, et al. 2-[4-[(5,6-diphenylpyrazin-2-yl)(isopropyl)amino] butoxy]-N-(methylsulfonyl)acetamide (NS-304), an orally available and long-acting prostacyclin receptor agonist prodrug. J Pharmacol Exp Ther. 2007;322:1181–8.
33. Morrison K, Studer R, Ernst R, et al. Differential effects of selexipag and prostacyclin analogs in rat pulmonary artery. J Pharmacol Exp Ther. 2012;343:547–55.

34. Sitbon O, Channick R, Chin KM, et al. Selexipag for the Treatment of Pulmonary Arterial Hypertension. N Engl J Med. 2015;373:2522–33.
35. Tran TA, Kramer B, Shin YJ, et al. Discovery of 2-(((1r,4r)-4-(((4-Chlorophenyl)(phenyl)carbamoyl)oxy)methyl)cyclohexyl)methoxy)a cetate (Ralinepag): an orally active prostacyclin receptor agonist for the treatment of pulmonary arterial hypertension. J Med Chem. 2017;60:913–27.
36. Clapp LH, Shen L, Patel J, et al. The single isomer beraprost-314d has disproportionate and superior prostacyclin (IP) receptor and antiproliferative activity compared with beraprost. Am J Respir Crit Care Med. 2015;191:A1940.
37. Shen L, Patel JA, Behan DP, et al. APD811, a novel and highly selective non-prostanoid IP receptor agonist in smooth muscle cells from patients with pulmonary hypertension. Circulation. 2018;134:A16601.
38. Gatfield J, Menyhart K, Wanner D, et al. Selexipag active metabolite ACT-333679 displays strong anticontractile and antiremodeling effects but low beta-arrestin recruitment and desensitization potential. J Pharmacol Exp Ther. 2017;362:186–99.
39. Bruderer S, Hurst N, Kaufmann P, et al. Multiple-dose up-titration study to evaluate the safety, tolerability, pharmacokinetics, and pharmacodynamics of selexipag, an orally available selective prostacyclin receptor agonist, in healthy subjects. Pharmacology. 2014;94:148–56.
40. Bazan IS, Fares WH. Hypercoagulability in pulmonary hypertension. Clin Chest Med. 2018;39:595–603.
41. Robbins IM, Kawut SM, Yung D, et al. A study of aspirin and clopidogrel in idiopathic pulmonary arterial hypertension. Eur Respir J. 2006;27:578–84.
42. Willis AL, Smith DL, Vigo C. Suppression of principal atherosclerotic mechanisms by prostacyclins and other eicosanoids. Prog Lipid Res. 1986;25:645–66.
43. Chin KM, Channick RN, de Lemos JA, et al. Hemodynamics and epoprostenol use are associated with thrombocytopenia in pulmonary arterial hypertension. Chest. 2009;135:130–6.
44. Patel JA, Shen L, Hall SM, et al. Prostanoid EP_2 receptors are up-regulated in human pulmonary arterial hypertension: A key anti-proliferative target for treprostinil in smooth muscle cells. Int J Mol Sci. 2018;19:2372.
45. Whittle BJ, Silverstein AM, Mottola DM, et al. Binding and activity of the prostacyclin receptor (IP) agonists, treprostinil and iloprost, at human prostanoid receptors: treprostinil is a potent DP_1 and EP_2 agonist. Biochem Pharmacol. 2012;84:68–75.
46. Syed NI, Jones RL. Assessing the agonist profiles of the prostacyclin analogues treprostinil and naxaprostene, particularly their DP_1 activity. Prostaglandins Leukot Essent Fatty Acids. 2015;95:19–29.
47. Lebender LF, Prunte L, Rumzhum NN, et al. Selectively targeting prostanoid E (EP) receptor-mediated cell signalling pathways: Implications for lung health and disease. Pulm Pharmacol Ther. 2018;49:75–87.
48. Woodward DF, Jones RL, Narumiya S. International union of basic and clinical pharmacology. LXXXIII: classification of prostanoid receptors, updating 15 years of progress. Pharmacol Rev. 2011;63:471–538.
49. Desai UA, Deo SK, Hyland KV, et al. Determination of prostacyclin in plasma through a bioluminescent immunoassay for 6-keto-prostaglandin $F_{1\alpha}$: implication of dosage in patients with primary pulmonary hypertension. Anal Chem. 2002;74:3892–8.
50. Norel X, Walch L, Labat C, et al. Prostanoid receptors involved in the relaxation of human bronchial preparations. Br J Pharmacol. 1999;126:867–72.
51. Fortner CN, Breyer RM, Paul RJ. EP_2 receptors mediate airway relaxation to substance P, ATP, and PGE_2. Am J Physiol Lung Cell Mol Physiol. 2001;281:L469–74.
52. Safholm J, Manson ML, Bood J, et al. Prostaglandin E2 inhibits mast cell-dependent bronchoconstriction in human small airways through the E prostanoid subtype 2 receptor. J Allergy Clin Immunol. 2015;136:1232–9.
53. Arthur G, Bradding P. New Developments in Mast Cell Biology: Clinical Implications. Chest. 2016;150:680–93.
54. Armour CL, Johnson PR, Alfredson ML, et al. Characterization of contractile prostanoid receptors on human airway smooth muscle. Eur J Pharmacol. 1989;165:215–22.

55. Walch L, Labat C, Gascard JP, et al. Prostanoid receptors involved in the relaxation of human pulmonary vessels. Br J Pharmacol. 1999;126:859–66.
56. Foudi N, Kotelevets L, Louedec L, et al. Vasorelaxation induced by prostaglandin E_2 in human pulmonary vein: role of the EP_4 receptor subtype. Br J Pharmacol. 2008;154:1631–9.
57. Jourdan KB, Evans TW, Curzen NP, et al. Evidence for a dilator function of 8-iso prostaglandin F-2 alpha in rat pulmonary artery. Br J Pharmacol. 1997;120:1280–5.
58. Kuwano K, Hashino A, Noda K, et al. A long-acting and highly selective prostacyclin receptor agonist prodrug, 2-{4-[(5,6-diphenylpyrazin-2-yl)(isopropyl)amino]butoxy}-N-(methylsulfonyl)acetamide (NS-304), ameliorates rat pulmonary hypertension with unique relaxant responses of its active form, {4-[(5,6-diphenylpyrazin-2-yl)(isopropyl)amino]butoxy}acetic acid (MRE-269), on rat pulmonary artery. J Pharmacol Exp Ther. 2008;326:691–9.
59. Fuchikami C, Murakami K, Tajima K, et al. A comparison of vasodilation mode among selexipag (NS-304; [2-{4-[(5,6-diphenylpyrazin-2-yl)(isopropyl)amino]butoxy}-N-(methylsulfonyl)aceta mide]), its active metabolite MRE-269 and various prostacyclin receptor agonists in rat, porcine and human pulmonary arteries. Eur J Pharmacol. 2017;795:75–83.
60. Norel X. Prostanoid receptors in the human vascular wall. ScientificWorldJournal. 2007;7:1359–74.
61. Walch L, de Montpreville V, Brink C, et al. Prostanoid EP_1 and TP-receptors involved in the contraction of human pulmonary veins. Br J Pharmacol. 2001;134:1671–8.
62. Orie NN, Ledwozyw A, Williams DJ, et al. Differential actions of the prostacyclin analogues treprostinil and iloprost and the selexipag metabolite, MRE-269 (ACT-333679) in rat small pulmonary arteries and veins. Prostaglandins Other Lipid Mediat. 2013;106:1–7.
63. Kennedy CR, Zhang Y, Brandon S, et al. Salt-sensitive hypertension and reduced fertility in mice lacking the prostaglandin EP_2 receptor. Nat Med. 1999;5:217–20.
64. Lai YJ, Pullamsetti SS, Dony E, et al. Role of the prostanoid EP_4 receptor in iloprost-mediated vasodilatation in pulmonary hypertension. Am J Respir Crit Care Med. 2008;178:188–96.
65. Orie NN, Clapp LH. Role of prostanoid IP and EP receptors in mediating vasorelaxant responses to PGI_2 analogues in rat tail artery: Evidence for $G_{i/o}$ modulation via EP_3 receptors. Eur J Pharmacol. 2011;654:258–65.
66. Norel X, Walch L, Gascard JP, et al. Prostacyclin release and receptor activation: differential control of human pulmonary venous and arterial tone. Br J Pharmacol. 2004;142:788–96.
67. Stenmark KR, Davie N, Frid M, et al. Role of the adventitia in pulmonary vascular remodeling. Physiology (Bethesda). 2006;21:134–45.
68. Tuder RM, Marecki JC, Richter A, et al. Pathology of pulmonary hypertension. Clin Chest Med. 2007;28:23–42.
69. Poloso NJ, Urquhart P, Nicolaou A, et al. PGE2 differentially regulates monocyte-derived dendritic cell cytokine responses depending on receptor usage (EP2/EP4). Mol Immunol. 2013;54:284–95.
70. Gomez-Arroyo J, Sakagami M, Syed AA, et al. Iloprost reverses established fibrosis in experimental right ventricular failure. Eur Respir J. 2015;45:449–62.
71. af Forselles KJ, Root J, Clarke T, et al. In vitro and in vivo characterization of PF-04418948, a novel, potent and selective prostaglandin EP_2 receptor antagonist. Br J Pharmacol. 2011;164:1847–56.
72. Lin H, Lee JL, Hou HH, et al. Molecular mechanisms of the antiproliferative effect of beraprost, a prostacyclin agonist, in murine vascular smooth muscle cells. J Cell Physiol. 2008;214:434–41.
73. Falcetti E, Flavell DM, Staels B, et al. IP receptor-dependent activation of PPARγ by stable prostacyclin analogues. Biochem Biophys Res Commun. 2007;360:821–7.
74. Burgess JK, Ge Q, Boustany S, et al. Increased sensitivity of asthmatic airway smooth muscle cells to prostaglandin E_2 might be mediated by increased numbers of E-prostanoid receptors. J Allergy Clin Immunol. 2004;113:876–81.

75. Zhu S, Xue R, Zhao P, et al. Targeted disruption of the prostaglandin E_2 E-prostanoid 2 receptor exacerbates vascular neointimal formation in mice. Arterioscler Thromb Vasc Biol. 2011;31:1739–47.
76. Tian M, Schiemann WP. PGE2 receptor EP2 mediates the antagonistic effect of COX-2 on TGF-beta signaling during mammary tumorigenesis. FASEB J. 2010;24:1105–16.
77. Dagouassat M, Gagliolo JM, Chrusciel S, et al. The cyclooxygenase-2-prostaglandin E2 pathway maintains senescence of chronic obstructive pulmonary disease fibroblasts. Am J Respir Crit Care Med. 2013;187:703–14.
78. Horikiri T, Hara H, Saito N, et al. Increased levels of prostaglandin E-major urinary metabolite (PGE-MUM) in chronic fibrosing interstitial pneumonia. Respir Med. 2017;122:43–50.
79. White ES, Atrasz RG, Dickie EG, et al. Prostaglandin E_2 inhibits fibroblast migration by E-prostanoid 2 receptor-mediated increase in PTEN activity. Am J Respir Cell Mol Biol. 2005;32:135–41.
80. Kolodsick JE, Peters-Golden M, Larios J, et al. Prostaglandin E_2 inhibits fibroblast to myofibroblast transition via E. prostanoid receptor 2 signaling and cyclic adenosine monophosphate elevation. Am J Respir Cell Mol Biol. 2003;29:537–44.
81. Moore BB, Ballinger MN, White ES, et al. Bleomycin-induced E prostanoid receptor changes alter fibroblast responses to prostaglandin E_2. J Immunol. 2005;174:5644–9.
82. Corboz MR, Zhang J, LaSala D, et al. Therapeutic administration of inhaled INS1009, a treprostinil prodrug formulation, inhibits bleomycin-induced pulmonary fibrosis in rats. Pulm Pharmacol Ther. 2018;49:95–103.
83. Lambers C, Roth M, Jaksch P, et al. Treprostinil inhibits proliferation and extracellular matrix deposition by fibroblasts through cAMP activation. Sci Rep. 2018;8:1087.
84. Lai YJ, Chen IC, Li HH, et al. EP4 agonist L-902,688 suppresses EndMT and attenuates right ventricular cardiac fibrosis in experimental pulmonary arterial hypertension. Int J Mol Sci. 2018;19:727.
85. Sieber P, Schafer A, Lieberherr R, et al. Novel high-throughput myofibroblast assays identify agonists with therapeutic potential in pulmonary fibrosis that act via EP2 and EP4 receptors. PLoS One. 2018;13:e0207872.
86. Lu A, Zuo C, He Y, et al. EP3 receptor deficiency attenuates pulmonary hypertension through suppression of Rho/TGF-beta1 signaling. J Clin Invest. 2015;125:1228–42.
87. Benyahia C, Ozen G, Orie N, et al. Ex vivo relaxations of pulmonary arteries induced by prostacyclin mimetics are highly dependent of the precontractile agents. Prostaglandins Other Lipid Mediat. 2015;121:46–52.
88. Christman BW, McPherson CD, Newman JH, et al. An imbalance between the excretion of thromboxane and prostacyclin metabolites in pulmonary hypertension. N Engl J Med. 1992;327:70–5.
89. Tuder RM, Archer SL, Dorfmuller P, et al. Relevant issues in the pathology and pathobiology of pulmonary hypertension. J Am Coll Cardiol. 2013;62:D4–12.
90. Ghigna MR, Guignabert C, Montani D, et al. BMPR2 mutation status influences bronchial vascular changes in pulmonary arterial hypertension. Eur Respir J. 2016;48:1668–81.
91. Dorfmuller P, Gunther S, Ghigna MR, et al. Microvascular disease in chronic thromboembolic pulmonary hypertension: a role for pulmonary veins and systemic vasculature. Eur Respir J. 2014;44:1275–88.
92. Chazova I, Loyd JE, Zhdanov VS, et al. Pulmonary artery adventitial changes and venous involvement in primary pulmonary hypertension. Am J Pathol. 1995;146:389–97.
93. Gerges C, Gerges M, Skoro-Sajer N, et al. Hemodynamic thresholds for precapillary pulmonary hypertension. Chest. 2016;149:1061–73.
94. Gao Y, Raj JU. Role of veins in regulation of pulmonary circulation. Am J Physiol Lung Cell Mol Physiol. 2005;288:L213–26.
95. Comellas AP, Briva A. Role of endothelin-1 in acute lung injury. Transl Res. 2009;153:263–71.
96. Goggel R, Hoffman S, Nusing R, et al. Platelet-activating factor-induced pulmonary edema is partly mediated by prostaglandin E(2), E-prostanoid 3-receptors, and potassium channels. Am J Respir Crit Care Med. 2002;166:657–62.

97. Califf RM, Adams KF, McKenna WJ, et al. A randomized controlled trial of epoprostenol therapy for severe congestive heart failure: The Flolan International Randomized Survival Trial (FIRST). Am Heart J. 1997;134:44–54.
98. Montani D, Lau EM, Dorfmuller P, et al. Pulmonary veno-occlusive disease. Eur Respir J. 2016;47:1518–34.
99. Sadushi-Kolici R, Jansa P, Kopec G, et al. Subcutaneous treprostinil for the treatment of severe non-operable chronic thromboembolic pulmonary hypertension (CTREPH): a double-blind, phase 3, randomised controlled trial. Lancet Respir Med. 2019;7(3):239–48. https://doi.org/10.1016/S2213-2600(18)30367-9.
100. Yang J, Li X, Al-Lamki RS, et al. Sildenafil potentiates bone morphogenetic protein signaling in pulmonary arterial smooth muscle cells and in experimental pulmonary hypertension. Arterioscler Thromb Vasc Biol. 2013;33:34–42.
101. Ogo T, Chowdhury HM, Yang J, et al. Inhibition of overactive transforming growth factor-β signaling by prostacyclin analogs in pulmonary arterial hypertension. Am J Respir Cell Mol Biol. 2013;48:733–41.
102. Chen Y, Yang S, Yao W, et al. Prostacyclin analogue beraprost inhibits cardiac fibroblast proliferation depending on prostacyclin receptor activation through a TGF beta-Smad signal pathway. PLoS One. 2014;9:e98483.
103. Olschewski A, Veale EL, Nagy BM, et al. TASK-1 (KCNK3) channels in the lung: from cell biology to clinical implications. Eur Respir J. 2017;50:700754.
104. Bohnen MS, Roman-Campos D, Terrenoire C, et al. The impact of heterozygous KCNK3 mutations associated with pulmonary arterial hypertension on channel function and pharmacological recovery. J Am Heart Assoc. 2017;6:e006465.
105. Gurney AM, Osipenko ON, MacMillan D, et al. Two-pore domain K channel, TASK-1, in pulmonary artery smooth muscle cells. Circ Res. 2003;93:957–64.
106. Olschewski A, Li Y, Tang B, et al. Impact of TASK-1 in human pulmonary artery smooth muscle cells. Circ Res. 2006;98:1072–80.
107. Ma L, Roman-Campos D, Austin ED, et al. A novel channelopathy in pulmonary arterial hypertension. N Engl J Med. 2013;369:351–61.
108. Navas TP, Tenorio CJ, Palomino DJ, et al. An homozygous mutation in KCNK3 is associated with an aggressive form of hereditary pulmonary arterial hypertension. Clin Genet. 2017;91:453–7.
109. Antigny F, Hautefort A, Meloche J, et al. Potassium channel subfamily K member 3 (KCNK3) contributes to the development of pulmonary arterial hypertension. Circulation. 2016;133:1371–85.
110. Li Y, Connolly M, Nagaraj C, et al. Peroxisome proliferator-activated receptor-beta/delta, the acute signaling factor in prostacyclin-induced pulmonary vasodilation. Am J Respir Cell Mol Biol. 2012;46:372–9.
111. Mant A, Elliott D, Eyers PA, et al. Protein kinase A is central for forward transport of two-pore domain potassium channels K2P3.1 and K2P9.1. J Biol Chem. 2011;286:14110–9.
112. Kilisch M, Lytovchenko O, Arakel EC, et al. A dual phosphorylation switch controls 14-3-3-dependent cell surface expression of TASK-1. J Cell Sci. 2016;129:831–42.
113. Cunningham KP, Veale EL, Abu-Hanna J, et al. The role of the K2P channels TASK-1, TREK-1 and TREK-2 in the use of treprostinil therapy in pulmonary arterial hypertension. FASEB J. 2018;32:567.6.
114. Davie NJ, Schermuly RT, Weissmann N, et al. The science of endothelin-1 and endothelin receptor antagonists in the management of pulmonary arterial hypertension: current understanding and future studies. Eur J Clin Invest. 2009;39(Suppl 2):38–49.
115. Tang B, Li Y, Nagaraj C, et al. Endothelin-1 inhibits background two-pore domain channel TASK-1 in primary human pulmonary artery smooth muscle cells. Am J Respir Cell Mol Biol. 2009;41:476–83.
116. Seyler C, Duthil-Straub E, Zitron E, et al. TASK1 (K(2P)3.1) K(+) channel inhibition by endothelin-1 is mediated through Rho kinase-dependent phosphorylation. Br J Pharmacol. 2012;165:1467–75.

117. Patel JA, Hall SM, Abraham DJ, et al. Comparison of current therapies to inhibit endothelin-induced growth of pulmonary artery smooth muscle cells (PASMCs) derived from patients with pulmonary arterial hypertension. Eur Respir J. 2014;44:P2355.
118. Schermuly RT, Yilmaz H, Ghofrani HA, et al. Inhaled iloprost reverses vascular remodeling in chronic experimental pulmonary hypertension. Am J Respir Crit Care Med. 2005;172:358–63.
119. Akagi S, Nakamura K, Matsubara H, et al. Intratracheal administration of prostacyclin analogue-incorporated nNanoparticles ameliorates the development of monocrotaline and sugen-hypoxia-induced pulmonary arterial hypertension. J Cardiovasc Pharmacol. 2016;67:290–8.
120. Bhat L, Hawkinson J, Cantillon M, et al. Evaluation of the effects of RP5063, a novel, multimodal, serotonin receptor modulator, as single-agent therapy and co-administrated with sildenafil, bosentan, and treprostinil in a monocrotaline-induced pulmonary arterial hypertension rat model. Eur J Pharmacol. 2018;827:159–66.
121. Pak O, Janssen W, Ghofrani HA, et al. Animal models of pulmonary hypertension: Role in translational research. Drug Discov Today. 2010;7:89–97.
122. Chaudhary KR, Deng Y, Suen CM, et al. Efficacy of treprostinil in the SU5416-hypoxia model of severe pulmonary arterial hypertension: haemodynamic benefits are not associated with improvements in arterial remodelling. Br J Pharmacol. 2018;175:3976–89.
123. Holmboe S, Andersen A, Johnsen J, et al. Inotropic effects of prostacyclins on the right ventricle are abolished in isolated rat hearts with right-ventricular hypertrophy and failure. J Cardiovasc Pharmacol. 2017;69:1–12.
124. Taraseviciene-Stewart L, Scerbavicius R, Choe KH, et al. Simvastatin causes endothelial cell apoptosis and attenuates severe pulmonary hypertension. Am J Physiol Lung Cell Mol Physiol. 2006;291:L668–76.
125. Kawut SM, Bagiella E, Lederer DJ, et al. Randomized clinical trial of aspirin and simvastatin for pulmonary arterial hypertension: ASA-STAT. Circulation. 2011;123:2985–93.
126. Aronoff DM, Peres CM, Serezani CH, et al. Synthetic prostacyclin analogs differentially regulate macrophage function via distinct analog-receptor binding specificities. J Immunol. 2007;178:1628–34.
127. Raychaudhuri B, Malur A, Bonfield TL, et al. The prostacyclin analogue treprostinil blocks NFκB nuclear translocation in human alveolar macrophages. J Biol Chem. 2002;277:33344–8.
128. Stenmark KR, Meyrick B, Galie N, et al. Animal models of pulmonary arterial hypertension: The hope for etiologic discovery and pharmacologic cure. Am J Physiol Lung Cell Mol Physiol. 2009;297:L1013–32.
129. Chida A, Shintani M, Yagi H, et al. Outcomes of childhood pulmonary arterial hypertension in BMPR2 and ALK1 mutation carriers. Am J Cardiol. 2012;110:586–93.

Endothelial-to-Mesenchymal Transition in Pulmonary Hypertension

6

Benoît Ranchoux, Virginie F. Tanguay, and Frédéric Perros

Abstract

Pulmonary arterial hypertension (PAH) is an incurable disease characterized by an intense thickening of the pulmonary arteries leading to their progressive obliteration. This vascular remodeling is a direct consequence of an aberrant accumulation of α-smooth muscle actin (α-SMA)-positive cells in the intravascular area. This process is multifactorial and complex. Recent studies have demonstrated that part of α-SMA-positive cells from intimal and plexiform lesions have an endothelial origin through a process called endothelial-to-mesenchymal transition (EndoMT). Interestingly most of molecular pathways implicated in PAH are known inducers of EndoMT. This review describes how EndoMT appears to play a crucial role in PAH progression.

Keywords

Pulmonary arterial hypertension · Endothelial-to-mesenchymal transition · Vascular remodeling · Endothelial dysfunction

6.1 Pulmonary Hypertension

Pulmonary arterial hypertension (PAH) is histologically characterized by an aberrant remodeling of the pulmonary arterial bed that includes adventitial, medial and intimal thickening as well as neo-muscularization of pre-capillary arterioles. These

B. Ranchoux (✉) · V. F. Tanguay
Research Center of the Institut Universitaire de Cardiologie et de Pneumologie de Québec,
Laval University, Quebec City, QC, Canada

F. Perros
INSERM UMR_S 999, Université Paris-Sud and Université Paris-Saclay,
Le Plessis-Robinson, France

© The Editor(s) (if applicable) and The Author(s) 2020
T. Nakanishi et al. (eds.), *Molecular Mechanism of Congenital Heart Disease
and Pulmonary Hypertension*, https://doi.org/10.1007/978-981-15-1185-1_6

63

modifications of the pulmonary vessels increase the vascular resistance and ultimately lead to the progressive occlusion of the lung vasculature. PAH is multifactorial and the underlying mechanisms that lead to the pathological accumulation of α-smooth muscle actin (α-SMA)-positive cells implicated in the remodeling process are yet under investigation. Among the possible explanations, it has been reported that the pathologic α-SMA cells were derived from circulating bone marrow–derived cells, pericytes or mesenchymal stem cells [1]. Growing evidence also suggest that part of α-SMA-positive cells may have an endothelial origin via a trans-differentiation mechanism called endothelial-to-mesenchymal transition (EndoMT).

6.2   Endothelial-to-Mesenchymal Transition

EndoMT is a key process in vascular development and tissue regeneration. In healthy vessels, the endothelial cells (ECs) are bound in a monolayer fashion by tight and adherens junctions that control EC polarity and barrier functions. During the EndoMT process, ECs lose their junctions and polarity to the endothelium and progressively switch from endothelial to mesenchymal markers. This phenotype switch is accompanied with invasive and proliferative properties that allow EndoMT cells to colonize the surrounding environment. The resultant mesenchymal cells become pluripotent and give rise to various lineages. EndoMT is crucial during embryonic development, angiogenesis and tissue regeneration but is also implicated in pathological process like cancer development, atherosclerosis and fibrotic diseases [2].

EndoMT is regulated by key transcription factors Snail/Slug/ZEB/Twist [3]. When expressed, these transcription factors primarily repress endothelial junctions. These junctions are composed of transmembrane proteins (such as VE-cadherin, CD31, Claudins and occludin) that are bound to the cytoskeleton and stabilized by cytoplasmic scaffold proteins (such as p120-cathenin, β-catenin or ZO-1) [4]. EndoMT-related transcription factors down-regulate the junction proteins, inducing the dissolution of the cell-cell junctions and the loss of EC polarity in the early stages of transition [3]. The disruption of the junctions also releases free scaffold proteins in the cytoplasm that, if not degraded, trigger secondary pathways promoting ECs proliferation and motility. For example, the inhibition of Claudins and occludin induces the release of ZO-1 from tight junction which promotes cell proliferation via CD1 and PCNA up-regulation [5]. Similarly, the inhibition of VE-cadherin leads to accumulation of free p120-catenin that promotes invasiveness by inhibiting RhoA activity, up-regulating mesenchymal cadherin and activating Rac1/MAPK and Ras/MAPK signaling pathways [6]. Therefore, the chronic activation of EndoMT pathways causes the loss of endothelium integrity (which directly regulates vascular homeostasis, angiogenesis and inflammation) and the invasion of the sub-endothelial area by proliferative mesenchymal cells.

6.3   EndoMT in PAH Pathogenesis

6.3.1   EndoMT in PAH Vascular Remodeling

Aberrant vascular remodeling with occlusive α-SMA-positive cell accumulation forming a neo-intima and endothelial dysfunction are hallmarks of PAH pathogenesis. Both features can be the results of an unresolved EndoMT process as suggested by Arciniegas and colleagues [7]. Our laboratory was the first to confirm the occurrence of EndoMT in situ in idiopathic PAH [8]. Using immunofluorescence, transmission electron microscopy and correlative light and electron microscopy, we provided phenotypic and ultrastructural evidences of ongoing EndoMT in remodeled PAH arteries. We were able to observe ongoing EndoMT in intimal and plexiform lesions where α-SMA-positive cells' accumulation contributed to vessel obliteration. These findings were associated with a loss of endothelial p120-catenin, which is essential for adherens junction and with an overexpression of Twist in PAH lungs. Similar results were observed in two established animal models of pulmonary hypertension (PH) induced by monocrotaline and Sugen/hypoxia. EndoMT was also observed in systemic sclerosis-associated PAH where cells expressing both endothelial and mesenchymal markers were found in 4% of the remodeled vessels [9]. Since then various studies have confirmed the occurrence of an ongoing EndoMT process in PAH with the overexpression of transcription factors Twist/Snail/Slug [10–12].

6.3.2   Molecular Pathways of EndoMT in PAH

The mechanisms that regulate EndoMT are complex and not fully understood but appear to be close of those involved in the epithelial-to-mesenchymal transition (EMT). Interestingly the main characteristics of PAH pathological environment are known inducers of EndoMT and EMT. Indeed, the ECs in PAH are locally exposed to chronic inflammation, hypoxia, mechanical stress and loss of endothelial junction. Inflammation is highly associated with EMT-associated tumor progression and EndoMT. Tumor necrosis factor (TNF)-α, interleukin (IL)-6, transforming growth factor (TGF)-β or IL-8 promote ZEB/Snail/Twist expression via NFκB and JAK/STAT signaling. Cells undergoing mesenchymal transition also induce local inflammation via increased secretion of cytokines such as IL-6, IL-8 and TNF-α [3, 9, 13]. Hypoxia is also a well-described inducer of EndoMT though hypoxia-inducible factor 2α (HIF-2α) activation. Tang et al. demonstrated that PAH ECs display an increased expression of HIF-2α even under normoxic conditions, and this leads to the up-regulation of Snail/Slug and therefore aberrant EndoMT [12]. Of note, HIF-1α, that is found up regulated in PAH smooth muscle cells, induces overexpression of Twist. The increased pressure and shear stress due to disturbed blood flow are known to trigger EndoMT to initiate adaptive muscularization of vessels but are also linked to neointimal hyperplasia in other vasculopathies like atherosclerosis [14]. Finally, the shear stress resulting from increased vascular resistances further damages the endothelial junctions. As presented above, it triggers EndoMT to overcome the mechanical stress by increasing vascular thickness. Nevertheless, as EndoMT reduces the overall endothelium integrity and increases the vascular remodeling, it may enter in a vicious circle of unresolved EndoMT. The pathological environment of chronic inflammation and increased pressure may then lead to an undesirable feedback loop leading to further endothelial dysfunction, inflammation and shear stress as the vascular remodeling progresses.

The main molecular pathways implicated in PAH development are also related to EndoMT molecular mechanisms. The TGF-β signaling pathways play a crucial role in PAH. TGF-β is found increased in serum and lungs from PAH patients and most of the genetic mutations related to PAH occur in genes encoding receptors of the TGF-β superfamily [1]. Interestingly TGF-β signaling is a key actor of EndoMT either via Smad-dependent or Smad-independent pathways. The activation of TGF-β receptors initiates Smad2/3/4 cascade which up-regulates Snail/Slug/Twist/ZEB. TGF-β also promotes EndoMT through various Smad-independent pathways leading, for example, to the inactivation of GSK-3β, a repressor of Snail- and β-catenin-induced EndoMT or to the PI3K/AKT-mediated up-regulation of Twist/Snail/Slug/ZEB expression through mTOR and NF-κB activation. Finally autocrine feedback loops appear in TGF-β-induced EndoMT since Twist overexpression in human pulmonary ECs also up-regulates TGF-β expression [11].

In addition, deficient signaling through bone morphogenetic protein receptor type 2 (BMPR-II), a member of the TGF-β receptor superfamily, plays a critical role in PAH. Indeed, mutations in the *BMPR2* gene are found in 70% of cases of familial PAH and in 10–40% of cases of idiopathic PAH. Moreover, in the absence of a *BMPR2* mutation, reduced expression of pulmonary vascular BMPR-II has also been observed in non-hereditary PAH. We created a rat strain with monoallelic mutations on *BMPR2*, which develops spontaneously PAH. In this animal model, altered BMPR-II signaling was associated with increased pulmonary Twist expression and EndoMT [8]. This link between the main genetic risk factor for PAH and unregulated EndoMT was confirmed by Hopper and colleagues as they found that reduced BMPR-II also promotes Slug overexpression via HMGA1 up-regulation [10].

The TGF-β pathways are not fully characterized, have feedback loops, talk to each other and have interactions with others signaling such as Notch, Wnt and receptor tyrosine kinases (RTKs), all involved in PAH pathogenesis and EndoMT [3, 15–20]. Notch1 was reported to be increased in lung from idiopathic PAH patient and Sugen/hypoxia rats [20], and Notch1/3 were found up-regulated in hypoxia- and MCT-induced PH [21]. Notch signaling also interacts with PAH-associated pathways such as HIF-1α and IL-6 [3, 15–19]. Notch activation up-regulates Snail/Slug expression [3]. In PAH, both canonical Wnt and non-canonical Wnt were found up-regulated [22, 23]. In the first one, activation of Wnt leads to GSK-3β inhibition and Snail- and β-catenin-induced EndoMT [3, 15, 16]. In the non-canonical one, Wnt activates GTPases Rac/Rho/cdc42, all involved in migration and cytoskeleton rearrangement [24]. Several growth factor signaling that act through RTKs are found up-regulated in PAH, including epidermal growth factor, fibroblast growth factor, vascular endothelial growth factor and platelet-derived growth factor [1]. Their roles are incompletely understood due to feedback loop regulations among given growth factor signaling and because of contradictory effects on pulmonary vasculature when used in vivo probably due to their numerous isoforms of receptor and ligand as well as the structural similarities and signaling versatility between different RTKs. Some RTK inhibitors like imatinib or sorafenib have been shown to exert beneficial effects in animal models of PH whereas others like dasatinib or Sugen are known inducers of PAH [25]. Interestingly the activation of most of those RTK signalings initiates the PI3K/AKT/NF-κB and Ras/MAPK pathways that ultimately up-regulate Twist/Snail/Slug/ZEB. RTKs signaling also cross talks with other EndoMT pathways like TGF-β-, β-catenin or Wnt-induced EndoMT via the common PI3K/AKT-dependant inhibition of GSK-3β [3]. Nevertheless despite improvements in haemodynamics and exercise capacity, the serious adverse events associated with RKT inhibitors in PAH therapies currently outweigh their beneficial role observed in animal models [1].

Other molecular actors of PAH pathogenesis might also contribute to EndoMT. For example, endothelin-1, which is overexpressed in PAH and contributes to vasoconstriction and vascular remodeling [1], has also been reported to induce EMT. It can trigger transdifferentiation either by activating both ET_A/ET_B receptors and subsequent PI3K/ILK/GSK-3β and AMPK pathways, or by repressing miR-300, a negative regulator of Twist or by inducing TGF-β overexpression [26–28]. Another hallmark of PAH is an increased level of serotonin in the patients' serum [25]. This neurotransmitter was reported to induce EMT in renal proximal tubular epithelial cells [29] and inhibition of its receptors 5-HT1B/5-HT1D down-regulates ZEB/Snail expression and undergoing EMT in human pancreatic cancer cells [30]. Finally, angiotensin-II which is increased in patients' blood with increased signaling through its type 1 receptor in PAH ECs [31] has also been implicated in EMT and EndoMT in cancer and diabetes-related cardiovascular diseases [32–34].

6.4 Conclusion

PAH has a multifactorial and complex pathobiology. Growing evidences support that an unresolved EndoMT process is actively implicated in the vascular remodeling and endothelial dysfunction involved in the disease progression. EndoMT can be the direct consequence of PAH pathological environment and dysregulated molecular pathways. As presented, EndoMT mechanisms are yet incompletely understood but their cross talk with most of PAH hallmarks leads us to believe that EndoMT might be a crucial actor in PAH progression and a promising therapeutic target.

6.5 Future Direction and Clinical Implications

EndoMT is a crucial actor in embryonic development and tissue regeneration in adult tissues. Numerous studies have demonstrated that the same cellular mechanisms of EndoMT are also implicated in the progression of cancers and cardiovascular diseases. Growing evidences support that EndoMT might play a central role in PAH pathogeny. These findings open exciting opportunities in the study of the initial triggers and the vascular remodeling process of PAH. A better understanding of EndoMT in PAH could lead to the development of novel anti-remodeling strategies in the management of PAH with potentially limited side effects on healthy tissues.

Acknowledgments F.P. received funding from the National Funding Agency for Research (ANR; grant: ANR-13-JSV1-0011-01) and from Fondation du Grand défi Pierre Lavoie. F.P. also received a PVRI BMPR2 Research Grant supported by the Dinosaur Trust.

References

1. Hemnes AR, Humbert M. Pathobiology of pulmonary arterial hypertension: understanding the roads less travelled. Eur Respir Rev. 2017;26:170093. https://doi.org/10.1183/16000617.0093-2017.
2. Yu W, Liu Z, An S, et al. The endothelial-mesenchymal transition (EndMT) and tissue regeneration. Curr Stem Cell Res Ther. 2014;9:196–204.
3. Lamouille S, Xu J, Derynck R. Molecular mechanisms of epithelial–mesenchymal transition. Nat Rev Mol Cell Biol. 2014;15:178–96. https://doi.org/10.1038/nrm3758.
4. Dejana E, Tournier-Lasserve E, Weinstein BM. The control of vascular integrity by endothelial cell junctions: molecular basis and pathological implications. Dev Cell. 2009;16:209–21. https://doi.org/10.1016/j.devcel.2009.01.004.
5. Huang RY-J, Guilford P, Thiery JP. Early events in cell adhesion and polarity during epithelial-mesenchymal transition. J Cell Sci. 2012;125:4417–22. https://doi.org/10.1242/jcs.099697.
6. Kourtidis A, Ngok SP, Anastasiadis PZ. p120 catenin: an essential regulator of cadherin stability, adhesion-induced signaling, and cancer progression. Prog Mol Biol Transl Sci. 2013;116:409–32. https://doi.org/10.1016/B978-0-12-394311-8.00018-2.
7. Arciniegas E, Frid MG, Douglas IS, Stenmark KR. Perspectives on endothelial-to-mesenchymal transition: potential contribution to vascular remodeling in chronic pulmonary hypertension. Am J Physiol Lung Cell Mol Physiol. 2007;293 (1):L1–L8.
8. Ranchoux B, Antigny F, Rucker-Martin C, et al. Endothelial-to-mesenchymal transition in pulmonary hypertension. Circulation. 2015;131:1006–18. https://doi.org/10.1161/CIRCULATIONAHA.114.008750.
9. Good RB, Gilbane AJ, Trinder SL, et al. Endothelial to mesenchymal transition contributes to endothelial dysfunction in pulmonary arterial hypertension. Am J Pathol. 2015;185:1850–8. https://doi.org/10.1016/j.ajpath.2015.03.019.
10. Hopper RK, Moonen J-RAJ, Diebold I, et al. In pulmonary arterial hypertension, reduced BMPR2 promotes endothelial-to-mesenchymal transition via HMGA1 and its target slug. Circulation. 2016;133:1783–94. https://doi.org/10.1161/CIRCULATIONAHA.115.020617.. Clinical Perspective.
11. Mammoto T, Muyleart M, Konduri GG, Mammoto A. Twist1 in hypoxia-induced pulmonary hypertension through transforming growth factor-β-Smad signaling. Am J Respir Cell Mol Biol. 2018;58:194–207. https://doi.org/10.1165/rcmb.2016-0323OC.

12. Tang H, Babicheva A, McDermott KM, et al. Endothelial HIF-2α contributes to severe pulmonary hypertension by inducing endothelial-to-mesenchymal transition. Am J Physiol Lung Cell Mol Physiol. 2017;00096:2017. https://doi.org/10.1152/ajplung.00096.2017.

13. Dominguez C, David JM, Palena C. Epithelial-mesenchymal transition and inflammation at the site of the primary tumor. Semin Cancer Biol. 2017;47:177–84. https://doi.org/10.1016/j.semcancer.2017.08.002.

14. Moonen J-RAJ, Lee ES, Schmidt M, et al. Endothelial-to-mesenchymal transition contributes to fibro-proliferative vascular disease and is modulated by fluid shear stress. Cardiovasc Res. 2015;108:377–86. https://doi.org/10.1093/cvr/cvv175.

15. Garg M. Epithelial-mesenchymal transition—activating transcription factors—multifunctional regulators in cancer. World J Stem Cells. 2013;5:188–95. https://doi.org/10.4252/wjsc.v5.i4.188.

16. Yang Y-M, Yang W-X. Epithelial-to-mesenchymal transition in the development of endometriosis. Oncotarget. 2017;8:41679–89. https://doi.org/10.18632/oncotarget.16472.

17. Yang J, Weinberg RA. Epithelial-mesenchymal transition: at the crossroads of development and tumor metastasis. Dev Cell. 2008;14:818–29. https://doi.org/10.1016/j.devcel.2008.05.009.

18. Derynck R, Muthusamy BP, Saeteurn KY. Signaling pathway cooperation in TGF-β-induced epithelial-mesenchymal transition. Curr Opin Cell Biol. 2014;31:56–66. https://doi.org/10.1016/j.ceb.2014.09.001.

19. Kalluri R, Weinberg RA. The basics of epithelial-mesenchymal transition. J Clin Invest. 2009;119:1420–8. https://doi.org/10.1172/JCI39104.

20. Dabral S, Tian X, Kojonazarov B, et al. Notch1 signalling regulates endothelial proliferation and apoptosis in pulmonary arterial hypertension. Eur Respir J. 2016;48(4):1137–49. https://doi.org/10.1183/13993003.00773-2015.

21. Xiao Y, Gong D, Wang W. Soluble JAGGED1 inhibits pulmonary hypertension by attenuating notch signaling. Arterioscler Thromb Vasc Biol. 2013;33:2733–9. https://doi.org/10.1161/ATVBAHA.113.302062.

22. Wu D, Talbot CC, Liu Q, et al. Identifying microRNAs targeting Wnt/β-catenin pathway in end-stage idiopathic pulmonary arterial hypertension. J Mol Med (Berl). 2016;94:875–85. https://doi.org/10.1007/s00109-016-1426-z.

23. Laumanns IP, Fink L, Wilhelm J, et al. The noncanonical WNT pathway is operative in idiopathic pulmonary arterial hypertension. Am J Respir Cell Mol Biol. 2009;40:683–91. https://doi.org/10.1165/rcmb.2008-0153OC.

24. de Jesus Perez V, Yuan K, Alastalo T-P, et al. Targeting the Wnt signaling pathways in pulmonary arterial hypertension. Drug Discov Today. 2014;19:1270–6. https://doi.org/10.1016/j.drudis.2014.06.014.

25. Guignabert C, Tu L, Le Hiress M, et al. Pathogenesis of pulmonary arterial hypertension: lessons from cancer. Eur Respir Rev. 2013;22:543–51. https://doi.org/10.1183/09059180.00007513.

26. Bagnato A, Rosanò L. Epithelial-mesenchymal transition in ovarian cancer progression: a crucial role for the endothelin axis. Cells Tissues Organs. 2007;185:85–94. https://doi.org/10.1159/000101307.

27. Wu M-H, Huang P-H, Hsieh M, et al. Endothelin-1 promotes epithelial-mesenchymal transition in human chondrosarcoma cells by repressing miR-300. Oncotarget. 2016;7:70232–46. https://doi.org/10.18632/oncotarget.11835.

28. Jain R, Shaul PW, Borok Z, Willis BC. Endothelin-1 induces alveolar epithelial-mesenchymal transition through endothelin type a receptor-mediated production of TGF-beta1. Am J Respir Cell Mol Biol. 2007;37:38–47. https://doi.org/10.1165/rcmb.2006-0353OC.

29. Erikci A, Ucar G, Yabanoglu-Ciftci S. Role of serotonin in the regulation of renal proximal tubular epithelial cells. Ren Fail. 2016;38:1141–50. https://doi.org/10.1080/0886022X.2016.1194165.

30. Gurbuz N, Ashour AA, Alpay SN, Ozpolat B. Down-regulation of 5-HT1B and 5-HT1D receptors inhibits proliferation, clonogenicity and invasion of human pancreatic cancer cells. PLoS One. 2014;9(8):e105245. https://doi.org/10.1371/journal.pone.0105245.

31. De Man F, Tu L, Handoko L, et al. Dysregulated renin-angiotensin-aldosterone system contributes to pulmonary arterial hypertension. Am J Respir Crit Care Med. 2012;186:780–9. https://doi.org/10.1164/rccm.201203-0411OC.
32. Tang R, Li Q, Lv L, et al. Angiotensin II mediates the high-glucose-induced endothelial-to-mesenchymal transition in human aortic endothelial cells. Cardiovasc Diabetol. 2010;9:31. https://doi.org/10.1186/1475-2840-9-31.
33. Nguyen L, Ager EI, Neo J, Christophi C. Regulation of colorectal cancer cell epithelial to mesenchymal transition by the renin angiotensin system. J Gastroenterol Hepatol. 2016;31:1773–82. https://doi.org/10.1111/jgh.13307.
34. Oh E, Kim JY, Cho Y, et al. Overexpression of angiotensin II type 1 receptor in breast cancer cells induces epithelial-mesenchymal transition and promotes tumor growth and angiogenesis. Biochim Biophys Acta. 2016;1863:1071–81. https://doi.org/10.1016/j.bbamcr.2016.03.010.

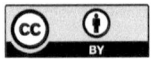

Extracellular Vesicles, MicroRNAs, and Pulmonary Hypertension

7

Tianji Chen and J. Usha Raj

Abstract

Pulmonary hypertension (PH) is a devastating disease that results in a progressive increase in pulmonary vascular resistance, right ventricular failure, and ultimately death of patients. Recent advances in our understanding of pathogenesis of diseases, including PH, have led to the study of extracellular vesicles (EV) as mediators of disease. Subsets of EV are microvesicles (MV), exosomes (Exo), and apoptotic bodies, and they are released from a variety of cell types and carry cargo such as proteins and microRNAs (miR). MicroRNAs contained within these EV play an important role in disease including in the pathogenesis of PH as well as other lung diseases.

Keywords

Extracellular vesicles · Pulmonary hypertension · Endothelial cells · Smooth muscle cells · microRNAs

7.1 Extracellular Vesicles (EV)

Extracellular vesicles (EV) are nano-sized, membrane-bound vesicles released from cells that can mediate intercellular communication [1]. Different EV types, including exosomes (Exo), microvesicles (MV), and apoptotic bodies, have been

T. Chen · J. U. Raj (✉)
Department of Pediatrics, University of Illinois, College of Medicine at Chicago, Chicago, IL, USA
e-mail: usharaj@uic.edu

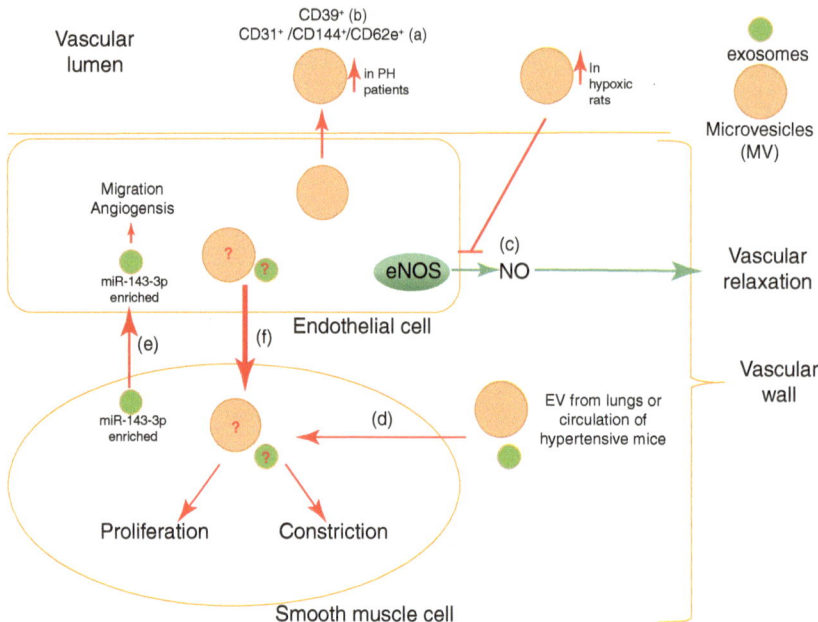

Fig. 7.1 Endothelial (EC) and smooth muscle (SMC) cells release extracellular vesicles (EV) and interact through transfer of EV. Increased circulating levels of endothelium-derived microvesicles (MV) have been documented in PH patients (*a*). Visovatti et al. demonstrated increased CD39 expression and function in circulating MV of idiopathic PAH patients, which may be associated with the increased ATPase/ADPase activity in MV (*b*). Tual-Chalot et al. showed that circulating MV from hypoxic rats can suppress endothelial-dependent vascular relaxation in rat aorta and pulmonary arteries by decreasing NO production (*c*). More recently, Aliotta et al. reported that healthy mice injected with circulating or lung EV isolated from MCT-treated mice show elevated right ventricular-to-body weight ratio and pulmonary arterial wall thickness-to-diameter ratio compared to that of mice injected with control EV (*d*). Deng et al. showed a high abundance of miR-143-3p in PASMC-derived exosomes and a paracrine pro-migratory and pro-angiogenic effect of these miR-143-3p-enriched PASMC-derived exosomes on PAEC (*e*). However, the cross talk between EC and SMC through EV transfer, especially from EC to SMC, and underlying molecular mechanisms remain unclear (*f*)

characterized on the basis of their biogenesis or release pathways: *Exosomes (Exo)* are 50–100 nm membrane vesicles of endocytic origin. They are released into the extracellular space by fusion with the plasma membrane. Exosomes contain endosome-specific proteins such as Alix and TSG101, components of microdomains in the plasma membrane such as cholesterol, ceramide, integrins, and tetraspanins, mRNAs, microRNA (miRNAs), and other non-coding RNAs. ExoCarta, an exosome database, provides a comprehensive list of exosomes identified (http://exocarta.org/) [2, 3]. *Microvesicles (MV)*, also referred to as microparticles (MP), especially in the cardiovascular field, are sized 20–1000 nm. They are formed through the outward budding and separation of the plasma membrane. During their formation, microvesicles retain surface molecules from parent cells and part of their cytosolic content (proteins, RNAs, microRNAs) [3, 4]. *Apoptotic bodies* are the largest vesicles of the EV with a size of 1–5 μm. They are formed through outward blebbing of the cell membrane during the late steps of apoptosis. Apoptotic bodies contain cellular organelles, proteins, DNAs, RNAs, and microRNAs [2, 3, 5].

7.2   EV in Pulmonary Hypertension (PH)

Pulmonary hypertension (PH) is a devastating disease that results in a progressive increase in pulmonary vascular resistance, right ventricular failure, and ultimately death of patients [6, 7]. Recent studies have shown that abnormal EV secretion is associated with the pathogenesis of PH, and increased circulating levels of endothelium-derived MV have been documented in various cardiovascular diseases including PH [4, 8]. In PH patients the levels of circulating endothelial CD31$^+$ (PECAM$^+$)/CD41$^-$, CD144$^+$(VE-cadherin$^+$), and CD62e$^+$ (E-selectin$^+$) positive microvesicles are increased compared with control subjects. Moreover, PAH patients exhibit higher values of endothelial PECAM$^+$ and VE-cadherin$^+$-positive MV versus those with chronic pulmonary disease-related PH [8]. Higher levels of endothelium-derived MV bearing E-selectin are also noted in thromboembolic PH as compared with non-thromboembolic PH subjects [9], suggesting that the etiology of the disease may influence MV levels [10].

MV are not only a biomarker of PH but rather actively contribute to development of PH [11, 12]. Visovatti and colleagues demonstrated increased CD39 expression and function in circulating MV of idiopathic PAH patients, which may be associated with the increased ATPase/ADPase activity in MV [13]. The endothelium-dependent relaxation of rat pulmonary arteries is suppressed after incubation with MV obtained from rats exposed to chronic hypoxia as compared to control arteries exposed to normoxia, accompanied by attenuated eNOS activity and increased ROS production [11]. In another study, Lee and colleagues demonstrated that mesenchymal stromal cell-derived exosomes exert a pleiotropic protective effect on the lung and inhibit vascular remodeling and hypoxic PH with suppression of STAT3/miR-17 levels and induction of miR-204 levels in the lung [14]. Moreover, a recent study reported that healthy mice injected with EV isolated from MCT-treated mice show elevated right ventricular-to-body weight ratio and pulmonary arterial wall thickness-to-diameter ratio compared to that of mice injected with control EV, providing direct in vivo evidence that EV contribute to pulmonary vascular remodeling and PH [12].

7.3   MicroRNA Transfer Through EV in PH

MicroRNAs (miRNAs, miRs) are small single-stranded non-coding RNAs that mediate post-transcriptional degradation or translation repression of target messenger RNAs (mRNAs) [15, 16]. Many miRNAs have been identified to play important roles in disease development, including PH [17–19]. In addition to the primary intracellular locations, miRNAs can be exported extracellularly into the circulation system [20–23] through the transfer of EV. A recent study by Aliotta et al. has reported dysregulated miRNA profiling in the circulating exosomes of monocrotaline (MCT)-induced PH in mice, as well in patients with idiopathic pulmonary artery hypertension (IPAH) [24], suggesting that exosome (and maybe also other EV)-mediated miRNA signaling may play a role in the pathogenesis of PH. This hypothesis is supported by their finding that healthy mice injected with EV isolated from MCT-treated mice show induced right ventricular hypertrophy and pulmonary vessel wall thickening [12].

In the pulmonary vasculature, endothelial and smooth muscle cells (EC and SMC) are the two key cell types that play a major role in the pathobiology of PH [25]. The miRNA cross talk between EC and SMC via EV in pulmonary vasculature is exemplified by a recent study by Deng et al. [26]. This study demonstrates that migration and angiogenesis of pulmonary arterial endothelial cells (PAEC) are induced not only by exosome-derived miR-143 but also by co-culture of PAEC with pulmonary arterial SMC (PASMC) under conditions where direct cell-cell contact is prevented. The miR-143-enriched exosomes derived from PASMC are internalized by PAEC which lead to increased EC migration and angiogenesis. This study also shows that miR-143 is upregulated in the pulmonary vasculature of murine models of PH and in patients with PH. Genetic deletion of miR-143 or pharmacological inhibition of miR-143 in mice prevented the development of hypoxiainduced pulmonary hypertension. Hence, cross talk between EC and SMC via miR-143-enriched exosomes may be involved in the pathogenesis of PH under in vivo conditions.

Our knowledge about the cross talk between EC and SMC through EV transfer, especially the information transfer from EC to SMC, is still very limited and further studies are warranted.

7.4 Future Direction and Clinical Implications

The release of extracellular vesicles (EV) is a phenomenon shared by most cell types, including EC and SMC [1]. EV released into the extracellular space can enter body fluids and/or potentially reach neighboring and/or distal cells. The cargo of EV includes the proteins, lipids, nucleic acids, and membrane receptors of the cells from which they originate. Hence, EV can function as the "mail carrier" and transfer information (microRNAs, proteins, etc.) to their target cells, thus representing an important mechanism for intercellular communications [3, 4, 27–32]. The EV-mediated intercellular communications are evolutionarily conserved [33]. Therefore, EV are rich sources of biomarkers for diagnosis and/or prognosis of human diseases [34–41] and provide us potential therapeutic approaches [42, 43].

Acknowledgment This work was supported in part by NIH R01HL123804 (JUR and GZ), an American Lung Association Biomedical Research Grant RG-416135 (TC) and a Gilead Sciences Research Scholars Program in Pulmonary Arterial Hypertension (TC).

References

1. Zaborowski MP, Balaj L, Breakefield XO, Lai CP. Extracellular Vesicles: composition, biological relevance, and methods of study. Bioscience. 2015;65:783–97.
2. Akers JC, Gonda D, Kim R, Carter BS, Chen CC. Biogenesis of extracellular vesicles (EV): exosomes, microvesicles, retrovirus-like vesicles, and apoptotic bodies. J Neurooncol. 2013;113:1–11.
3. van der Pol E, Boing AN, Harrison P, Sturk A, Nieuwland R. Classification, functions, and clinical relevance of extracellular vesicles. Pharmacol Rev. 2012;64:676–705.
4. Loyer X, Vion AC, Tedgui A, Boulanger CM. Microvesicles as cell-cell messengers in cardiovascular diseases. Circ Res. 2014;114:345–53.
5. Taylor RC, Cullen SP, Martin SJ. Apoptosis: controlled demolition at the cellular level. Nat Rev Mol Cell Biol. 2008;9:231–41.
6. Humbert M, Sitbon O, Simonneau G. Treatment of pulmonary arterial hypertension. N Engl J Med. 2004;351:1425–36.
7. McLaughlin VV, Archer SL, Badesch DB, Barst RJ, Farber HW, Lindner JR, Mathier MA, McGoon MD, Park MH, Rosenson RS, et al. ACCF/AHA 2009 expert consensus document on pulmonary hypertension: a report of the American College of Cardiology Foundation Task Force on Expert Consensus Documents and the American Heart Association: developed in collaboration with the American College of Chest Physicians, American Thoracic Society, Inc., and the Pulmonary Hypertension Association. Circulation. 2009;119:2250–94.
8. Amabile N, Heiss C, Real WM, Minasi P, McGlothlin D, Rame EJ, Grossman W, De Marco T, Yeghiazarians Y. Circulating endothelial microparticle levels predict hemodynamic severity of pulmonary hypertension. Am J Respir Crit Care Med. 2008;177:1268–75.
9. Diehl P, Aleker M, Helbing T, Sossong V, Germann M, Sorichter S, Bode C, Moser M. Increased platelet, leukocyte and endothelial microparticles predict enhanced coagulation and vascular inflammation in pulmonary hypertension. J Thromb Thrombolysis. 2011;31:173–9.
10. Amabile N, Guignabert C, Montani D, Yeghiazarians Y, Boulanger CM, Humbert M. Cellular microparticles in the pathogenesis of pulmonary hypertension. Eur Respir J. 2013;42:272–9.
11. Tual-Chalot S, Guibert C, Muller B, Savineau JP, Andriantsitohaina R, Martinez MC. Circulating microparticles from pulmonary hypertensive rats induce endothelial dysfunction. Am J Respir Crit Care Med. 2010;182:261–8.
12. Aliotta JM, Pereira M, Amaral A, Sorokina A, Igbinoba Z, Hasslinger A, El-Bizri R, Rounds SI, Quesenberry PJ, Klinger JR. Induction of pulmonary hypertensive changes by extracellular vesicles from monocrotaline-treated mice. Cardiovasc Res. 2013;100:354–62.
13. Visovatti SH, Hyman MC, Bouis D, Neubig R, McLaughlin VV, Pinsky DJ. Increased CD39 nucleotidase activity on microparticles from patients with idiopathic pulmonary arterial hypertension. PLoS One. 2012;7:e40829.
14. Lee C, Mitsialis SA, Aslam M, Vitali SH, Vergadi E, Konstantinou G, Sdrimas K, Fernandez-Gonzalez A, Kourembanas S. Exosomes mediate the cytoprotective action of mesenchymal stromal cells on hypoxia-induced pulmonary hypertension. Circulation. 2012;126:2601–11.
15. Bartel DP. MicroRNAs: genomics, biogenesis, mechanism, and function. Cell. 2004;116:281–97.
16. Bartel DP. MicroRNAs: target recognition and regulatory functions. Cell. 2009;136:215–33.
17. Boucherat O, Potus F, Bonnet S. microRNA and pulmonary hypertension. Adv Exp Med Biol. 2015;888:237–52.
18. Grant JS, White K, MacLean MR, Baker AH. MicroRNAs in pulmonary arterial remodeling. Cell Mol Life Sci. 2013;70:4479–94.
19. Zhou G, Chen T, Raj JU. MicroRNAs in pulmonary arterial hypertension. Am J Respir Cell Mol Biol. 2015;52:139–51.
20. Fichtlscherer S, De Rosa S, Fox H, Schwietz T, Fischer A, Liebetrau C, Weber M, Hamm CW, Roxe T, Muller-Ardogan M, et al. Circulating microRNAs in patients with coronary artery disease. Circ Res. 2010;107:677–84.

21. Turchinovich A, Weiz L, Langheinz A, Burwinkel B. Characterization of extracellular circulating microRNA. Nucleic Acids Res. 2011;39:7223–33.
22. Vickers KC, Palmisano BT, Shoucri BM, Shamburek RD, Remaley AT. MicroRNAs are transported in plasma and delivered to recipient cells by high-density lipoproteins. Nat Cell Biol. 2011;13:423–33.
23. Wang K, Zhang S, Weber J, Baxter D, Galas DJ. Export of microRNAs and microRNA-protective protein by mammalian cells. Nucleic Acids Res. 2010;38:7248–59.
24. Aliotta JM, Pereira M, Wen S, Dooner MS, Del Tatto M, Papa E, Goldberg LR, Baird GL, Ventetuolo CE, Quesenberry PJ, Klinger JR. Exosomes induce and reverse monocrotaline-induced pulmonary hypertension in mice. Cardiovasc Res. 2016;110:319–30.
25. Gao Y, Chen T, Raj JU. Endothelial and smooth muscle cell interactions in the pathobiology of pulmonary hypertension. Am J Respir Cell Mol Biol. 2016;54:451–60.
26. Deng L, Blanco FJ, Stevens H, Lu R, Caudrillier A, McBride MW, McClure JD, Grant JS, Thomas M, Frid MG, et al. miR-143 activation regulates smooth muscle and endothelial cell crosstalk in pulmonary arterial hypertension. Circ Res. 2015;117(10):870–83.
27. Schiro A, Wilkinson FL, Weston R, Smyth JV, Serracino-Inglott F, Alexander MY. Endothelial microparticles as conveyors of information in atherosclerotic disease. Atherosclerosis. 2014;234:295–302.
28. Kim DK, Lee J, Kim SR, Choi DS, Yoon YJ, Kim JH, Go G, Nhung D, Hong K, Jang SC, et al. EVpedia: a community web portal for extracellular vesicles research. Bioinformatics. 2015;31:933–9.
29. Antonyak MA, Cerione RA. Microvesicles as mediators of intercellular communication in cancer. Methods Mol Biol. 2014;1165:147–73.
30. Cocucci E, Racchetti G, Meldolesi J. Shedding microvesicles: artefacts no more. Trends Cell Biol. 2009;19:43–51.
31. Simons M, Raposo G. Exosomes—vesicular carriers for intercellular communication. Curr Opin Cell Biol. 2009;21:575–81.
32. Thery C, Ostrowski M, Segura E. Membrane vesicles as conveyors of immune responses. Nat Rev Immunol. 2009;9:581–93.
33. Deatherage BL, Cookson BT. Membrane vesicle release in bacteria, eukaryotes, and archaea: a conserved yet underappreciated aspect of microbial life. Infect Immun. 2012;80:1948–57.
34. Caby MP, Lankar D, Vincendeau-Scherrer C, Raposo G, Bonnerot C. Exosomal-like vesicles are present in human blood plasma. Int Immunol. 2005;17:879–87.
35. Choi DS, Lee J, Go G, Kim YK, Gho YS. Circulating extracellular vesicles in cancer diagnosis and monitoring: an appraisal of clinical potential. Mol Diagn Ther. 2013;17:265–71.
36. D'Souza-Schorey C, Clancy JW. Tumor-derived microvesicles: shedding light on novel microenvironment modulators and prospective cancer biomarkers. Genes Dev. 2012;26:1287–99.
37. Mullier F, Minet V, Bailly N, Devalet B, Douxfils J, Chatelain C, Elalamy I, Dogne JM, Chatelain B. Platelet microparticle generation assay: a valuable test for immune heparin-induced thrombocytopenia diagnosis. Thromb Res. 2014;133:1068–73.
38. Sarlon-Bartoli G, Bennis Y, Lacroix R, Piercecchi-Marti MD, Bartoli MA, Arnaud L, Mancini J, Boudes A, Sarlon E, Thevenin B, et al. Plasmatic level of leukocyte-derived microparticles is associated with unstable plaque in asymptomatic patients with high-grade carotid stenosis. J Am Coll Cardiol. 2013;62:1436–41.
39. Shedden K, Xie XT, Chandaroy P, Chang YT, Rosania GR. Expulsion of small molecules in vesicles shed by cancer cells: association with gene expression and chemosensitivity profiles. Cancer Res. 2003;63:4331–7.
40. Simpson RJ, Lim JW, Moritz RL, Mathivanan S. Exosomes: proteomic insights and diagnostic potential. Expert Rev Proteomics. 2009;6:267–83.

41. Hergenreider E, Heydt S, Treguer K, Boettger T, Horrevoets AJ, Zeiher AM, Scheffer MP, Frangakis AS, Yin X, Mayr M, et al. Atheroprotective communication between endothelial cells and smooth muscle cells through miRNAs. Nat Cell Biol. 2012;14:249–56.
42. EL Andaloussi S, Mäger I, Breakefield XO, Wood MJ. Extracellular vesicles: biology and emerging therapeutic opportunities. Nat Rev Drug Discov. 2013;12:347–57.
43. Chaput N, Taieb J, Andre F, Zitvogel L. The potential of exosomes in immunotherapy. Expert Opin Biol Ther. 2005;5:737–47.

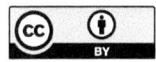

Roles of Tbx4 in the Lung Mesenchyme for Airway and Vascular Development

8

Keiko Uchida, Yu Yoshida, Kazuki Kodo,
and Hiroyuki Yamagishi

Keywords
Lung · Mesenchyme · Vascular development · Transcription factor

The T-box family genes are evolutionarily conserved transcription factors. In particular, Tbx4 and Tbx5 are closely conserved and play crucial roles in development and organogenesis. Tbx4 is essential for hindlimb and allantoic vessel formation [1]. Our data show that it is also highly expressed in the lung mesenchyme (Fig. 8.1), initially expressed at embryonic day (E) 9.25 and later expressed throughout murine embryogenesis [2].

Lung mesenchyme is stromal tissue that surrounds the epithelium and consists of undifferentiated progenitor cells, which give rise to various cell types, such as smooth muscle, cartilage, fibroblasts, endothelium, pericytes, and mesothelium. Although the behavior of epithelial progenitors has been elucidated, much less is known about the identity and behavior of mesenchymal progenitors in the lungs. Mesenchymal cells are generally thought to have highly proliferative, migratory, and multipotent potential. Lung-specific mesenchymal Tbx4 and Tbx5 deficiency revealed that these transcription factors cooperatively regulated branching morphogenesis, likely through the activation of fibroblast growth factor (Fgf) 10

K. Uchida (✉)
Department of Pediatrics, Keio University School of Medicine, Shinjuku, Tokyo, Japan

Health Center, Keio University, Minato, Tokyo, Japan
e-mail: keiuchid@keio.jp

Y. Yoshida · K. Kodo
Department of Pediatrics, Keio University School of Medicine, Shinjuku, Tokyo, Japan

H. Yamagishi (✉)
Division of Pediatric Cardiology, Department of Pediatrics,
Keio University School of Medicine, Tokyo, Japan
e-mail: hyamag@keio.jp

© The Editor(s) (if applicable) and The Author(s) 2020
T. Nakanishi et al. (eds.), *Molecular Mechanism of Congenital Heart Disease and Pulmonary Hypertension*, https://doi.org/10.1007/978-981-15-1185-1_8

79

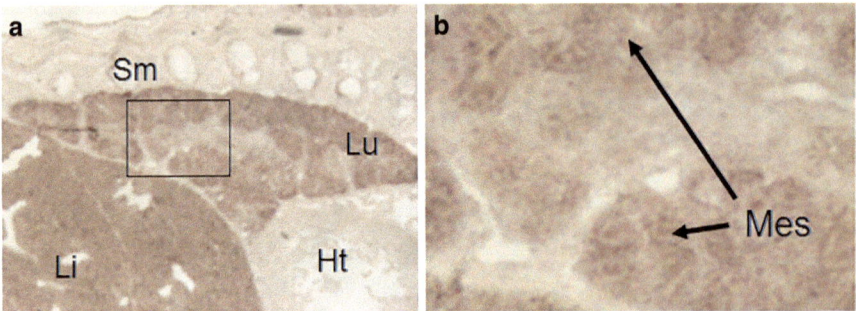

Fig. 8.1 Tbx4 is expressed in the lung mesenchyme. Section ISH with Tbx4 anti-sense riboprobe (**a** low magnification, **b** high magnification of the square area in **a**) shows Tbx4 is expressed throughout the lung mesenchyme at E14.5. *Ht* heart, *Li* liver, *Lu* lung, *Mes* mesenchyme, *Sm* somite

signaling during the lung development [2]. Tbx4 is detectable at earlier stages of lung development compared to other mesenchymal transcription factors [3], suggesting that Tbx4 functions upstream from them. Cell lineage tracing using transgenic mice harboring the lung-specific mesenchyme enhancer (LME) from the mouse Tbx4 locus (Tbx4-LME)-specific Cre transgene showed that Tbx4-expressing cells give rise to all cell types of the lung mesenchyme [3]. Although it remains controversial whether they become pulmonary vascular endothelial cells or not, Tbx4 lung enhancer-driven Tet-On inducible Cre reporter mice showed that both of pulmonary endothelium and vascular smooth muscle were targeted from E11.5; it was also found that the expression level of Tbx4 decreased once the pulmonary vascular cells were differentiated [4].

From these reports, Tbx4 in undifferentiated mesenchymal progenitor cells may be involved in the formation of both airways and vessels in the lungs. The roles of Tbx4 in the lung mesenchyme may pave the way for novel mechanisms underlying pulmonary vascular development.

Acknowledgment This work was supported by JSPS KAKENHI Grant Numbers JP17K10153 and JP23591583 to KU, and 16H05359 to HY.

References

1. Naiche LA, Papaioannou VE. Tbx4 is not required for hindlimb identity or post-bud hindlimb outgrowth. Development. 2007;134:93–103.
2. Arora R, Metzger RJ, Papaioannou VE. Multiple roles and interactions of Tbx4 and Tbx5 in development of the respiratory system. PLoS Genet. 2012;8:e1002866.
3. Kumar ME, Bogard PE, Espinoza FH, et al. Defining a mesenchymal progenitor niche at single-cell resolution. Science. 2014;346:1258810.
4. Zhang W, Menke DB, Jiang M, et al. Spatial-temporal targeting of lung-specific mesenchyme by a Tbx4 enhancer. BMC Biol. 2013;11:111.

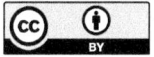

A lacZ Reporter Transgenic Mouse Line Revealing the Development of Pulmonary Artery

9

Reina Ishizaki, Keiko Uchida, Akimichi Shibata,
Takatoshi Tsuchihashi, Jun Maeda, Katsuhiko Mikoshiba,
and Hiroyuki Yamagishi

Keywords

Vasculogenesis · Angiogenesis · Cardiovascular system · Pulmonary arterial smooth muscle cell

Pulmonary vasculature in mice develops through two main mechanisms, namely angiogenesis and vasculogenesis. At embryonic day (E) 9.5, vascular endothelial marker Tie2-driven LacZ expression in whole-mount transgenic lungs showed continuity between the primitive lung vasculature and the aortic sac [1]. Scanning electron microscopic study of vascular casts and graphic reconstruction in the 32- and 34-somite (E10) embryos demonstrated that the primordium of the pulmonary artery (PA) arose from the proximal portion of the sixth pharyngeal arch artery and ran straight in the caudal direction [2]. At E10.5, though the afferent vessels were not yet defined as vascular tubes, they resembled two plexiform networks that coalesce alongside the trachea. From these observations, "distal angiogenesis" was proposed as a model for the pulmonary vascular morphogenesis where PAs arise from the pharyngeal arch artery and elongate into the lung buds [1]. Another study provided evidence to support vasculogenesis as the mechanism of both proximal and distal vessel formation during the development of murine lungs [3]. Detailed

R. Ishizaki · K. Uchida · A. Shibata · T. Tsuchihashi · J. Maeda
Department of Pediatrics, Keio University School of Medicine, Shinjuku, Tokyo, Japan

K. Mikoshiba
SIAIS (Shanghai Institute for Advanced Immunochemical Studies), ShanghaiTech University, Shanghai, China

H. Yamagishi (✉)
Division of Pediatric Cardiology, Department of Pediatrics,
Keio University School of Medicine, Tokyo, Japan
e-mail: hyamag@keio.jp

analysis using Mercox vascular casts revealed that vasculogenesis occurred periph- erally in the lungs to form isolated blood islands and that angiogenesis centrally forms the axial and lateral arteries and veins. The fusion and coalescence of these central and peripheral systems lead to the development of the pulmonary circuit [4]. The earliest connection between the peripheral and central spaces was identified between E13 and E14.

Muscularization is part of the gradual maturation process of airways and vessels in the lungs [1]. Cells positive for α-smooth muscle actin in the vascular wall of PA are evident at E11.5 [1, 5]. In terms of local development of vascular smooth mus- cle, the PA wall is constructed radially, from the inside out, by two separate, but coordinated processes: one is the sequential induction and recruitment of successive cell layers from surrounding mesenchymal progenitor cells and the other is the con- trolled invasion of the surrounding layer by inner layer cells. Later on in the process, inner layer cells initially divide and migrate extensively within the layer before radi- ally reorienting to either migrate into the second layer or radially divide to send daughter cells into the next developing layer [6].

Through the recent analysis of a transgenic mouse line harboring the lacZ reporter gene in a certain targeted locus, we found that the lacZ marker was spe- cifically expressed in PA smooth muscle cells using whole-mount staining during the lung development (Fig. 9.1). Our results suggest that PA smooth muscle may elongate gradually from the proximal pulmonary trunk to the peripheral pulmo- nary arteries similar to the "distal angiogenesis" model during development [7].

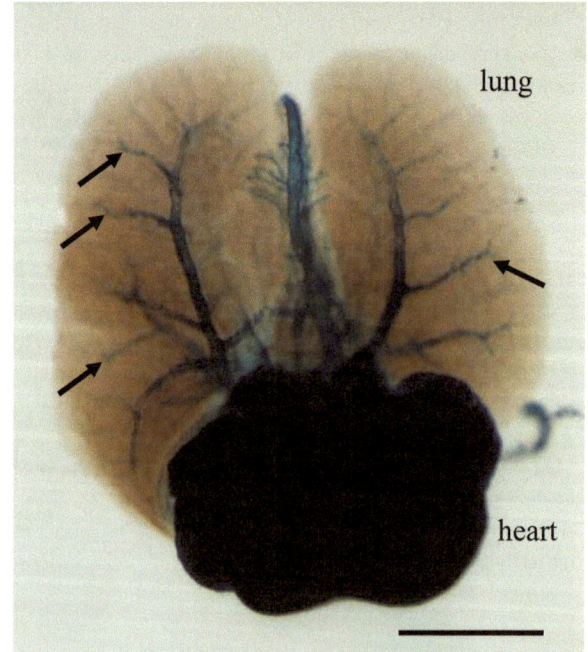

Fig. 9.1 Visualization of pulmonary artery using a reporter transgenic mouse. Whole-mount β-galactosidase staining heart and lungs at embryonic day (E) 15.5. The β-galactosidase- positive pulmonary arteries continuously elongate from the central pulmonary trunk to peripheral small arteries (arrows). Scale bar, 1 mm

References

1. Parera MC, van Dooren M. Distal angiogenesis: a new concept for lung vascular morphogenesis. Am J Physiol Lung Cell Mol Physiol. 2005;288(1):L141–9.
2. Hiruma T, Nakajima Y, Nakamura H. Development of pharyngeal arch arteries in early mouse embryo. J Anat. 2002;201(1):15–29.
3. Schachtner SK, Wang Y, Baldwin HS. Qualitative and quantitative analysis of embryonic pulmonary vessel formation. Am J Respir Cell Mol Biol. 2000;22(2):157–65.
4. deMello DE, Sawyer D, Galvin N, et al. Early fetal development of lung vasculature. Am J Respir Cell Mol Biol. 1997;16(5):568–81.
5. Tollet J, Everett AW, Sparrow MP. Spatial and temporal distribution of nerves, ganglia, and smooth muscle during the early pseudoglandular stage of fetal mouse lung development. Dev Dyn. 2001;221(1):48–60.
6. Greif DM, Kumar M, Lighthouse JK, et al. Radial construction of an arterial wall. Dev Cell. 2012;23(3):482–93. https://doi.org/10.1016/j.devcel.2012.07.009.
7. Ishizaki-Asami R, Uchida K, Tsuchihashi T, et al. Inositol 1,4,5-trisphosphate receptor 2 as a novel marker of vasculature to delineate processes of cardiopulmonary development. Dev Biol. 2020;458(2):237–45. https://doi.org/10.1016/j.ydbio.2019.11.011

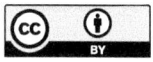

Roles of Stem Cell Antigen-1 in the Pulmonary Endothelium

10

Jun Maeda, Keiko Uchida, Kazuki Kodo, and Hiroyuki Yamagishi

Keywords
Resident progenitor cell · Pulmonary vessels · Sca-1 · Angiogenesis

There is growing evidence that resident progenitor cell populations exist in murine lung tissues and differentiate into a mesenchymal cell lineage [1, 2]. Stem cell antigen-1 (Sca-1) is a cell surface glycoprotein, initially found in murine bone marrow–derived stem cell subtypes, such as hematopoietic stem cells. Some studies showed Sca-1 expression in the pulmonary vascular endothelium of adult murine lungs [3], while a subset of Sca-1-expressing cells formed vascular-like structures under specific conditions [1].

We previously performed DNA microarray analysis using murine lung cells positive for vascular endothelial marker, CD31, selected by fluorescence-activated cell sorting (FACS) at embryonic and postnatal stages. Sca-1 was found to be more robustly expressed in postnatal pups than in embryos (Uchida K, unpublished observation), suggesting that a subset of Sca-1-expressing cells may be related to the formation of the capillary network during later development.

First, we performed immunohistochemistry using eight-week-old murine lung sections where Sca-1 immunostaining was found in the vascular wall of pulmonary vessels and alveolar capillaries. Some of these Sca-1-positive cells showed overlapping expression with vascular endothelial marker, vWF. Cell populations were then

J. Maeda · K. Uchida · K. Kodo
Department of Pediatrics, Keio University School of Medicine, Shinjuku, Tokyo, Japan

H. Yamagishi (✉)
Division of Pediatric Cardiology, Department of Pediatrics,
Keio University School of Medicine, Tokyo, Japan
e-mail: hyamag@keio.jp

T. Nakanishi et al. (eds.), *Molecular Mechanism of Congenital Heart Disease and Pulmonary Hypertension*, https://doi.org/10.1007/978-981-15-1185-1_10

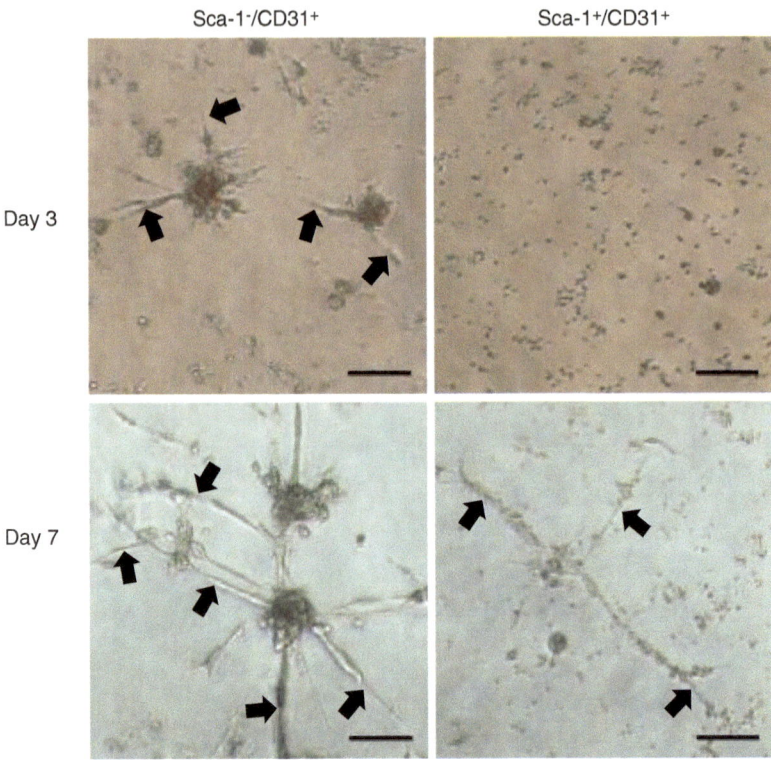

Fig. 10.1. The tube formation assay. The tube formation (arrows) reflecting angiogenesis is more robustly observed in Sca-1 (−) CD31 (+) cells than in Sca-1 (+) CD31 (+) cells. Scale bars, 100 μm

isolated from whole-lung cells by FACS, using antibodies for Sca-1 and CD31, following the depletion of CD45-positive cells. We investigated the tube formation ability of these sorted cells cultured in endothelial growth media and found that Sca-1 (−) CD31 (+) cells were more robust in tube formation than Sca-1 (+) CD31 (+) cells (Fig. 10.1).

These results suggest that though Sca-1 (+) CD31 (+) cells form vascular tube structures, they have lower tube formation activity than Sca-1 (−) CD31 (+) cells. Sca-1 may possibly repress angiogenesis activity in the endothelial cells and potentially make progenitor cell populations stay resident in adult murine lungs. Further analysis would delineate the physiological function of Sca-1 in developing lungs through embryonic to adult stages.

Acknowledgment This work was supported by JSPS KAKENHI Grant Number JP16K10074 to J.M.

References

1. Summer R, Kotton DN, Liang S, et al. Embryonic lung side population cells are hematopoietic and vascular precursors. Am J Respir Cell Mol Biol. 2005;33:32–40.
2. McQualter JL, Brouard N, Williams B, et al. Endogenous fibroblastic progenitor cells in the adult mouse lung are highly enriched in the Sca-1 positive cell fraction. Stem Cells. 2009;27:623–33.
3. Kotton DN, Summer RS, Sun X, et al. Stem cell antigen-1 expression in the pulmonary vascular endothelium. Am J Physiol Lung Cell Mol Physiol. 2003;284:L990–6.

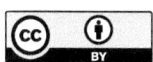

Morphological Characterization of Pulmonary Microvascular Disease in Bronchopulmonary Dysplasia Caused by Hyperoxia in Newborn Mice

11

Hidehiko Nakanishi, Shunichi Morikawa, Shuji Kitahara, Asuka Yoshii, Atsushi Uchiyama, Satoshi Kusuda, and Taichi Ezaki

Keywords

Bronchopulmonary dysplasia · Pulmonary hypertension · Pulmonary microvascular disease

Bronchopulmonary dysplasia (BPD) is one of the most significant medical complications in preterm infants, and pulmonary microvascular injury is associated with the pathogenesis of BPD [1]. Furthermore, impairments of developing pulmonary vasculature may cause secondary pulmonary hypertension (PH), which contributes significantly to morbidity and mortality among preterm infants [2]. To characterize the mechanisms of pulmonary vascular disease resulting from BPD, we studied the ultrastructural changes affecting pulmonary microvasculature.

Newborn ICR mice were exposed to 85% hyperoxia or normoxia for 14 days, and then normal air replacement conditions for the following 7 days. At postnatal day (P)14 and P21, lungs were harvested for ultrastructural examination and assessment of PH. To this end, we studied ultrastructural changes in pulmonary microvasculature, such as endothelial cells (ECs) and blood-air barriers (BABs), and examined the structure of pulmonary arteries associated with terminal and respiratory bronchioles as well as right ventricular hypertrophy (RVH).

H. Nakanishi (✉) · A. Uchiyama · S. Kusuda
Maternal and Perinatal Center Neonatal Division, Tokyo Women's Medical University, Tokyo, Japan
e-mail: hidehiko@qf6.so-net.ne.jp

S. Morikawa · S. Kitahara · A. Yoshii · T. Ezaki
Department of Anatomy and Developmental Biology, Tokyo Women's Medical University School of Medicine, Tokyo, Japan

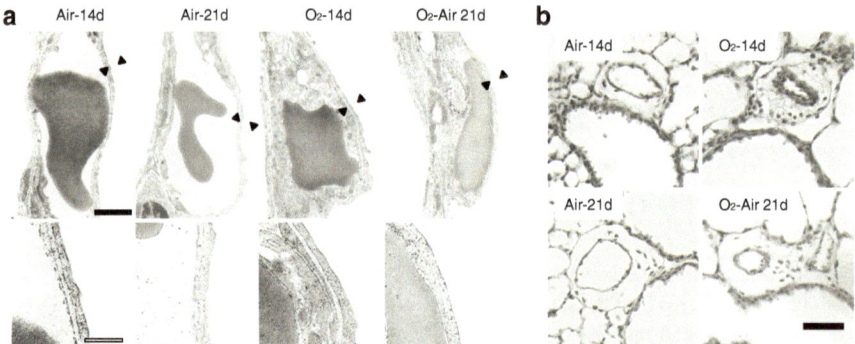

Fig. 11.1 (**a**) Pulmonary capillaries and blood-air barriers in Air-14d, Air-21d, O2-14d, and normal air replacement conditions after hyperoxia (O2-Air-21d). Scale bar black, 1.0 μm; white, 0.35 μm. Black arrowheads denote the parts of BABs magnified in the lower panels. (**b**) H&E-stained lung sections indicating the thickness of pulmonary arteries associated with terminal and respiratory bronchioles. Scale bar (black), 50 μm

ECs presented a heterogeneously thick and irregular cytoplasm with well-developed basal infoldings (Fig. 11.1a). Moreover, red blood cells inside the alveolar capillary seemed to be stuck in the capillary lumen, suggesting collapsed capillaries and altered pulmonary microcirculation. BABs from injured lungs, comprising EC, alveolar epithelial cells, and the basal lamina, were much thicker than those of air-exposed lungs, and most BABs were filled with abnormal mitochondria-rich EC layers. In contrast, BAB basal lamina layers in hyperoxia-exposed lungs were not significantly different from those in controls. Even in the lungs of animals exposed to normal air replacement conditions, ECs presented a heterogeneously thick cytoplasm rich in organelles, collapsed alveolar capillaries, and EC layers occupying most of the BABs. Structural changes were accompanied by increased pulmonary artery medial thickness and RVH (Fig. 11.1b). Results were confirmed by morphometric quantification.

Pulmonary capillaries in the injured newborn mouse lung presented thick BABs consisting of ECs with abnormal morphology, which persisted following subsequent exposure to normal air replacement conditions. These ultrastructural changes might cause abnormal pulmonary microcirculation and finally lead to secondary PH in BPD.

Acknowledgment This study was supported by the Ministry of Education, Culture, Sports, Science and Technology (MEXT) KAKENHI (Grant Number 16K10111).

References

1. Abman SH. Bronchopulmonary dysplasia: "a vascular hypothesis". Am J Respir Crit Care Med. 2001;164:1755–6.
2. Nakanishi H, Uchiyama A, Kusuda S. Impact of pulmonary hypertension on neurodevelopmental outcome in preterm infants with bronchopulmonary dysplasia: a cohort study. J Perinatol. 2016;36:890–6.

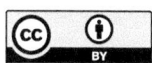

Involvement of CXCR4 and Stem Cells in a Rat Model of Pulmonary Arterial Hypertension

12

Tingting Zhang, Nanako Kawaguchi, Emiko Hayama, Yoshiyuki Furutani, and Toshio Nakanishi

Keywords

Pulmonary arterial hypertension · CXCR4 · Mesenchymal stem cells · Pulmonary vascular remodeling

Pulmonary arterial hypertension (PAH) is a severe and fatal clinical syndrome. C-X-C chemokine receptor type 4 (CXCR4) is known to be expressed in cancer and stem/progenitor cells. In the present study, PAH was induced in a rat model by 5 weeks of 10% hypoxia and treatment with a single subcutaneous injection of monocrotaline (60 mg/kg) [1] to investigate the involvement of CXCR4 in PAH development [2].

The successful establishment of the PAH model was confirmed by significant differences in the right ventricular systolic pressure, Fulton index, wall thickness, vascular occlusion score determined by immunohistochemical staining, and the expression of inflammatory markers measured by reverse transcription quantitative polymerase chain reaction (RT-qPCR) between the PAH and control groups We compared the expression of CXCR4 and other stem cell markers in the PAH and control groups. The results of RT-qPCR revealed that the expression of CXCR4, SCF, c-Kit, and CD29 was significantly higher in the PAH group. Immunohistochemical staining also showed that the numbers of CXCR4-, c-Kit-, and CD90-positive cells were significantly higher in the PAH group. We hypothesized that these markers play important roles in chemotaxis, proliferation, and survival of smooth muscle cells or endothelial cells, leading to pulmonary vascular remodeling. Further studies to clarify the role of CXCR4 and stem cells in PAH development may provide additional treatment options, such as CXCR4 inhibitors.

T. Zhang · N. Kawaguchi · E. Hayama · Y. Furutani · T. Nakanishi (✉)
Department of Pediatric Cardiology, Tokyo Women's Medical University, Tokyo, Japan
e-mail: nakanishi.toshio@twmu.ac.jp

Acknowledgment The authors would like to acknowledge Mr. Kenji Yoshihara and Mr. Hiroaki Nagao at Tokyo Women's Medical University for their excellent technical assistance.

References

1. Lan B, Hayama E, Kawaguchi N, et al. Therapeutic efficacy of valproic acid in a combined monocrotaline and chronic hypoxia rat model of severe pulmonary hypertension. PLoS One. 2015;10:e0117211.
2. Zhang T, Kawaguchi N, Hayama E, et al. High expression of CXCR4 and stem cell markers in a monocrotaline and chronic hypoxia-induced rat model of pulmonary arterial hypertension. Exp Ther Med. 2018;15(6):4615–22. https://doi.org/10.3892/etm.2018.6027.

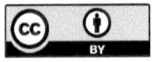

Ca²⁺ Signal Through Inositol Trisphosphate Receptors for Cardiovascular Development and Pathophysiology of Pulmonary Arterial Hypertension

Akimichi Shibata, Keiko Uchida, Katsuhiko Mikoshiba, and Hiroyuki Yamagishi

Keywords

Inositol trisphosphate receptor · Calcium signaling · Cardiovascular system Pulmonary arterial hypertension

Inositol triphosphate receptor (IP_3R) is an intracellular Ca^{2+} release channel located on the membrane of the sarco/endoplasmic reticulum (SR/ER), a major intracellular storage site for Ca^{2+}. There are three subtypes of IP_3R (IP_3R1, 2, and 3), each of which is known to have versatile roles in the pathophysiology of many organs [1].

In the cardiovascular system, all subtypes of IP_3Rs are expressed from embryonic to postnatal periods. We previously reported that IP_3R1-IP_3R2 or IP_3R1-IP_3R3 double-knockout (DKO) mice died around embryonic day (E) 11.5 due to disorder of cardiovascular development (Fig. 13.1). IP_3R1-IP_3R2 DKO mice showed developmental defects of the myocardium and endocardial cushion, resulting from the disturbance of calcineurin/NFAT signaling [2]. IP_3R1-IP_3R3 DKO mice demonstrated hypoplasia of the outflow tract and the right ventricle of embryonic heart

A. Shibata · K. Uchida (✉)
Department of Pediatrics, Keio University School of Medicine, Shinjuku, Tokyo, Japan
e-mail: keiuchid@keio.jp

K. Mikoshiba
SIAIS (Shanghai Institute for Advanced Immunochemical Studies), ShanghaiTech University, Shanghai, China

H. Yamagishi (✉)
Division of Pediatric Cardiology, Department of Pediatrics,
Keio University School of Medicine, Tokyo, Japan
e-mail: hyamag@keio.jp

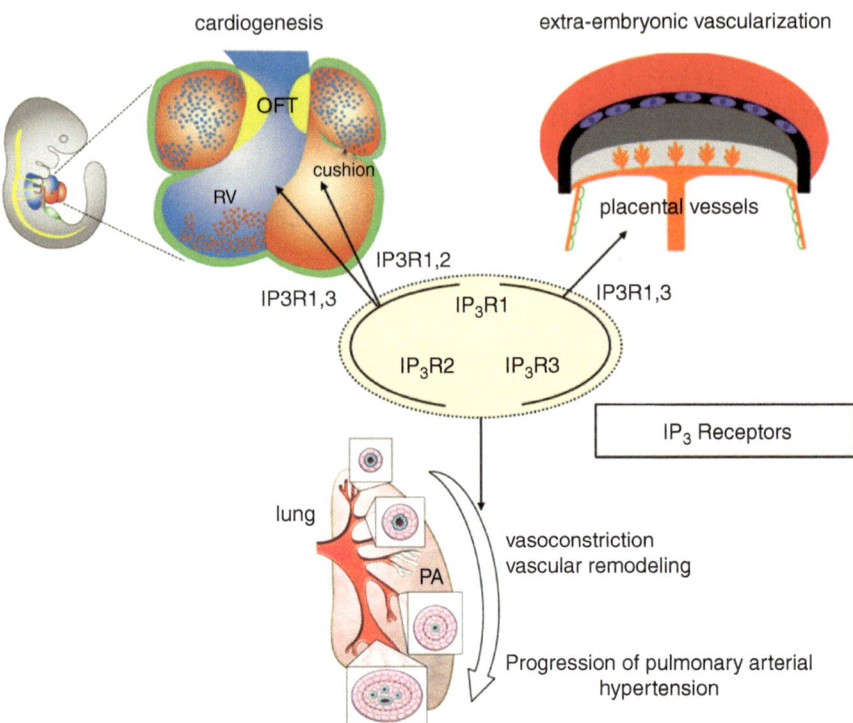

Fig. 13.1 The role of IP₃Rs for cardiogenesis, extra-embryonic vascularization, and suppression of pulmonary arterial hypertension. *RV* right ventricle, *OFT* outflow tract, *PA* pulmonary artery

with reduced expression levels of molecular markers for the second heart field [3]. In addition, IP$_3$R1-IP$_3$R3 DKO embryos exhibited defects in the vasculature of the labyrinth layers of the placenta, allantois, and yolk sac. Therefore, this suggests the essential redundant roles of endothelial IP$_3$R1 and 3 for angiogenesis during embryonic and extra-embryonic vascular development [4].

Recently, we found the specific expression of IP$_3$R in the pulmonary artery smooth muscle cells (PASMCs) of murine lungs. Although there are some reports that implicated IP$_3$R1 in vasoconstriction or remodeling in vascular smooth muscle cells [5], the precise role of IP$_3$Rs in PASMCs remains unknown. Since intracellular Ca^{2+} signaling in PASMCs is a major regulator for pulmonary vasoconstriction and remodeling, its dysregulation leads to the progression of pulmonary arterial hypertension (PAH). It was reported that store-operated Ca^{2+} (SOC) entry was upregulated in PASMCs with PAH patients. Our results suggest that intracellular Ca^{2+} depletion through Ca^{2+} release by IP$_3$R from the SR/ER may lead to the opening of SOC channels, a mechanism potentially involved in the pathophysiology of PAH (Fig. 13.1) [6].

Acknowledgment This work was supported by Acterion Academia Prize 2015 to A.S. and JSPS KAKENHI Grant Numbers JP19390288 to H.Y. and JP26461619 to K.U.

References

1. Mikoshiba K. Role of IP3 receptor signaling in cell functions and diseases. Adv Biol Regul. 2015;57:217–27.
2. Uchida K, Aramaki M, Nakazawa M, et al. Gene knock-outs of inositol 1,4,5-trisphosphate receptors types 1 and 2 result in perturbation of cardiogenesis. PLoS One. 2010;5(9):e12500.
3. Nakazawa M, Uchida K, Aramaki M, et al. Inositol 1,4,5-trisphosphate receptors are essential for the development of the second heart field. J Mol Cell Cardiol. 2011;51(1):58e66.
4. Uchida K, Nakazawa M, Yamagishi C, et al. Type 1 and 3 inositol trisphosphate receptors are required for extra-embryonic vascular development. Dev Biol. 2016;418(1):89–97.
5. Narayanam D, Adebiyi A, Jaggar JH, et al. Inositol trisphosphate receptors in smooth muscle cells. Am J Physiol Heart Circ Physiol. 2012;302:H2190–210.
6. Shibata A, Uchida K, Kodo K, et al. Type 2 inositol 1,4,5-trisphosphate receptor inhibits the progression of pulmonary arterial hypertension via calcium signaling and apoptosis. Heart and Vessels. 2019;34(4):724–734.

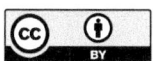

Part II

Abnormal Pulmonary Circulation in the Developing Lung and Heart

Perspective for Part II

14

Toshio Nakanishi

Pulmonary blood flow increases gradually during fetal life, and dramatic changes in the pulmonary circulation occur from the fetus to newborn, including decrease in pulmonary arterial resistance, increase in pulmonary blood flow, and closure of ductus arteriosus. Upon initiation of breathing after birth, pulmonary circulation is important for gas exchange between the alveoli and capillary vessels. Presence of congenital heart disease modifies development of the lung and pulmonary vessels, even before birth. For example, enlarged right atrium due to severe Ebstein's anomaly compresses the fetal lung and compromises lung development. Decreases in pulmonary blood flow during fetal life and especially after birth, for example, due to pulmonary stenosis or outflow stenosis may compromise the development of pulmonary arteries. In the research of morphogenesis of congenital heart disease, it is important to understand normal and abnormal lung and pulmonary vessel developments.

14.1   Idiopathic Pulmonary Arterial Hypertension (IPAH)

IPAH was discussed in this symposium because genetic background plays an important role and, therefore, IPAH is sort of a congenital disease. In IPAH, pulmonary smooth muscle cells and endothelial cells proliferate and obstruct small pulmonary arteries. Gene mutations such as bone morphogenic protein receptor II (BMPR II) are found in some patients with IPAH but the mechanisms how these gene mutations cause proliferation of pulmonary smooth muscle cells are still not clear. In addition to the genetic background, other factors such as inflammation may be involved because penetration rate of gene mutation is low.

T. Nakanishi (✉)
Department of Pediatric Cardiology, Tokyo Women's Medical University, Tokyo, Japan
e-mail: nakanishi.toshio@twmu.ac.jp

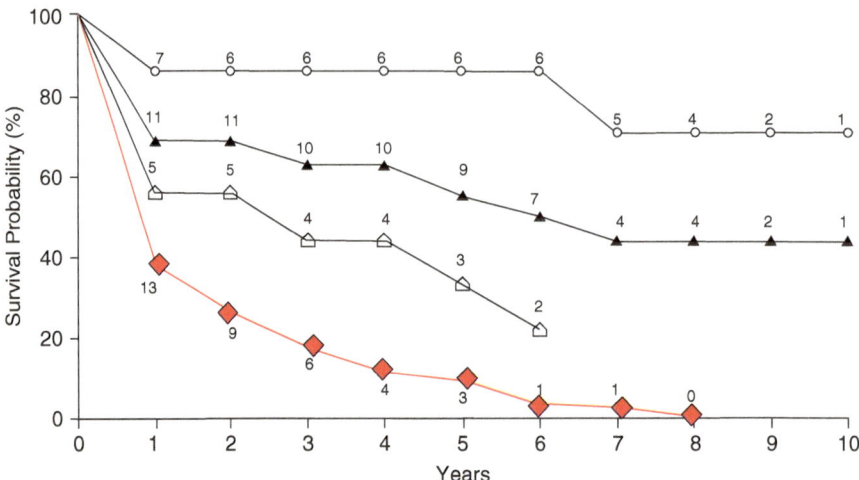

Fig. 14.1 Prognosis of pediatric IPAH. Red diamond: historical data before 1963. Open triangle: non-responders to acute prostanlandin I$_2$ testing. Open sun: responders to acute prostanlandin I$_2$ testing. Closed triangle: Patients who received pulmonary vasodilator therapy

Before pulmonary vasodilators were developed, calcium antagonists were the only drugs to treat IPAH, and prognosis of IPAH, especially pediatric IPAH, was very poor [1] (Fig. 14.1). In 1986, nitric oxide was found as a vasodilator, and after that various pulmonary vasodilators have been developed and used in patients with IPAH (Table 14.1). Time of government approval for clinical use differed in each country (Fig. 14.2). For example, intravenous epoprostenol was approved for clinical use in 1995 by FDA and in 1999 in Japan. It has not been approved in China at this moment in 2019. Prognosis of IPAH has improved depending on the time when a certain vasodilator could be used [2] (Fig. 14.3).

Use of pulmonary vasodilators improves prognosis of patients, but these drugs may not change the background pathophysiology of IPAH. Research to clarify the pathophysiology of IPAH is important to further improve prognosis of patients. Good animal models of IPAH are important to study the pathophysiology of IPAH and to develop a treatment strategy for IPAH. iPS cells have the potential to establish a good IPAH model in vitro.

To understand molecular mechanisms of IPAH, it may be important to clarify normal pathways governing morphogenesis of the lung and pulmonary vessels. If we can clarify how the lung and pulmonary vessels are formed, how each gene is involved, and how each signal transduction is involved, then we may be able know the precise mechanisms how pulmonary smooth muscle cells and endothelial cells start to proliferate and obstruct small pulmonary arteries in IPAH in the presence of gene mutations.

Table 14.1   Pulmonary vasodilators

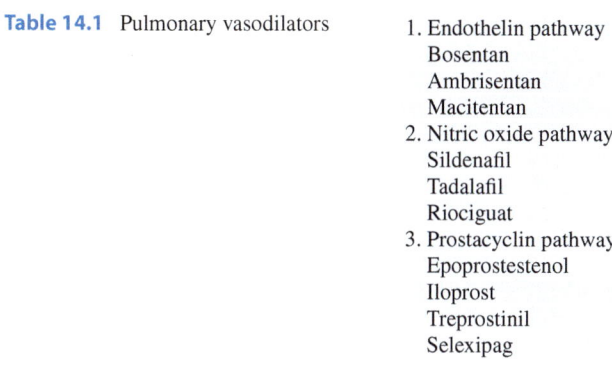

1. Endothelin pathway
   Bosentan
   Ambrisentan
   Macitentan
2. Nitric oxide pathway
   Sildenafil
   Tadalafil
   Riociguat
3. Prostacyclin pathway
   Epoprostestenol
   Iloprost
   Treprostinil
   Selexipag

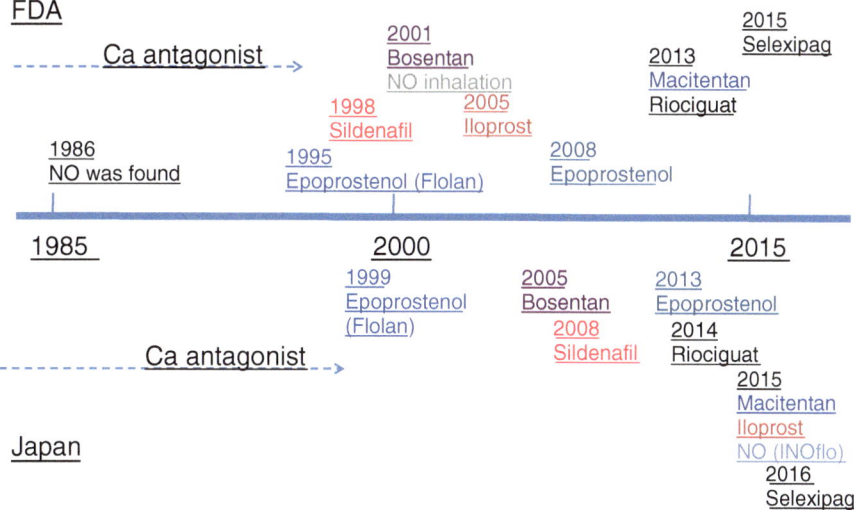

Fig. 14.2   Time of government approval for clinical use in USA (FDA) and in Japan. In 1986, nitric oxide was found as a vasodilator, and after that various pulmonary vasodilators have been developed and used in patients with IPAH

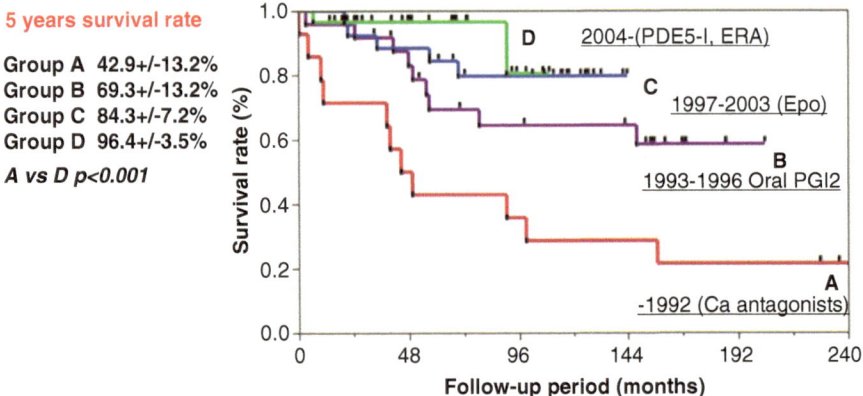

Fig. 14.3 Prognosis of pediatric IPAH in Japan. Prognosis of IPAH has been improved depending on the time when certain vasodilator could be used

14.2 Pulmonary Hypertension with Congenital Heart Disease

Fish has only one atrium and one ventricle. Frog and turtle have basically one ventricle and truncus, and yet it looks like they do not develop pulmonary hypertension although their blood pressure is low. Mammals have two ventricles and two circulations, systemic (left) and pulmonary (right) circulation, and if pulmonary blood flow is more than the systemic blood flow due to left to right shunt and if the pulmonary artery is exposed to high pressure, pulmonary smooth muscle cells and endothelial cells start to proliferate and obstruct vessels. We still do knot know the precise mechanisms for the proliferation of the pulmonary smooth muscle cells and endothelial cells in these conditions. The threshold of the "high pressure" is unclear but in human the pulmonary artery systolic pressure higher than 50 mmHg can induce irreversible pulmonary obstructive disease. Once this condition has been established with the shunt remaining open, a relatively stable clinical condition continues until patients die earlier than a normal lifespan.

In IPAH and pulmonary hypertension with congenital heart disease, the right ventricle should tolerate increased afterload. Management of right ventricular contractile force is important in the treatment of patients with Eisenmenger syndrome and IPAH.

14.3 Pulmonary Circulation in Patients with Congenital Heart Disease

Fontan operation is performed if only one ventricle is functional in conditions such as tricuspid atresia, hypoplastic left heart syndrome, or single ventricle. Pulmonary circulation after Fontan operation is unique. In this operation, the right atrium is

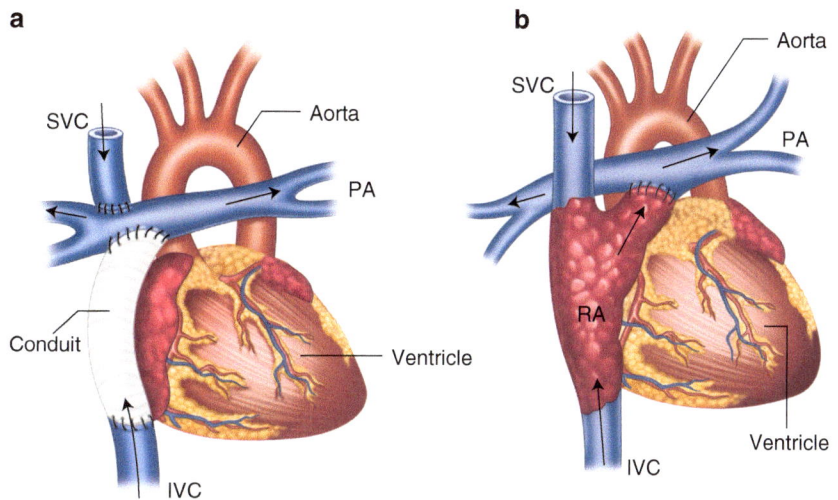

Fig. 14.4 Two types of Fontan operation. (**a**) Total cavo-pulmonary connection (TCPC). (**b**) Atrio pulmonary connection (APC). In TCPC, superior vena cava (SVC) is connected to the pulmonary artery (PA) and inferior vena cava (IVC) is connected with PA using conduit. In APC, right atrial appendage is connected with PA

connected to the pulmonary artery directly, or the superior vena cava and the inferior vena cava are connected to the pulmonary artery (Fig. 14.4). There is no pulsatile flow in the pulmonary artery after Fontan operation. After Fontan operation, pulmonary resistance can be slightly higher (3–5 Wood unit.m^2) than normal (less than 3 Wood unit.m^2). This slightly higher pulmonary resistance may compromise quality of life and lifespan of patients. The high pulmonary resistance may decrease pulmonary venous return, decrease cardiac output, increase central venous pressure, induce atrial ahhrythmia, increase liver congestion, induce liver cihhrosis, and/or induce protein losing enteropathy. Whether pulmonary vasodilators are effective in the management of Fontan patients is not yet clear. More importantly, molecular and cellular mechanisms of abnormal pulmonary circulation after Fontan operation have not been investigated and should be clarified in future.

References

1. Barst RJ. Primary pulmonary hypertension in children. In: Rubin LJ, Rich S, editors. Primary pulmonary hypertension. Marcel Dekker: New York; 1977. p. 179–225.
2. Saji T. Update on pediatric pulmonary arterial hypertension. Circ J. 2013;77:2639–50.

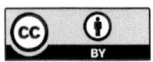

Pathophysiology of Pulmonary Circulation in Congenital Heart Disease

15

Megumi Hashimoto, Masahiro Kaneko, Naohisa Nishida, Hina Serizawa, Kohei Kawata, Rika Sekiya, and Hideaki Senzaki

Abstract

There are several types of abnormalities in the integrated physiology of pulmonary circulation in congenital heart disease. The main pathology of Eisenmenger syndrome involves a change in pulmonary resistance and is the most commonly observed pathophysiology in pulmonary hypertension. Other diseases also present with the main pathophysiological characteristic of reduced pulmonary compliance, such as tetralogy of Fallot and multiple peripheral pulmonary stenosis. In addition, the cavo-pulmonary connection has the unique feature of both pulmonary circulation and regulation. According to the differences in the pathophysiological features of pulmonary circulation, therapeutic approaches may considerably differ between diseases and conditions. Physiology-based clinical insights with regard to pulmonary circulation in congenital heart disease will be discussed in this chapter.

Keywords

Impedance · Wave reflection · Characteristic impedance · Compliance · Pressure-volume relationships

M. Hashimoto · M. Kaneko · N. Nishida · H. Serizawa · K. Kawata
R. Sekiya · H. Senzaki (✉)
Pediatric Cardiology and Pediatrics, Kitasato University School of Medicine, Kanagawa, Japan

15.1   Introduction

This chapter discusses the pathophysiology of pulmonary circulation in congenital heart disease. This refers to the macrophysiology of cardiovascular hemodynamics, an understanding of which is essential for the treatment of patients with abnormal pulmonary circulation and congenital heart disease. We hope this chapter can provide some hints and insights for use in future research on pulmonary hypertension in congenital disease as well as in the fields of physiology and molecular and cellular biology.

We will first discuss how we comprehensively assess integrated pulmonary circulation in congenital heart disease in vivo. Subsequently, using methodology for comprehensive assessment, we will discuss the pathophysiological characteristics of pulmonary circulation in patients with various types of congenital heart disease.

15.2   Comprehensive Assessment of Integrated Pulmonary Circulation

15.2.1 Physiologic Components of Pulmonary Circulation

Pulmonary circulation consists of the following three major components: resistive, elastic, and reflective components. The resistive component is described as pulmonary vascular resistance (PVR). PVR acts in opposition to mean or non-pulsatile steady flow and is analogous to electric resistance, which acts in opposition to direct current in an electronic circuit. Thus, PVR can be calculated as the ratio of mean pulmonary flow to mean pulmonary arterial pressure according to Ohm's law for an electric circuit. In other words, PVR only determines mean pulmonary pressure according to the amount of pulmonary blood flow. An increase in PVR causes an increase in mean pulmonary arterial pressure without a marked change in pulse pressure (Fig. 15.1a).

The elastic component is vascular compliance or capacitance. The pulmonary artery is not a rigid tube but has elasticity to buffer intermittent pulsatile flow ejected by the right ventricle. Pulmonary arterial capacitance is a vascular property in this buffering system and is determined by both arterial wall elasticity and vascular size or volume. Pulmonary compliance/capacitance is analogous to a capacitor or condenser in an electric circuit. An alternating current but not a direct current goes in and out of the capacitor. Similarly, only pulsatile flow goes in and out of the pulmonary vascular bed with capacitance and is associated with a change in pulse pressure. When pulmonary capacitance is decreased, in other words, when the pulmonary arterial wall is stiff and/or pulmonary vascular bed is small, blood pressure increases through an increase in pulse pressure without a change in mean blood pressure (Fig. 15.1b).

There is yet another property of the elastic component of the pulmonary vascular bed. This is termed characteristic impedance and represents wall stiffness in the proximal artery. In an electric circuit, characteristic impedance is described as

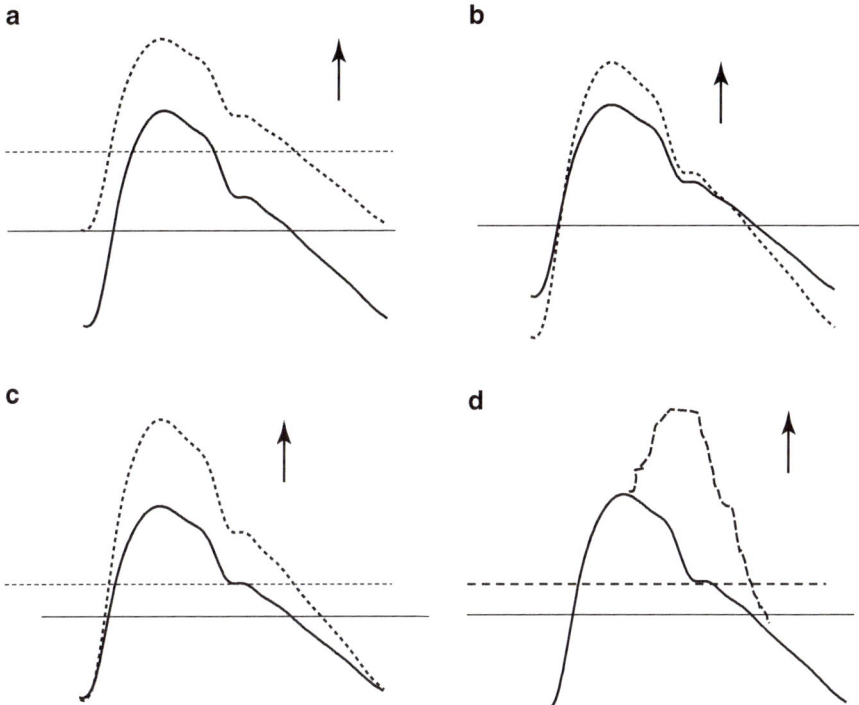

Fig. 15.1 Effects of changes in resistance (**a**), compliance (**b**), characteristic impedance (**c**), and wave reflection (**d**) on pulmonary artery pressure

resistance upstream of the resistor-capacitor parallel circuit. When characteristic impedance increases, in other words, when the proximal pulmonary arterial wall stiffens, blood pressure increases by an increase in pulse pressure above the diastolic pressure as shown in Fig. 15.1c.

The last major component is a reflective component. The pulmonary vascular bed is not an infinite system but has an end at the left atrium. The pulmonary vascular bed also has many bifurcations with caliber changes. In this type of system, blood flow and pressure waves produce reflections at the site of a bifurcation or vessel caliber change [1, 2]. Therefore, the measured pressure or flow we observe is the sum of forward and reflected waves, and thus augmentation of reflected waves causes significant pressure elevation (Fig. 15.1d).

Therefore, abnormalities in each component contribute differently to pressure elevation in patients with pulmonary hypertension. Resistance change increases pulmonary arterial pressure (PAP) by increasing mean arterial pressure, changes in capacitance and characteristic impedance increase arterial pressure by increasing pulse pressure, and wave reflection increases PAP by adding reflected pressure. Therefore, to better understand the pathophysiology of pulmonary hypertension, it is very important to identify to what extent each of these components is abnormal and contributes to pressure elevation in pulmonary hypertension.

15.2.2 Impedance Analysis

Impedance analysis is an ideal method for this purpose by providing comprehensive information regarding the vascular system, including vascular compliance and wave reflection as well as vascular resistance [3, 4]. To briefly explain (Fig. 15.2), instantaneously measured pressure and flow data are mathematically transformed as the sum of pressure and flow waves at each frequency of the integer multiple of a fundamental frequency. The fundamental frequency corresponds to the heart rate. The ratio of pressure to flow at each frequency yields impedance spectra. Fig. 15.3 shows examples of impedance spectra. Impedance at 0 frequency, or zero oscillation, represents pulmonary resistance. Characteristic impedance is calculated as the average impedance at higher frequencies. Compliance is calculated from lower frequency impedance or the time constant of diastolic pressure decay. Wave reflection increases oscillation of the impedance spectra at higher frequencies and is directly calculated using the formula described in Fig. 15.3. Thus, all other vascular components, including characteristic impedance, pulmonary arterial compliance, and wave reflection, are obtained from these spectra.

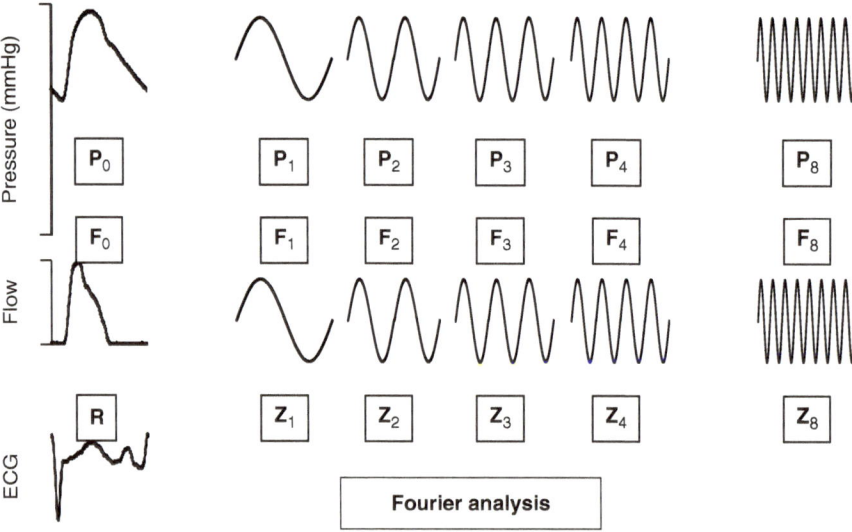

Fig. 15.2 Fourier transformation of pressure and flow data, yielding impedance spectra in the frequency domain

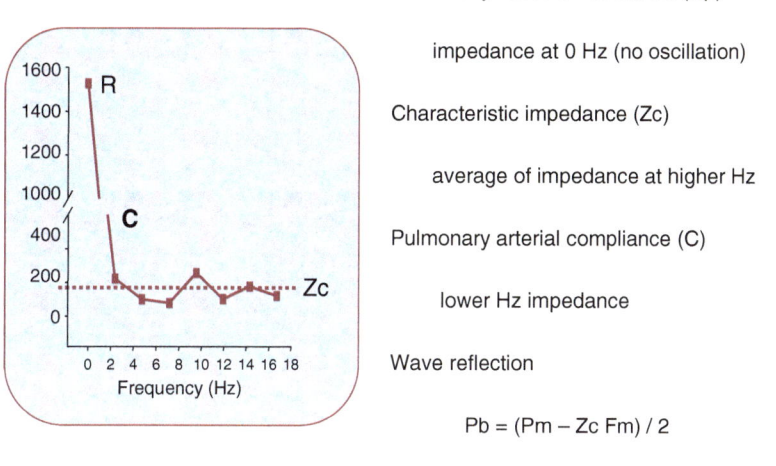

Impedance

Pulmonary vascular resistance (Rp)

impedance at 0 Hz (no oscillation)

Characteristic impedance (Zc)

average of impedance at higher Hz

Pulmonary arterial compliance (C)

lower Hz impedance

Wave reflection

$$Pb = (Pm - Zc\ Fm) / 2$$

Pm and Fm: measured pressure and flow

Fig. 15.3 Example of impedance spectra, which provide comprehensive measurements of vascular properties, including pulmonary vascular resistance, characteristic impedance, pulmonary arterial compliance, and wave reflection

15.3 Pathophysiological Characteristics of Pulmonary Circulation in Congenital Heart Disease

Using impedance analysis, let us discuss the pathophysiological characteristics of pulmonary circulation in patients with various types of congenital heart disease.

15.3.1 Abnormal Resistance Is the Main Pathophysiology

In the disease entity of abnormal pulmonary circulation, increased pulmonary resistance is the main pathophysiology. Eisenmenger syndrome due to high pulmonary flow and idiopathic pulmonary arterial hypertension (PAH) are examples. Fig. 15.4 shows an example of PAH due to patent ductus arteriosus in a 1-year-old patient with trisomy 21. PAP is 80/40 mmHg. Compared to a control patient with normal pulmonary arterial pressure, wave reflection (shown via the dashed lines) is augmented in this patient. Impedance spectra exhibit an upward shift in this patient, particularly at 0 frequency or pulmonary resistance. There are also mild abnormalities in characteristic impedance (Zc), compliance (C), and wave reflection. In this patient, oral administration of sildenafil markedly reduced PAP as shown by the yellow lines. This is mainly the result of reduction of pulmonary vascular resistance, with some degree of improvement in vascular compliance and wave reflection.

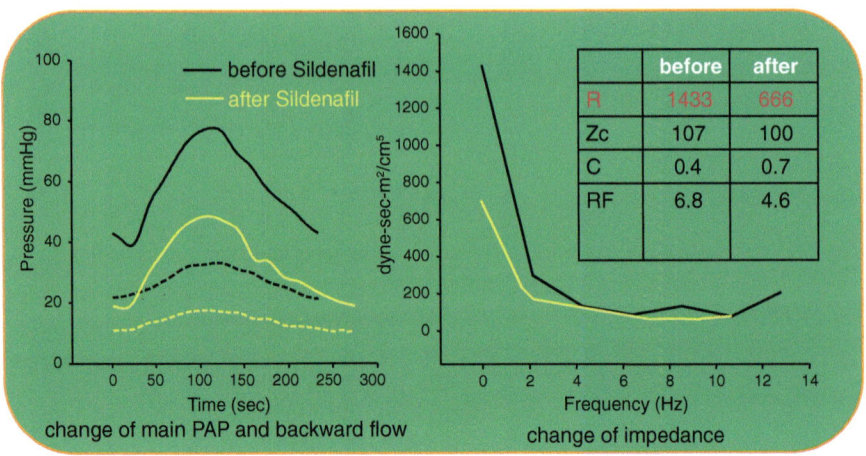

Fig. 15.4 Pressure (left) and impedance (right) data before and after oral administration of silde-nafil. R, Zc, C, and RF represent resistance, characteristic impedance, compliance, and reflection factor

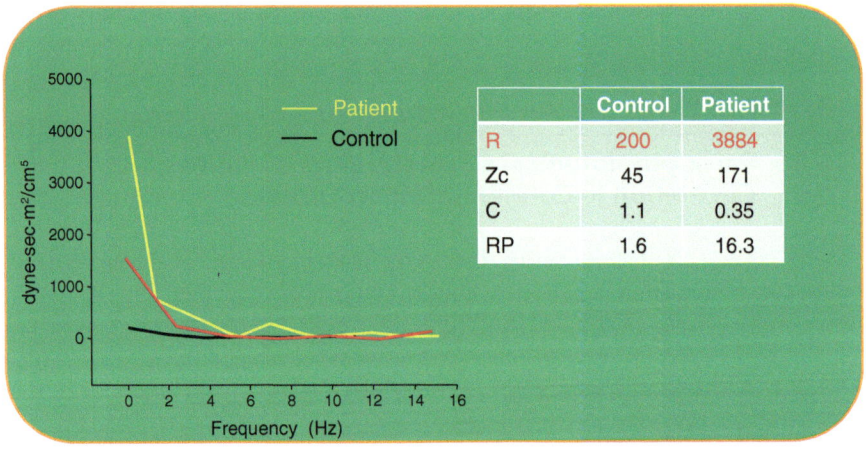

Fig. 15.5 Impedance data before and after oral administration of sildenafil. R, Zc, C, and RF represent resistance, characteristic impedance, compliance, and reflection factor

Here is another example of PAH in a 9-year-old girl after repair of transposition of the great arteries. PAP is 125/68 mmHg. Impedance spectra in this patient are characterized by a further upward shift of the yellow line compared to those in controls and the previous case of PAH, indicating a more advanced stage of PAH (Fig. 15.5). Interestingly, oral administration of sildenafil, as shown by the yellow line, did not have a marked effect on pulmonary vascular resistance but still reduced PAP by 20 mmHg. This was mainly owing to the change in characteristic imped-ance, which caused the reduction of pulse pressure (Fig. 15.6). These data show that

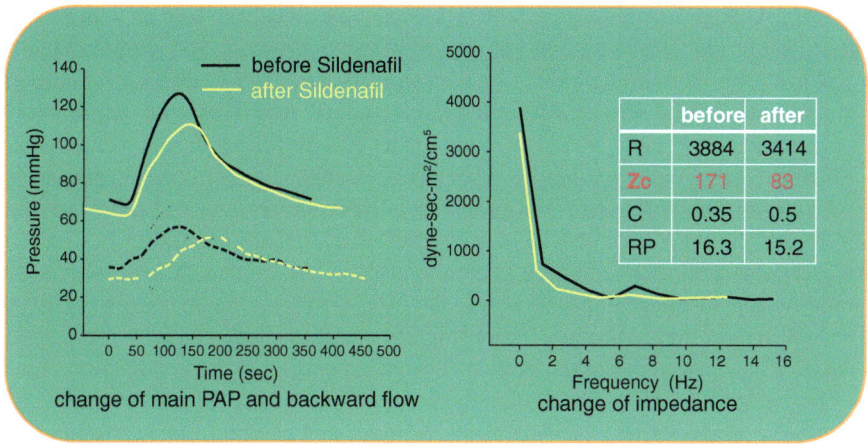

Fig. 15.6 Pressure (left) and impedance (right) data before and after oral administration of silde-nafil. R, Zc, C, and RF represent resistance, characteristic impedance, compliance, and reflection factor

pharmacologic effects and the mechanism of action of pulmonary dilators can be different according to the disease stage and condition and that impedance analysis enables detailed assessment about where the main lesions of pathologic change are and how the vascular bed responds to medications.

In addition to each parameter of impedance, combining resistance and compliance as their product, RC, also provides useful information about the pulmonary circulation. RC represents the time required for diastolic pressure decay, and a longer RC indicates that the blood does not go through the pulmonary vascular bed smoothly [5].

Therefore, advanced PAH should be associated with higher RC values. In fact, although PVR alone could not clearly distinguish pulmonary hypertension patients with irreversible pulmonary vascular disease from those whose PAP normalized after ventricular septal defect closure, plots of RC against Qp/Qs clearly distinguished the two groups [5].

15.3.2 Right Ventricular Function and Coupling to PA Load

In addition to the precise assessment and understanding of pathophysiological changes in the pulmonary vascular bed as shown thus far, an accurate assessment of intrinsic right ventricular (RV) contractility and its relation to the pulmonary artery (PA) load is essential for refining risk stratification and optimizing treatment in pulmonary hypertension because prognosis in PAH is now known to be strongly related to RV compensation rather than to the degree of the vascular injury itself as reported by many investigators [6–8]. Therefore, we will briefly introduce the method of assessing RV-PA interaction or RV-PA coupling.

The ventricular pressure-volume relationship is the best way to demonstrate this [9–11]. An instantaneous plot of ventricular pressure and volume change yields a pressure-volume loop [12]. We can further construct successive ventricular pressure-volume loops during transient preload reduction with inferior vena cava occlusion [11, 13, 14]. The slope of the end-systolic pressure-volume relationship, called end-systolic elastance (Ees), represents ventricular contractility, whereas arterial elastance (Ea) represents ventricular afterload and provides information on PA impedance [14, 15]. Therefore, the simple ratio of Ees/Ea represents ventricular-arterial (V-A) coupling status [16]. Figure 15.7a shows the PV relationship in the normal left ventricle (LV). Compared to that for the LV, the normal RV pressure-volume relationship has, as shown in Fig. 15.7b, a triangular shape with a low ventricular contractility corresponding to the low PA impedance or low ventricular afterload. With progression of pulmonary hypertension, the RV generally adapts to increased afterload by increasing contractility, preserving V-A coupling status and, thereby, cardiac output (Fig. 15.8a, b). However, once the RV contractile adaptation begins to fail, the RV needs to increase its volume to preserve cardiac output, leading to a course of progressive failure and poor outcome as shown in the yellow lines. The PV relationship is also useful to predict treatment response. Because Ees represents ventricular systolic stiffness, it predicts pressure variation at a given change in loading condition and, thereby, treatment response [17, 18].

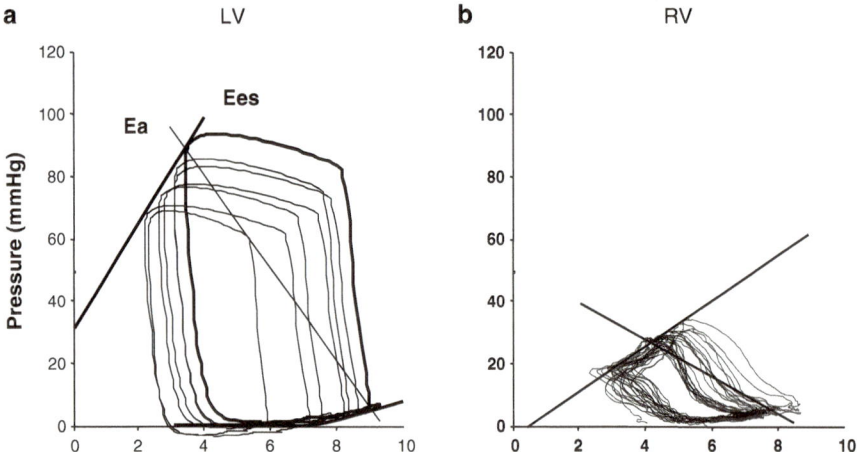

Fig. 15.7 Examples of pressure-volume relationships in normal left ventricle (**a**) and right ventricle (**b**)

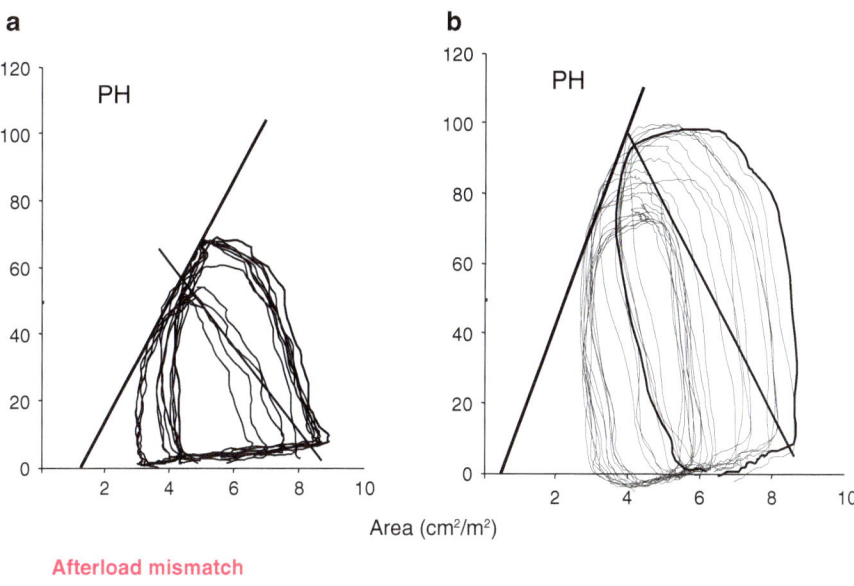

Fig. 15.8 Changes in pressure-volume relationships with progression (**a**, **b**) of pulmonary hypertension (PH). Afterload-mismatched right ventricle (RV) represented by red lines (**c**)

15.3.3 Abnormalities of Compliance Is the Main Pathophysiology

Next, we will discuss another disease entity of abnormal pulmonary circulation in which change in arterial compliance is the predominant pathophysiology of pulmonary hypertension. Tetralogy of Fallot (TOF) and multiple peripheral pulmonary stenosis are representative of this group. We measured pulmonary vascular impedance in 29 pediatric patients with repaired TOF [19]. Impedance spectra of TOF shifted upward compared to those of control patients, and PA exhibited augmented pulse pressure with increased wave reflection [19]. As summarized in Fig. 15.9, the abnormality of pulmonary vasculature in TOF is more evident in elastic components than in resistive components as shown by the increased characteristic impedance and decreased arterial compliance. Wave reflection is also augmented, contributing to the change in pulsatile nature of the pulmonary circulation in TOF. These data indicating enhanced pulmonary arterial stiffness are consistent with a previous histologic examination of the pulmonary artery in patients with TOF [20, 21]. Bedard et al. reported abnormal elastic tissue configuration and a high proportion of medionecrosis and elastic fragmentation [20]. These changes suggest decreased distensibility of the pulmonary arteries. Importantly, we also found that decreased pulmonary compliance was associated with RV dilation independent of the severity of pulmonary regurgitation [19]. Therefore, decreased pulmonary compliance in TOF serves as a pulsatile afterload to the RV and contributes to the progression of RV failure.

15.3.4 Non-pulsatile Pulmonary Flow Is the Main Pathophysiology

Lastly, cavo-pulmonary connection, as in Fontan or Glenn circulation, is another disease entity of abnormal pulmonary circulation in congenital heart disease. Although Fontan circulation does not cause apparent pulmonary hypertension,

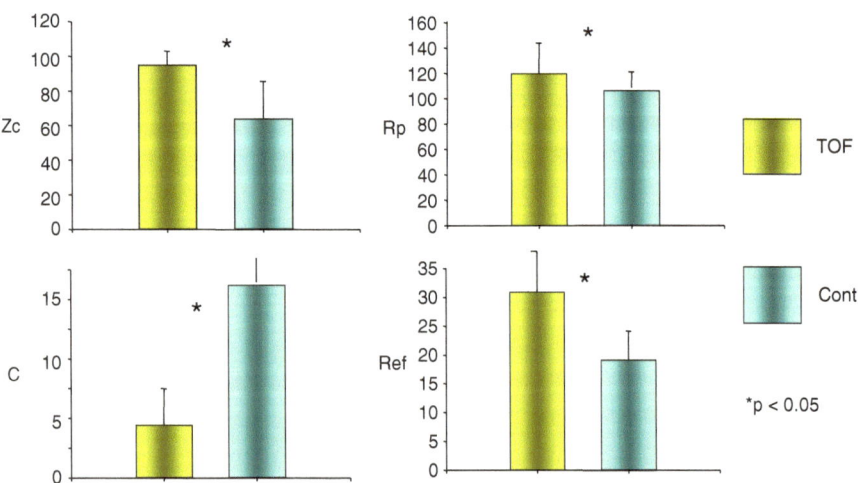

Fig. 15.9 Comparison of characteristic impedance (Zc), pulmonary resistance (Rp), compliance (C), and wave reflection (Ref) between tetralogy of Fallot (TOF) and control patients (Cont)

unique pulmonary hemodynamics are characterized by non-pulsatile flow due to lack of a pulmonary ventricle [22]. The pulsatile nature of pulmonary blood flow is important for shear stress-mediated release of endothelium-derived nitric oxide (NO) and lowering of PVR, thereby reducing NO-cGMP-mediated vasodilatory capacity [23–25]. In addition, low cardiac output and elevated central venous pressure (CVP) in Fontan circulation can activate vasoconstrictive hormones, including endothelin and angiotensin II [22, 26, 27]. Therefore, PVR is generally slightly but significantly higher than normal even in good Fontan status. In fact, we can decrease PVR using exogenous NO in patients late after Fontan surgery. Redington's group examined NO responsiveness in 15 Fontan patients with a median postoperative period of 9 years and demonstrated significant reduction of PVR with inhaled NO. [28] Interestingly, the effect was even more evident in patients with total cavo-pulmonary connection (TCPC) than in those with atrio-pulmonary connection (APC) and some degree of pulmonary flow pulsatility, suggesting the importance of pulsatility [28]. Our own data also indicated significant reduction of PAP using sildenafil or tadalafil in 26 patients with Glenn circulation (Fig. 15.10).

There are many studies indicating activation of endothelin-1 or the renin-angiotensin system in Fontan circulation [29–31]. A significant correlation between endothelin-1 and PVR after the Fontan operation was also reported [31]. In addition, an endothelin receptor antagonist effectively reduced PVR in Fontan patients and improved exercise tolerance and quality of life [32]. Therefore, even in good Fontan status, pulmonary dilators targeting NO and endothelin pathways may have some role in improving Fontan pulmonary circulation and thereby improving the long-term outcome.

Let us briefly think about the role of pulmonary compliance or capacitance in the Fontan circulation. Theoretically, as we explained earlier, only pulsatile flow goes into capacitance, and thus, in the Fontan pulmonary circulation where pulmonary flow is basically non-pulsatile, PAP is determined predominantly by the PVR [22].

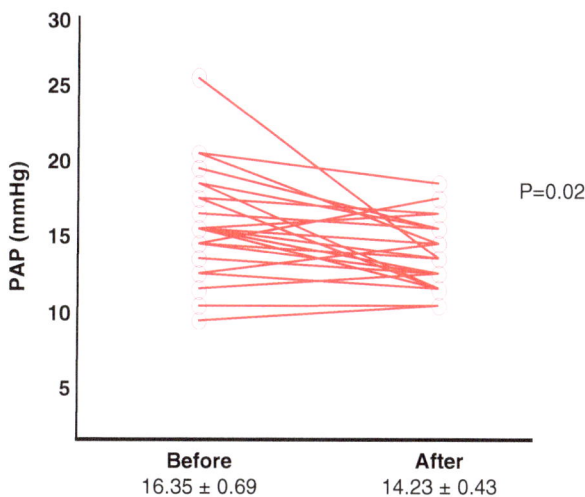

Fig. 15.10 Changes in pulmonary artery pressure (PAP) before and after oral administration of sildenafil in Glenn patients

P=0.02

Before
16.35 ± 0.69

After
14.23 ± 0.43

Nonetheless, pulmonary vascular capacitance still possesses important pathophysiological roles in the Fontan circulation. First, because of the direct connection of systemic and pulmonary circulation, pulmonary vascular capacitance serves as part of the total vascular impedance from the aorta to the pulmonary vascular bed [22]. Total vascular impedance is afterload to the Fontan single ventricle. As shown here, total vascular impedance, or ventricular afterload, increases with an increase in pulmonary vascular capacitance [22]. Second, perhaps more importantly, our computer simulation clearly indicated that smaller pulmonary vascular capacitance is related to a more marked increase in CVP in response to changes in pulmonary blood volume, which can occur with exercise and excessive water intake [33, 34]. Therefore, CVP variation during daily life should be pronounced in Fontan patients with decreased pulmonary capacitance. As in the original "10 Commandments" or indications for Fontan surgery [35], pulmonary arterial size, which is related to pulmonary capacitance, is important, independent of PVR, for the establishment of stable Fontan hemodynamics.

Similar to the effects of pulmonary artery capacitance, systemic venous capacitance is important and is an even more important hemodynamic parameter to establish lower levels of CVP in the Fontan circulation [34, 36].

Figure 15.11 shows the effects of changes in each vascular parameter in Fontan hemodynamics [33]. Each parameter was changed by 50% from the baseline values and their effects on CVP were examined by computer simulation. As shown, venous capacitance has the strongest influence on the change in CVP, followed by pulmonary capacitance and pulmonary resistance [33]. The importance of venous capacitance is realized by our "super-Fontan" strategy, which is an aggressive venodilation therapy with nitrates and angiotensin-converting enzyme (ACE) inhibitors, and pulmonary dilators if necessary, to achieve supernormal, extremely good Fontan circulation [37]. In fact, this strategy significantly increases venous capacitance as measured by the dye-dilution technique [37–39]. As shown in Fig. 15.11, eight consecutive patients who received super-Fontan therapy soon after Fontan surgery had

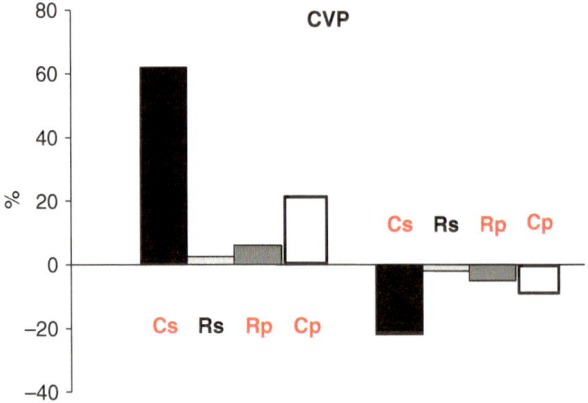

Fig. 15.11 The effects of changes in each vascular parameter in Fontan. *Cs* systemic venous compliance, *Rs* systemic resistance, *Rp* pulmonary resistance, *Cp* pulmonary compliance

significantly lower CVP values than patients without super-Fontan strategy at cardiac catheterization 1 year after Fontan surgery; however, the cardiac index (CI) was comparable in both groups. Six patients who received super-Fontan therapy had CVP values of <10 mmHg.

In addition, we newly applied this strategy to 20 patients at an average 7 years postoperatively. The venous capacitance measured by the dye-dilution technique significantly increased after 6 months of this therapy. Importantly, with this change in venous capacitance, CVP again significantly and consistently decreased after the therapy without changes in heart rate and cardiac index.

We will close this chapter by presenting a case of protein-losing enteropathy (PLE) in which super-Fontan strategy was very effective. The patient was a 16-year-old boy with asplenia syndrome, major atrio-pulmonary collateral arteries, and atrioventricular valve regurgitation who underwent TCPC at the age of 7 but developed PLE after the TCPC. Every possible medication had been prescribed. He was referred to our hospital and underwent the super-Fontan strategy, which effectively reduced CVP from 21 to 15 mmHg and, more importantly, resolved the PLE.

In summary, comprehensive assessment of changes in the pulmonary vascular bed and their coupling to RV function is important. Impedance analysis and determination of pressure-volume relationships are ideal methods for this purpose. There are several disease entities with abnormal pulmonary circulation in congenital heart disease characterized by abnormalities of resistance, compliance, and flow pulsatility. Venous capacitance as well as pulmonary resistance can be an important therapeutic target to improve Fontan prognosis.

References

1. Murgo JP, Westerhof N, Giolma JP, Altobelli SA. Aortic input impedance in normal man: Relationship to pressure wave forms. Circulation. 1980;62:105–16.
2. Senzaki H, Chen CH, Ishido H, Masutani S, Matsunaga T, Taketazu M, Kobayashi T, Sasaki N, Kyo S, Yokote Y. Arterial hemodynamics in patients after Kawasaki disease. Circulation. 2005;111:2119–25.
3. Newman DL, Walesby RK, Bowden NL. Hemodynamic effects of acute experimental aortic coarctation in the dog. Circ Res. 1975;36:165–72.
4. Senzaki H, Isoda T, Ishizawa A, Hishi T. Reconsideration of criteria for the fontan operation. Influence of pulmonary artery size on postoperative hemodynamics of the fontan operation. Circulation. 1994;89:1196–202.
5. Senzaki H, Kato H, Akagi M, Hishi T, Yanagisawa M. New criteria for the radical repair of congenital heart disease with pulmonary hypertension. In order to avoid postoperative residual pulmonary hypertension. Jpn Heart J. 1995;36:49–59.
6. Vanderpool RR, Pinsky MR, Naeije R, Deible C, Kosaraju V, Bunner C, Mathier MA, Lacomis J, Champion HC, Simon MA. Rv-pulmonary arterial coupling predicts outcome in patients referred for pulmonary hypertension. Heart. 2015;101:37–43.
7. Inuzuka R, Kass DA, Senzaki H. Novel, single-beat approach for determining both end-systolic pressure-dimension relationship and preload recruitable stroke work. Open Heart. 2016;3:e000451.

8. Sugimoto M, Masutani S, Seki M, Kajino H, Fujieda K, Senzaki H. High serum levels of procollagen type III-n-terminal amino peptide in patients with congenital heart disease. Heart. 2009;95(24):2023–8.

9. Senzaki H, Naito C, Masutani S, Nogaki M, Ohono A, Kobayashi J, Sasaki N, Asano H, Shunei K, Yokote Y, Kobayashi T. Hemodynamic evaluation for closing interatrial communication after fenestrated fontan operation. J Thorac Cardiovasc Surg. 2001;121:1200–2.

10. Senzaki H, Chen CH, Masutani S, Taketazu M, Kobayashi J, Kobayashi T, Sasaki N, Asano H, Kyo S, Yokote Y. Assessment of cardiovascular dynamics by pressure-area relations in pediatric patients with congenital heart disease. J Thorac Cardiovasc Surg. 2001;122:535–47.

11. Senzaki H, Chen H, Kass D. Single-beat estimation of end-systolic pressure-volume relation in humans a new method with the potential for noninvasive application. Circulation. 1996;94:2497–506.

12. Senzaki H, Gluzband YA, Pak PH, Crow MT, Janicki JS, Kass DA. Synergistic exacerbation of diastolic stiffness from short-term tachycardia-induced cardiodepression and angiotensin ii. Circ Res. 1998;82:503–12.

13. Senzaki H, Miyagawa K, Kishigami Y, Sasaki N, Masutani S, Taketazu M, Kobayashi J, Kobyashi T, Asano H, Kyo S, Yokote Y. Inferior vena cava occlusion catheter for pediatric patients with heart disease: For more detailed cardiovascular assessments. Catheter Cardiovasc Interv. 2001;53:392–6.

14. Senzaki H, Isoda T, Paolocci N, Ekelund U, Hare JM, Kass DA. Improved mechanoenergetics and cardiac rest and reserve function of in vivo failing heart by calcium sensitizer emd-57033. Circulation. 2000;101:1040–8.

15. Senzaki H, Masutani S, Ishido H, Taketazu M, Kobayashi T, Sasaki N, Asano H, Katogi T, Kyo S, Yokote Y. Cardiac rest and reserve function in patients with fontan circulation. J Am Coll Cardiol. 2006;47:2528–35.

16. Senzaki H, Fetics B, Chen CH, Kass DA. Comparison of ventricular pressure relaxation assessments in human heart failure: Quantitative influence on load and drug sensitivity analysis. J Am Coll Cardiol. 1999;34:1529–36.

17. Senzaki H, Iwamoto Y, Ishido H, Masutani S, Taketazu M, Kobayashi T, Katogi T, Kyo S. Ventricular-vascular stiffening in patients with repaired coarctation of aorta: Integrated pathophysiology of hypertension. Circulation. 2008;118:S191–8.

18. Khono K, Tamai A, Kobayashi T, Senzaki H. Effects of stent implantation for peripheral pulmonary artery stenosis on pulmonary vascular hemodynamics and right ventricular function in a patient with repaired tetralogy of fallot. Heart Vessels. 2011;26(6):672–6.

19. Inuzuka R, Seki M, Sugimoto M, Saiki H, Masutani S, Senzaki H. Pulmonary arterial wall stiffness and its impact on right ventricular afterload in patients with repaired tetralogy of fallot. Ann Thorac Surg. 2013;96:1435–41.

20. Bedard E, McCarthy KP, Dimopoulos K, Giannakoulas G, Gatzoulis MA, Ho SY. Structural abnormalities of the pulmonary trunk in tetralogy of fallot and potential clinical implications: A morphological study. J Am Coll Cardiol. 2009;54:1883–90.

21. Senzaki H, Iwamoto Y, Ishido H, Matsunaga T, Taketazu M, Kobayashi T, Asano H, Katogi T, Kyo S. Arterial haemodynamics in patients after repair of tetralogy of fallot: Influence on left ventricular after load and aortic dilatation. Heart. 2008;94:70–4.

22. Senzaki H, Isoda T, Ishizawa A, Hishi T. Reconsideration of criteria for the fontan operation. Influence of pulmonary artery size on postoperative hemodynamics of the fontan operation. Circulation. 1994;89:266–71.

23. Recchia FA, Senzaki H, Saeki A, Byrne BJ, Kass DA. Pulse pressure-related changes in coronary flow in vivo are modulated by nitric oxide and adenosine. Circ Res. 1996;79:849–56.

24. Peng X, Haldar S, Deshpande S, Irani K, Kass DA. Wall stiffness suppresses akt/enos and cytoprotection in pulse-perfused endothelium. Hypertension. 2003;41:378–81.

25. Masutani S, Saiki H, Kurishima C, Ishido H, Tamura M, Senzaki H. Heart failure with preserved ejection fraction in children: Hormonal imbalance between aldosterone and brain natriuretic peptide. Circ J. 2013;77:2375–82.

26. Ohuchi H, Takasugi H, Ohashi H, Yamada O, Watanabe K, Yagihara T, Echigo S. Abnormalities of neurohormonal and cardiac autonomic nervous activities relate poorly to functional status in fontan patients. Circulation. 2004;110:2601–8.
27. Saiki H, Kuwata S, Kurishima C, Iwamoto Y, Ishido H, Masutani S, Senzaki H. Aldosterone-cortisol imbalance immediately after fontan operation with implications for abnormal fluid homeostasis. Am J Cardiol. 2014;114:1578–83.
28. Khambadkone S, Li J, de Leval MR, Cullen S, Deanfield JE, Redington AN. Basal pulmonary vascular resistance and nitric oxide responsiveness late after fontan-type operation. Circulation. 2003;107:3204–8.
29. Ishida H, Kogaki S, Ichimori H, Narita J, Nawa N, Ueno T, Takahashi K, Kayatani F, Kishimoto H, Nakayama M, Sawa Y, Beghetti M, Ozono K. Overexpression of endothelin-1 and endothelin receptors in the pulmonary arteries of failed fontan patients. Int J Cardiol. 2012;159(1):34–9.
30. Inai K, Nakanishi T, Nakazawa M. Clinical correlation and prognostic predictive value of neurohumoral factors in patients late after the fontan operation. Am Heart J. 2005;150:588–94.
31. Hiramatsu T, Imai Y, Takanashi Y, Seo K, Terada M, Aoki M, Nakazawa M. Time course of endothelin-1 and adrenomedullin after the fontan procedure. Ann Thorac Surg. 1999;68:169–72.
32. Agnoletti G, Gala S, Ferroni F, Bordese R, Appendini L, Pace Napoleone C, Bergamasco L. Endothelin inhibitors lower pulmonary vascular resistance and improve functional capacity in patients with fontan circulation. J Thorac Cardiovasc Surg. 2017;153:1468–75.
33. Liang F, Senzaki H, Yin Z, Fan Y, Sughimoto K, Liu H. Transient hemodynamic changes upon changing a bcpa into a tcpc in staged fontan operation: A computational model study. ScientificWorldJournal. 2013;2013:486815.
34. Liang F, Senzaki H, Kurishima C, Sughimoto K, Inuzuka R, Liu H. Hemodynamic performance of the fontan circulation compared with a normal biventricular circulation: A computational model study. Am J Physiol. 2014;307:H1056–72.
35. Fontan F, Baudet E. Surgical repair of tricuspid atresia. Thorax. 1971;26:240–8.
36. Saiki H, Sugimoto M, Kuwata S, Kurishima C, Iwamoto Y, Ishido H, Masutani S, Senzaki H. Novel mechanisms for cerebral blood flow regulation in patients with congenital heart disease. Am Heart J. 2016;172:152–9.
37. Kurishima C, Saiki H, Masutani S, Senzaki H. Tailored therapy for aggressive dilatation of systemic veins and arteries may result in improved long-term fontan circulation. J Thorac Cardiovasc Surg. 2015;150(5):1367–70.
38. Masutani S, Kurishima C, Yana A, Kuwata S, Iwamoto Y, Saiki H, Ishido H, Senzaki H. Assessment of central venous physiology of fontan circulation using peripheral venous pressure. J Thorac Cardiovasc Surg. 2017;153:912–20.
39. Kim J, Kuwata S, Kurishima C, Iwamoto Y, Ishido H, Masutani S, Senzaki H. Importance of dynamic central venous pressure in fontan circulation. Heart Vessels. 2018;33(6):664–70.

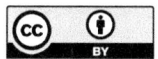

Development of Novel Therapies for Pulmonary Hypertension by Clinical Application of Basic Research

16

Kimio Satoh and Hiroaki Shimokawa

Abstract

Pulmonary hypertension is a lethal disease in which inflammation and oxidative stress are deeply involved in the disease state. We have recently screened novel pathogenic molecules and have performed drug discovery targeting those molecules. To confirm its clinical significance, we used patient-derived blood samples to evaluate the potential as a biomarker for diagnosis and prognosis. Finally, we conducted a high-throughput screening and found inhibitors for the pathogenic proteins. In this chapter, we would like to introduce the recent progress on the basic and clinical research focusing on the screening of pathogenic proteins in pulmonary hypertension.

Keywords

Pulmonary hypertension · Transnational research · Drug discovery · Biomarker Diagnosis

16.1 Introduction

Pulmonary arterial hypertension (PAH) is characterized by intimal/medial thickening and perivascular inflammation and fibrotic change. In addition to genetic backgrounds, many environmental factors as well as volume overload due to heart disease and inflammation due to collagen disease are involved in the development of PAH. The identification of pathogenic genes, which induce the abnormal characteristics of pulmonary artery smooth muscle cells (PASMCs), should be useful for

K. Satoh (✉) · H. Shimokawa
Department of Cardiovascular Medicine, Tohoku University Graduate School of Medicine, Sendai, Japan
e-mail: satoh-k@cardio.med.tohoku.ac.jp

the development of novel therapies for PAH. The characteristics of PASMCs of patients with PAH (PAH-PASMCs) are different from those of healthy controls. In this chapter, we would like to summarize our recent progress on the basic and clinical research focusing on the screening of pathogenic proteins in PAH.

16.2   Endothelial Function in the Development of PAH

Endothelial dysfunction triggers a variety of vascular disorders such as PAH. We have reported a protective role of the endogenous erythropoietin (Epo)/Epo receptor (EpoR) system against the development of PH [12]. This system also plays a crucial role in the functional recovery of ischemic heart [20] and ischemic lower limb [6], demonstrating the importance of endothelial function [4, 10]. Additionally, we found that pravastatin and metformin protect pulmonary endothelial function and ameliorate hypoxia-induced PH in animals [8, 11]. AMP-activated protein kinase (AMPK) is a serine/threonine kinase that functions as an important energy sensor. AMPK has an anti-apoptotic effect in endothelial cells and a pro-apoptotic effect in vascular smooth muscle cells (VSMCs). Both endothelial nitric oxide (NO) production and NO-mediated signaling in VSMCs are targets of the AMPK. In endothelial cells, AMPK positively regulates NO production. In VSMCs, AMPK reduces secretion of growth factors that promote VSMC proliferation and vascular remodeling. Indeed, we have demonstrated that endothelial AMPK plays an important role in microvascular homeostasis in mice in vivo [2]. Additionally, AMPK activators (e.g., statins, metformin, and apelin) are protective against the development of PAH. We also demonstrated that endothelial AMPK plays protective roles against hypoxia-induced PH in mice [8, 11]. Circulating inflammatory cytokines downregulate AMPK and induce endothelial dysfunction in pulmonary circulation [9, 17]. Thus, endothelial AMPK as well as circulating inflammatory cytokines may be therapeutic targets for the treatment of PAH. Thus, AMPK is a key molecule at the crossroad of inflammation and pulmonary artery endothelial dysfunction in the pathogenesis of PAH.

16.3   PASMCs in the Development of PAH

Pulmonary vascular inflammation plays a crucial role for the development of hypoxia-induced PH [11, 12], for which Rho-kinase plays a crucial role [1, 3, 16]. Excessive and continuous activation of Rho-kinase promotes secretion of cyclophilin A (CyPA) from VSMCs and extracellular CyPA stimulates VSMC proliferation [13]. Additionally, extracellular CyPA induces endothelial cell adhesion molecule expression and endothelial apoptosis [7]. Basigin (Bsg) is an extracellular CyPA receptor. Bsg is also known as an essential receptor for Malaria, which disrupts NO metabolism and causes harmful endothelial activation, including the Rho/Rho-kinase activation. Based on these backgrounds, we have demonstrated that CyPA and Bsg promote hypoxia-induced PH [15]. More importantly, plasma CyPA was significantly increased in patients with PAH and well correlated with the disease severity and long-term survival. Thus, extracellular CyPA and its signaling through Bsg are novel therapeutic targets for PAH. We have previously reported that statins and Rho-kinase inhibitors reduce CyPA secretion from VSMCs [14, 19]. Thus, inhibition of CyPA secretion by Rho-kinase inhibitors may have therapeutic efficacy in PAH. In addition, Bsg is strongly expressed in the pulmonary arteries of patients with PAH [15]. Thus, pharmacological agents that prevent the interaction of extracellular CyPA and vascular Bsg could be useful for the treatment of PAH. Indeed, our drug discovery research demonstrated that celastrol significantly inhibits CyPA and Bsg, inhibiting proliferation of PAH-PASMCs [18]. Here, we used PASMCs and high-throughput screening to identify novel agents to inhibit both CyPA and Bsg. PASMCs in the remodeled pulmonary arteries have special characteristics with pro-proliferative features. Importantly, celastrol suppressed CyPA and Bsg expressions in the heart and lung and ameliorated both heart failure (HF) and post-capillary PH. Taken together, inhibiting both CyPA and Bsg may represent a novel therapeutic strategy for the treatment of HF patients with post-capillary PH [18]. As patients with HF and coexisting post-capillary PH show poor clinical outcomes, targeting both cardiac dysfunction and pulmonary vascular remodeling could be a novel concept for the treatment of HF.

16.4   Selenoprotein P in the Development of PAH

Since conventional pulmonary vasodilators have limited efficacy for the treatment of severe PAH, we have performed a series of screens and tried to find a novel therapeutic target. To identify a novel pathogenic protein, we performed microarray analyses using PAH-PASMCs and found 32-fold upregulation of selenoprotein P (SeP) as compared with control PASMCs [5]. Indeed, SeP is highly upregulated in the distal pulmonary arteries of PAH patients. SeP is a secreted protein mainly produced by hepatocytes, which contains 10 selenocysteine residues and transports selenium to maintain cellular metabolism. SeP is upregulated in the liver of patients with type 2 diabetes and downregulates the metabolic switch, AMPK. Additionally, single-nucleotide polymorphisms in the *SEPP1* gene have been reported to be associated with abdominal aortic aneurysm formation. Based on these backgrounds, we further demonstrated that SeP in PASMCs promotes cell proliferation through increased oxidative stress and mitochondrial dysfunction in an autocrine/paracrine manner [5]. Moreover, we demonstrated a pathogenic role of SeP in the development of hypoxia-induced PH in vivo. Since there is a limited efficacy in the treatment of patients with severe PAH, we performed a series of screening to find a novel therapeutic target. Finally, we identified that sanguinarine, an orally active small molecule, reduces SeP expression and PASMC proliferation and ameliorates PH in mice and rats. When we consider the pro-proliferative role of SeP in PAH-PASMCs, the anti-proliferative effect of sanguinarine in several kinds of cancer in vivo could be attributed to the suppression of SeP. Actually, sanguinarine administration to the animal models of PH revealed therapeutic effects on PH and RV failure without any adverse effects [5]. Moreover, serum levels of SeP were significantly elevated in PAH patients in whom higher serum levels of SeP predicted a poor outcome. Based on these results, serum levels of SeP can be used as a novel biomarker for PAH and are useful to evaluate the therapeutic effect of SeP inhibitors (companion diagnostics). Using a combination of SeP inhibitors and serum levels of SeP, we may find good candidates among PAH patients that can be used to demonstrate the effectiveness of this strategy.

16.5 Conclusion

In this chapter, we introduced our recent findings on Epo, AMPK, Rho-kinase, CyPA, Bsg, and SeP, all of which are substantially involved in the pathogenesis of PAH. Additionally, we have also mentioned as to the screening of inhibitors for those pathogenic proteins. By using the novel biomarkers and therapeutic agents, we will continue translational research for the early diagnosis and the development of fundamental therapy in PAH patients.

Acknowledgments This work was supported in part by the grants-in-aid for Scientific Research (15H02535, 15H04816, and 15K15046) from the Ministry of Education, Culture, Sports, Science and Technology, Tokyo, Japan; the Ministry of Health, Labour, and Welfare, Tokyo, Japan (10102895); and the Japan Agency for Medical Research and Development, Tokyo, Japan (15ak0101035h0001, 16ek0109176h0001, and 17ek0109227h0001).

References

1. Elias-Al-Mamun M, Satoh K, Tanaka S, et al. Combination therapy with fasudil and sildenafil ameliorates monocrotaline-induced pulmonary hypertension and survival in rats. Circ J. 2014;78:967–76.
2. Enkhjargal B, Godo S, Sawada A, et al. Endothelial AMP-activated protein kinase regulates blood pressure and coronary flow responses through hyperpolarization mechanism in mice. Arterioscler Thromb Vasc Biol. 2014;34:1505–13.
3. Ikeda S, Satoh K, Kikuchi N, et al. Crucial role of Rho-kinase in pressure overload-induced right ventricular hypertrophy and dysfunction in mice. Arterioscler Thromb Vasc Biol. 2014;34:1260–71.
4. Kagaya Y, Asaumi Y, Wang W, et al. Current perspectives on protective roles of erythropoietin in cardiovascular system: erythropoietin receptor as a novel therapeutic target. Tohoku J Exp Med. 2012;227:83–91.
5. Kikuchi N, Satoh K, Kurosawa R, et al. Selenoprotein p promotes the development of pulmonary arterial hypertension. Circulation. 2018;138:600–23.
6. Nakano M, Satoh K, Fukumoto Y, et al. Important role of erythropoietin receptor to promote VEGF expression and angiogenesis in peripheral ischemia in mice. Circ Res. 2007;100:662–9.
7. Nigro P, Satoh K, O'dell MR, et al. Cyclophilin A is an inflammatory mediator that promotes atherosclerosis in apolipoprotein E-deficient mice. J Exp Med. 2011;208:53–66.
8. Omura J, Satoh K, Kikuchi N, et al. Protective roles of endothelial AMP-activated protein kinase against hypoxia-induced pulmonary hypertension in mice. Circ Res. 2016;119:197–209.
9. Rabinovitch M, Guignabert C, Humbert M, et al. Inflammation and immunity in the pathogenesis of pulmonary arterial hypertension. Circ Res. 2014;115:165–75.

10. Satoh K, Fukumoto Y, Nakano M, et al. Emergence of the erythropoietin/erythropoietin receptor system as a novel cardiovascular therapeutic target. J Cardiovasc Pharmacol. 2011;58:570–4.
11. Satoh K, Fukumoto Y, Nakano M, et al. Statin ameliorates hypoxia-induced pulmonary hypertension associated with down-regulated stromal cell-derived factor-1. Cardiovasc Res. 2009;81:226–34.
12. Satoh K, Kagaya Y, Nakano M, et al. Important role of endogenous erythropoietin system in recruitment of endothelial progenitor cells in hypoxia-induced pulmonary hypertension in mice. Circulation. 2006;113:1442–50.
13. Satoh K, Matoba T, Suzuki J, et al. Cyclophilin A mediates vascular remodeling by promoting inflammation and vascular smooth muscle cell proliferation. Circulation. 2008;117:3088–98.
14. Satoh K, Nigro P, Matoba T, et al. Cyclophilin A enhances vascular oxidative stress and the development of angiotensin II-induced aortic aneurysms. Nat Med. 2009;15:649–56.
15. Satoh K, Satoh T, Kikuchi N, et al. Basigin mediates pulmonary hypertension by promoting inflammation and vascular smooth muscle cell proliferation. Circ Res. 2014;115:738–50.
16. Shimizu T, Fukumoto Y, Tanaka S, et al. Crucial role of ROCK2 in vascular smooth muscle cells for hypoxia-induced pulmonary hypertension in mice. Arterioscler Thromb Vasc Biol. 2013;33:2780–91.
17. Soon E, Holmes AM, Treacy CM, et al. Elevated levels of inflammatory cytokines predict survival in idiopathic and familial pulmonary arterial hypertension. Circulation. 2010;122:920–7.
18. Sunamura S, Satoh K, Kurosawa R, et al. Different roles of myocardial ROCK1 and ROCK2 in cardiac dysfunction and postcapillary pulmonary hypertension in mice. Proc Natl Acad Sci U S A. 2018;115:E7129–38.
19. Suzuki J, Jin ZG, Meoli DF, et al. Cyclophilin A is secreted by a vesicular pathway in vascular smooth muscle cells. Circ Res. 2006;98:811–7.
20. Tada H, Kagaya Y, Takeda M, et al. Endogenous erythropoietin system in non-hematopoietic lineage cells plays a protective role in myocardial ischemia/reperfusion. Cardiovasc Res. 2006;71:466–77.

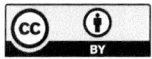

Using Patient-Specific Induced Pluripotent Stem Cells to Understand and Treat Pulmonary Arterial Hypertension

17

Mingxia Gu

Abstract

Pulmonary arterial hypertension (PAH) is characterized by endothelial cell (EC) dysfunction, loss of peripheral pulmonary arterial (PA) microvessels, and proliferation of vascular cells in proximal PAs, leading to occlusion of the lumen. Loss of function mutations in bone morphogenetic protein receptor (BMPR)2 occur in over 70% of heritable form of PAH (HPAH) patients. Intriguingly, only 20% of the mutation carriers develop clinical symptoms, suggesting that genetic variation may provide modifiers that alleviate the disease. Induced pluripotent stem cell (iPSC)-derived vascular cells provide a new opportunity to further understand the disease mechanisms in a personalized manner. In our study, we demonstrated that iPSC-derived endothelial cell (iPSC-EC) recapitulates the functional and gene expression abnormalities in native PAEC from the same PAH patients compared with healthy controls. Interestingly, PAH PAEC and iPSC-EC also respond similarly to potential PAH therapies elafin and FK506 in terms of improved angiogenesis. We then used iPSC-ECs to further understand the reduced penetrance of the BMPR2 mutation. iPSC-EC was generated from three families with unaffected mutation carriers (UMC), HPAH patients, and gender-matched controls. We identified patient-specific features of preserved function in UMC iPSC-EC attributed to the regulators of BMPR2 signaling or to cell survival gene revealed by RNA-Seq analyses. Our findings therefore highlight

M. Gu (✉)

Vera Moulton Wall Center for Pulmonary Vascular Diseases, Stanford University School of Medicine, Stanford, CA, USA

Stanford Cardiovascular Institute, Stanford University School of Medicine, Stanford, CA, USA

Department of Pediatrics, Stanford University School of Medicine, Stanford, CA, USA

Department of Medicine, Stanford University School of Medicine, Stanford, CA, USA
e-mail: Mingxia@stanford.edu

© The Editor(s) (if applicable) and The Author(s) 2020
T. Nakanishi et al. (eds.), *Molecular Mechanism of Congenital Heart Disease and Pulmonary Hypertension*, https://doi.org/10.1007/978-981-15 1185 1_17

protective modifiers for HPAH that could help inform development of future treatment strategies. Despite the site of disease in the lung and the particular vulnerability of the PA vasculature, iPSC-EC is a good surrogate for PAH modeling and drug testing.

Keywords
Induced pluripotent stem cell · Endothelial cell · BMPR2 · Genome editing Pulmonary arterial hypertension

17.1   Introduction

PAH is a progressive disease in which small peripheral arteries are lost or obliterated and more proximal vessels narrow and stiffen, progressively increasing resistance to flow and eventually leading to right heart failure [1, 2]. While the cause of PAH remains poorly understood, the last two decades have shed light on genetic and cellular abnormalities responsible for predisposition to vascular remodeling in PAH. In particular, it has been shown that the endothelial cells (ECs) in PAH are dysfunctional, as evidenced by susceptibility to apoptosis associated with loss of peripheral arteries [3], reduced adhesion related to impaired regeneration [4], decreased migration [5] and tube formation in angiogenesis assays [3] as well as heightened glycolysis, and emergence of apoptosis-resistant cells [6].

One of the major genetic mechanisms driving the endothelial dysfunctions is the loss of function mutations in bone-morphogenetic-protein receptor 2 (BMPR2), which is seen in 70% of patients with the heritable form of PAH (HPAH) and in 20% of sporadic cases of idiopathic PAH (IPAH). Intriguingly, in HPAH families, only 20% of the BMPR2 mutation carriers develop clinical symptoms. Various factors have been linked to the low penetrance: a TGF-β1 polymorphism [7], lower BMPR2 expression from the wild-type allele [8], and reduced expression of the estrogen metabolizing gene *CYP1B1* [9]. However, due to lack of a reliable source of tissues or cells from affected and unaffected BMPR2 mutation carriers to perform in depth genetic and functional studies, our understanding of the protective modifiers or risk factors for BMPR2 mutation carriers remains incomplete.

Induced pluripotent stem cells (iPSC) reprogrammed from somatic cells provide a new resource to understand both personal and common genetic underpinnings as well as cellular dysfunction related to the pathogenesis of IPAH/HPAH. iPSC can be propagated indefinitely, differentiated into EC [10] and smooth muscle cells (SMC) [11], and used for vascular disease modeling [12] and drug testing [13] (Fig. 17.1). In our studies, we applied an iPSCs-based model to systematically study the EC abnormalities in PAH and to further understand the reduced penetrance of the BMPR2 mutation in causing the disease phenotype. By correcting the BMPR2 mutation using CRISPR/Cas9 technology, we demonstrated that in the absence of protective modifiers, the BMPR2 mutation is sufficient for EC dysfunction associated with PAH. Our studies pave the way for using iPSC-derived vascular cells, integrative "omics," and genome editing to better understand patient-specific disease mechanisms for developing precision medicine.

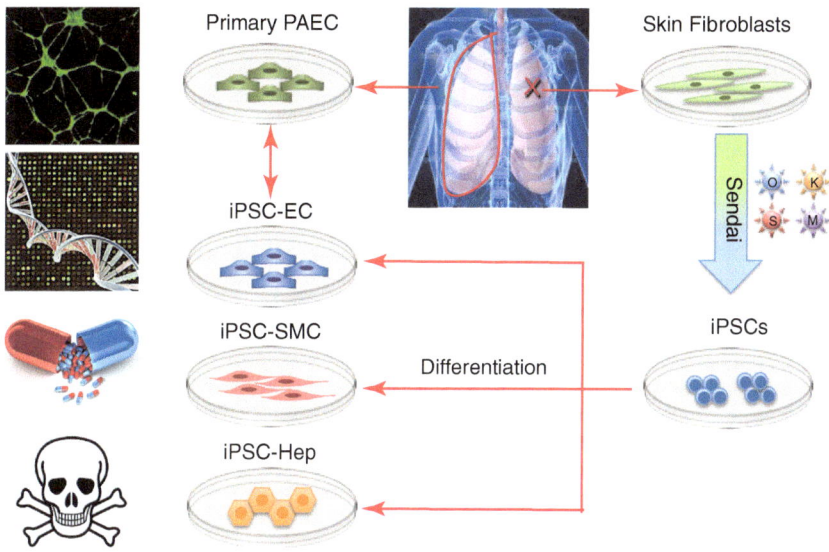

Fig. 17.1 Disease modeling and drug screening using patient-specific iPSC in PAH. At the time of lung transplantation, both skin fibroblasts and primary PAEC were isolated from the same patient. Skin fibroblasts were then reprogramed to iPSC using Sendai virus overexpressing four Yamanaka factors. To model PAH phenotype "in a dish," patient-specific iPSCs were further differentiated into EC and SMC. By comparing primary PAEC and iPSC-EC, we identified disease phenotypes, gene expression abnormalities, and screened for compounds that could reverse EC and SMC dysfunctions associated with PAH. IPSC also has the potential to give rise to hepatocyte, which can be used to test drug toxicity in a personalized manner. *PAEC* pulmonary artery endothelial cells. *EC* endothelial cell, *SMC* smooth muscle cell

17.2   Patient-Specific iPSC-Derived Endothelial Cells to Model PAH

The mechanism underlying PAH vary in individuals, perhaps because of genetic factors and environmental exposures. IPSC-EC that preserves the gene variants from the patient could be a good surrogate for native PAEC to understand the genotype-phenotype correlation, and to increase the opportunity to individualized therapy.

17.2.1 iPSC-EC Recapitulates Native Pulmonary Arterial Endothelial Cell (PAEC)

To investigate the use of iPSC-EC as a surrogate for native EC to better understand and treat PAH, we compared PAH PAEC, harvested and cultured from lungs removed at the time of transplantation, with PAH EC differentiated from iPSC (iPSC-EC) that had been reprogrammed from skin fibroblasts obtained from a small biopsy taken at the incision site of the same patients. Control fibroblasts and PAEC were obtained from unused donor lungs [13].

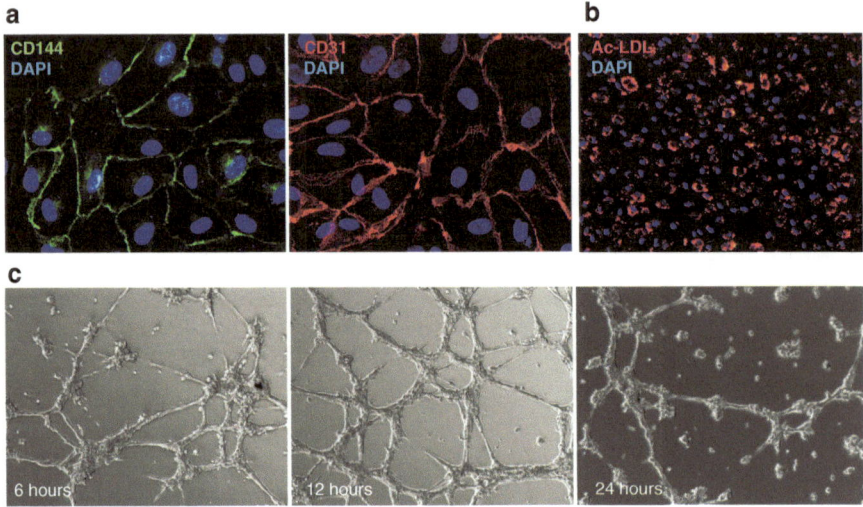

Fig. 17.2 Characterization of iPSC-EC from healthy control. (**a**) iPSC-EC differentiated from skin fibroblast-derived iPSC express the endothelial surface marker CD144 (green) and CD31 (red). Nuclear staining using DAPI is in blue. (**b**) iPSC-ECs incorporate acetylated low-density lipoprotein (Ac-LDL, red; DAPI, Blue). (**c**) Angiogenesis assays: representative images of tube formation 6, 12, and 24 h after seeding cells in growth factor reduced Matrigel. iPSC-ECs start forming tubes at 6 h and will regress after 24 h

We found that there was marked similarity between iPSC-EC and native PAEC judged by the typical EC cobblestone morphology, acetylated low-density lipoprotein uptake, and expression of endothelial cell surface marker VE-cadherin (CD144) (Fig. 17.2). Interestingly, compared with HUVEC, iPSC-ECs from both control and PAH patients expressed increased arterial EC gene ephrin-B2 (EFNB2) and reduced venous EC gene ephrin type-B receptor 4 (EPHB4) and nuclear receptor subfamily 2 (NR2F2), possibly due to the high dose of VEGF added during the EC differentiation from iPSCs.

Additionally, PAH PAEC and iPSC-EC compared with those from control lungs showed reduced adhesion to laminin, decreased migration detected by wound closure scratch assay, increased vulnerability to apoptosis with serum withdrawal analyzed by caspase3/7 activity asssay, and impaired angiogenesis judged by the inability to form capillary-like tubes when seeded onto growth factor reduced Matrigel. These functional abnormalities could attribute to the impaired pSmad-ID1 pathway in both PAH PAEC and iPSC-EC compared with respective control cells. However, two abnormalities in PAH PAEC could not be recapitulated by iPSC-EC: an increase in unrepaired DNA damage judged by the "comet tails" of nuclear DNA following alkali digestion and higher mitochondrial membrane potential measured by the JC-1 assay after serum starvation in PAH PAEC compared with control subjects. This indicates that DNA damage and increased mitochondrial membrane potential in PAH EC might be related to the environment exposure in the lung, and once the cells are being reprogrammed and re-differentiated, they may lose these features.

17.2.2 Patient-Specific Drug Response in IPSC-EC and PAEC

Recent advances in iPSC technology also provide a new paradigm for drug screening by permitting the use of human cells with the same genetic background as the patients without the typical quantity constraints associated with patient primary cells. Thus, we compared drug response in PAH PAEC and iPSC-EC from the same group of patients using new promising treatments for PAH, FK506, and elafin. FK506 is an immunosuppressant identified as an activator of BMPR2 signaling [14], and elafin is a neutrophil elastase inhibitor that enhances BMPR2 signaling in a caveolin-1-dependent manner and improves angiogenesis in PAH [3]. In three patients with IPAH/HPAH, elafin and FK506 improved angiogenesis as judged by capillary-like tubes formed on Matrigel in both PAEC and iPSC-EC whereas in the other three patients, there was no change in either cell type. Our data indicates that PAH iPSC-EC could recapitulate the drug response in native PAEC based on in vitro EC functional assays.

17.3   Modeling Reduced Penetrance of BMPR2 Mutation in PAH

Due to the limited access to native PAEC from HPAH patients and no access from unaffected BMPR2 mutation carriers (UMCs), iPSC-EC could provide a unique platform to model the propensity to HPAH "in-a-dish." The compensatory mechanisms in UMC shed light on the protective modifiers for HPAH that could help inform development of future therapeutic strategies.

17.3.1 Preserved EC Function in Unaffected BMPR2 Mutation Carrier (UMC)

To determine if the lack of clinic manifestation of the disease can be recapitulated in UMC iPSC-EC, we recruited 11 individuals from three HPAH families, with HPAH patients, UMC, and gender-matched controls [15]. We observed that cell adhesion to a wide variety of extracellular matrix substrates and cell survival measured by caspase3/7 activity either after serum withdrawal or following reoxygenation after hypoxia were preserved in UMC iPSC-EC in that values were similar to those in control cells, whereas these functions were significantly impaired in HPAH iPSC-EC. Cell migration and tube formation in Matrigel were similarly impaired in iPSC-ECs from both UMCs and HPAH patients compared with controls. However, when iPSC-EC was stimulated with BMPR2 ligand BMP4, cell migration and angiogenesis were significantly improved in UMC iPSC-EC with values similar to those in control iPSC-EC whereas these features remained impaired in iPSC-EC from HPAH patients. Our study revealed that UMC iPSC-EC showed preserved EC functions that were similar to control iPSC-EC and different from HPAH iPSC-EC.

17.3.2 Preserved pP38 Signaling Pathway in Unaffected BMPR2 Mutation Carrier

To determine whether compensatory BMPR2 signaling was responsible for preservation of normal UMC iPSC-EC functions, we tested both canonical and noncanonical BMP signaling pathways including pSMAD1/5-ID1, pErk, pAkt, and pP38. Interestingly, the only pathway that could distinguish UMC versus HPAH iPSC-EC is the pP38 pathway, which was consistently activated in response to BMP4 or under cell adhesion condition in iPSC-ECs from both controls and UMCs, but not in the HPAH iPSC-EC from all three families. Further studies showed that the compensatory pP38 signaling in UMC iPSC-EC was due to an increase in BMPR2 activators LRP1 and caveolin1 as well as a reduction in BMPR2 inhibitors gremlin1 and FKBP12, which could be assessed prospectively to determine whether they are biomarkers that reduce the risk of HPAH in UMC.

17.4   Gene Editing in PAH IPSCs

Genome editing in human iPSCs represents an opportunity to examine the contribution of pathogenic and disease-modifying mutations to molecular and cellular phenotypes [16]. Here, we summarized recent studies that utilized CRISPR/Cas9 gene editing in iPSCs to address the controversial question of whether BMPR2 mutation alone is necessary and/or sufficient for establishing the major cellular phenotypes associated with PAH.

17.4.1 Correction of the BMPR2 Mutation in PAH iPSCs

To determine the extent to which the BMPR2 mutation accounts for the iPSC-EC dysfunction in HPAH, we corrected the BMPR2 missense mutation in one of the HPAH iPSC lines we previously characterized using CRISPR/Cas9-mediated homology directed repair. Upon differentiation, the corrected HPAH iPSC-EC line showed control levels of cell adhesion and survival in response to either serum withdrawal or after hypoxia and reoxygenation. The pP38 signaling pathway was also rescued in the edited iPSC-EC. Tube formation and cell migration were still impaired under baseline following editing of the BMPR2 mutation; however, these were improved to control levels with BMP4 stimulation. This suggests that both protective modifiers and a corrected BMPR2 mutation are necessary to fully normalize EC function in HPAH patients.

17.4.2 Generation of iPSC Line with BMPR2 Mutation

To assess the effect of a BMPR2 mutation without the confounding effects of genetic differences between cell lines, Kiskin et al. generated two isogenic lines carrying either a known causal BMPR2 mutation (W9X; referred to as C2 W9X$^{+/-}$) or a deletion of exon 1 (C2 ΔExon1) from a wild-type iPSC line [17]. Subsequently, these iPSCs were differentiated into SMC expressing smooth muscle actin, calponin, and myosin heavy chain 11 that had a contractile phenotype as well as iPSC-EC, which were enriched for arterial-specific EC markers. Under serum-free, chemically defined conditions, BMPR2 heterozygosity alone was sufficient to cause reduced apoptosis and increased proliferation in iPSC-SMCs, which has been shown in native PASMCs. Additionally, after serum exposure for 1 week for iPSC-ECs and serum + TNFα exposure for 1 week or serum-only for 2 weeks for iPSC-SMCs, these cells acquire inner mitochondrial membrane hyperpolarization. Although the generation of pulmonary SMC and EC from iPSC is yet to be achieved, the differentiation protocols used in this study produced cells that recapitulated key phenotypes found in diseased adult PASMCs and PAECs.

17.5   Future Directions and Clinical Implications

The studies summarized here demonstrate that iPSC-EC and PAEC from the same group of PAH patients showed similar functional impairment, reduced BMPR2 signaling, and subgroup responsiveness to potential PAH therapy, suggesting that despite the site of disease in the lung and the particular vulnerability of the PA vasculature, iPSC-EC are good surrogates for native PAEC to study the fundamental pathobiology in PAH. The results of these studies also suggest the potential of using of iPSC-derived vascular cells to model other vascular diseases where the phenotype may be variable, e.g., Marfan, Williams, or Alagille syndromes.

Because patient-specific iPSC has the potential to give rise to unlimited number of all the cell types in the vasculature including EC, SMC and fibroblasts, it holds great promise for screening compounds that reverse the cellular phenotype associated with PAH in a high-throughput manner, which may ultimately change the current paradigm of treating PAH with "one size fits all" strategy to precision medicine.

Additionally, since PAH iPSC-EC does not recapitulate all the phenotypes in native EC from the lung such as increased DNA damage and higher mitochondrial membrane potential, the next step would be to generate tissue-specific, functionally distinct endothelial cell subtypes from iPSCs. This will allow us to study fundamental questions about lineage specification during development and provide a scalable cell-specific source for tissue engineering, cell therapy, disease modeling, and drug discovery.

Acknowledgment This work was supported by funding from NIH HL135258 (M.G.)

References

1. Rabinovitch M. Molecular pathogenesis of pulmonary arterial hypertension. J Clin Invest. 2012;122:4306–13. https://doi.org/10.1172/JCI60658.
2. Tuder RM, et al. Relevant issues in the pathology and pathobiology of pulmonary hypertension. J Am Coll Cardiol. 2013;62:D4–12. https://doi.org/10.1016/j.jacc.2013.10.025.
3. Nickel NP, et al. Elafin Reverses Pulmonary Hypertension via Caveolin-1-Dependent Bone Morphogenetic Protein Signaling. Am J Respir Crit Care Med. 2015;191:1273–86. https://doi.org/10.1164/rccm.201412-2291OC.

4. de Jesus Perez VA, et al. Loss of adenomatous poliposis coli-alpha3 integrin interaction promotes endothelial apoptosis in mice and humans. Circ Res. 2012;111:1551–64. https://doi.org/10.1161/CIRCRESAHA.112.267849.
5. Rhodes CJ, et al. RNA sequencing analysis detection of a novel pathway of endothelial dysfunction in pulmonary arterial hypertension. Am J Respir Crit Care Med. 2015;192:356–66. https://doi.org/10.1164/rccm.201408-1528OC.
6. Masri FA, et al. Hyperproliferative apoptosis-resistant endothelial cells in idiopathic pulmonary arterial hypertension. Am J Physiol Lung Cell Mol Physiol. 2007;293:L548–54. https://doi.org/10.1152/ajplung.00428.2006.
7. Phillips JA 3rd, et al. Synergistic heterozygosity for TGFbeta1 SNPs and BMPR2 mutations modulates the age at diagnosis and penetrance of familial pulmonary arterial hypertension. Genet Med. 2008;10:359–65. https://doi.org/10.1097/GIM.0b013e318172dcdf.
8. Hamid R, Cogan JD, Hedges LK, Austin E, Phillips JA 3rd, Newman JH, Loyd JE. Penetrance of pulmonary arterial hypertension is modulated by the expression of normal BMPR2 allele. Hum Mutat. 2009;30:649–54. https://doi.org/10.1002/humu.20922.
9. West J, et al. Gene expression in BMPR2 mutation carriers with and without evidence of pulmonary arterial hypertension suggests pathways relevant to disease penetrance. BMC Med Genomics. 2008;1:45. https://doi.org/10.1186/1755-8794-1-45.
10. Gu M. Efficient differentiation of human pluripotent stem cells to endothelial cells. Curr Protoc Hum Genet. 2018;6:e64. https://doi.org/10.1002/cphg.64.
11. Patsch C, et al. Generation of vascular endothelial and smooth muscle cells from human pluripotent stem cells. Nat Cell Biol. 2015;17:994–1003. https://doi.org/10.1038/ncb3205.
12. Theodoris CV, et al. Human disease modeling reveals integrated transcriptional and epigenetic mechanisms of NOTCH1 haploinsufficiency. Cell. 2015;160:1072–86. https://doi.org/10.1016/j.cell.2015.02.035.
13. Sa S, et al. Induced pluripotent stem cell model of pulmonary arterial hypertension reveals novel gene expression and patient specificity. Am J Respir Crit Care Med. 2017;195:930–41. https://doi.org/10.1164/rccm.201606-1200OC.
14. Spiekerkoetter E, et al. FK506 activates BMPR2, rescues endothelial dysfunction, and reverses pulmonary hypertension. J Clin Invest. 2013;123:3600–13. https://doi.org/10.1172/JCI65592.
15. Gu M, et al. Patient-specific iPSC-derived endothelial cells uncover pathways that protect against pulmonary hypertension in bmpr2 mutation carriers. Cell stem cell. 2017;20:490–504e495. https://doi.org/10.1016/j.stem.2016.08.019.
16. Hockemeyer D, Jaenisch R. Induced pluripotent stem cells meet genome editing. Cell Stem Cell. 2016;18:573–86. https://doi.org/10.1016/j.stem.2016.04.013.
17. Kiskin FN, et al. Contributions of BMPR2 mutations and extrinsic factors to cellular phenotypes of pulmonary arterial hypertension revealed by induced pluripotent stem cell modeling. Am J Respir Crit Care Med. 2018;198:271–5. https://doi.org/10.1164/rccm.201801-0049LE.

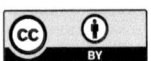

Modeling Pulmonary Arterial Hypertension Using Induced Pluripotent Stem Cells

18

Amer A. Rana, Fedir N. Kiskin, and C.-Hong Chang

Abstract

Heritable pulmonary arterial hypertension belongs to a group of pulmonary vascular diseases for which there is currently no cure other than a heart and lung transplantation. Increased endothelial and smooth muscle cell proliferation leads to vascular remodeling, resulting in increased blood pressure in the lungs which ultimately causes right heart failure. Understanding the molecular mechanisms implicated in the establishment and progression of pulmonary arterial hypertension is hampered due to a lack of disease models, including a limited availability of patient-derived cells and the low penetrance of *BMPR2,* the major disease-associated gene. Induced pluripotent stem cells provide a series of advantages for disease modeling that could potentially allow theses issues to be overcome. These include (1) a limitlessly self-renewing capacity that overcomes the restricted supply of cells from diseased patients, (2) an epigenome that has been wiped of pathogenic modifications which have accumulated during the disease process, (3) an amenability to gene editing which allows the introduction of specific pathogenic mutations in an otherwise isogenic background to facilitate the dissection of the precise contribution of disease-associated genetic mutations, and (4) the generation of isogenic cell, tissue, and organ-specific disease models.

A. A. Rana (✉)
Division of Respiratory Medicine, Department of Medicine, University of Cambridge, Cambridge, UK

British Heart Foundation Oxford and Cambridge Centre of Regenerative Medicine, Cambridge, UK

British Heart Foundation Cambridge Centre of Research Excellence, Cambridge, UK
e-mail: ar332@cam.ac.uk

F. N. Kiskin · C.-H. Chang
Division of Respiratory Medicine, Department of Medicine, University of Cambridge, Cambridge, UK

© The Editor(s) (if applicable) and The Author(s) 2020
T. Nakanishi et al. (eds.), *Molecular Mechanism of Congenital Heart Disease and Pulmonary Hypertension*, https://doi.org/10.1007/978-981-15-1185-1_18

139

Keywords
Pulmonary arterial hypertension · BMPR2 · Induced pluripotent stem cells · Smooth muscle and endothelial cells · Disease modeling

18.1 Heritable Pulmonary Arterial Hypertension

Heritable pulmonary arterial hypertension (HPAH) is a debilitating, often fatal disease caused by increased proliferation and apoptotic resistance of smooth muscle and endothelial cells which drive the vascular remodeling of small pulmonary arterioles and results in their narrowing and obliteration. This causes increased pulmonary vascular resistance and hence increased blood pressure in the pulmonary vessels, eventually leading to right-heart failure [1]. Although currently available therapies have improved life expectancy, they do not prevent disease progression.

18.1.1 Insights into the Pathobiology of PAH

Major insights into PAH pathobiology followed the identification of causal heterozygous germline mutations in the gene encoding the bone morphogenetic protein type II receptor (*BMPR2*) in over 80% of cases of families with PAH [2]. BMPR2 is a receptor for bone morphogenetic proteins (BMPs), which are members of the transforming growth factor-β superfamily. Furthermore, around 20% of cases of sporadic or idiopathic PAH harbor mutations in *BMPR2* [2]. The *BMPR2* locus is marked by considerable allelic heterogeneity with over 660 germline variants identified to date. Approximately 70% of mutations lead to haploinsufficiency due to nonsense-mediated mRNA decay of the mutant transcript. Additional mutations include missense mutations that lead to substitutions in highly conserved amino acids in important functional domains of the receptor [2].

The central role of the BMPR2 pathway in PAH is supported by the identification of causal mutations in other members of this pathway including *ACVRL1*, *ENG*, *GDF2* (BMP9), and *SMAD9* [3]. In addition, loss of BMPR2 signaling appears to play a critical role in non-genetic forms of PAH in humans and in preclinical rodent models. Furthermore, treatment with the selective BMPR2/ALK1 ligand BMP9 has been shown to increase lung endothelial BMPR2 expression and reverse PAH in rodent models [4]

18.1.2 Reduced Penetrance of *BMPR2* in PAH

An important observation in heritable PAH is that *BMPR2* mutations exhibit low penetrance (approximately 20–30% in families), suggesting a requirement for additional environmental or genetic triggers necessary for disease initiation and progression [5]. Interestingly, identical twins carrying mutations in *BMPR2*, where only one sibling presents with PAH, have been identified [6]. Together, these argue that environmental factors must have a critical role in disease establishment, and in some contexts, these may be more important than the presence of particular genetic modifiers of *BMPR2*.

Insights into potential environmental factors that interact with BMPR2 to cause PAH have come from animal models free of genetic mutations in *BMPR2*, including lipopoly-saccharide-, monocrotaline-, Sugen-5416/hypoxia-, and chronic hypoxia–induced mouse and rat models, as well as from mice with lung-specific overexpression of tumor necrosis factor (TNFα) [7]. However, a common and important feature of these non-genetic models of PAH is the general reduction in BMPR2 at the protein level, which further supports a central role of BMPR2 in the establishment of PAH. In recent work from our labs, we have dissected the mechanism of how inflammatory signaling in the form of TNFα can cause a reduction in BMPR2 signaling [8]. This is achieved by via the shedding of BMPR2 extracellular domain at the cell surface, which reduces intact receptor expression, as well as by the transcriptional repression of *BMPR2*, which reduces the total overall expression of BMPR2 in cells. Taken together, these changes ultimately lead to hyper-proliferation of pulmonary artery smooth muscle cells.

18.2 Modeling Pulmonary Arterial Hypertension with Induced Pluripotent Stem Cells

The limited availability of human tissue from PAH patients with end-stage disease and only at the time of transplantation has hampered progress in understanding the initiation and progression of PAH. In addition, mouse knockout or transgenic models of *BMPR2* deficiency fail to fully recapitulate the pathology observed in humans [7]. Hence, there is a pressing need for alternative human models of PAH to accelerate the development of new treatments for this devastating disease.

Induced pluripotent stem cells (iPSCs) provide major opportunities for disease modeling because they can be derived from specific patients, possess a limitless ability to self-renew, differentiate into all somatic cell lineages, and are amenable to targeted genetic engineering [9]. Their epigenetic memory is also reset during the reprogramming process, wiping epigenetic remodeling marks accumulated during the disease process and therefore potentially providing a naïve non-diseased system which can be used to induce a disease state and thus elucidate hitherto unknown mechanisms of disease progression.

However, an important consideration is whether iPSC-derived cells resemble the relevant adult cell types closely enough. In the case of PAH, the goal is to mimic pulmonary arterial endothelial and distal smooth muscle cells. For example, fundamental differences in responses to hypoxia exist between the pulmonary vasculature and the systemic vasculature and also between the BMP responsiveness of proximal and peripheral (distal) portions of the pulmonary vascular branch.

While systemic arteries relax in response to tissue hypoxia in order to improve blood flow and oxygen supply in hypoxic tissues, pulmonary arteries respond by contracting, thereby diverting blood flow from poorly ventilated regions toward the more oxygenated areas of the lungs [10]. Furthermore, previous work has demonstrated that in contrast to proximal cells, peripheral PASMCs are not growth-suppressed and exhibit reduced apoptosis when treated with BMP4 [11].

18.2.1 Embryological Origins of the Pulmonary Vasculature

In order to differentiate iPSCs toward pulmonary vascular lineages we must consider the embryological origins of the pulmonary vascular cells and the developmental pathways that have directed them toward their specific fate. For example, the differences in responsiveness to hypoxia and BMP signaling might be due to cells of the pulmonary vasculature having different embryological origins. Lineage tracing has shown that four major embryonic lineages contribute to the pulmonary vasculature: (1) Wnt1+ neural crest, which contributes to the SMCs at the root of the pulmonary artery, (2) cardiopulmonary progenitors (CPPs), which contribute ECs and SMCs to the proximal pulmonary artery and vein, (3) WT1+ mesothelium, which surrounds the lung and contributes widely to both ECs and SMCs throughout the vasculature, and (4) lateral plate mesoderm, which contributes to the PASMCs in peripheral pulmonary arteries [12]. The ability to recapitulate specific lineages and their vascular derivatives is likely to be critical for generating a high-fidelity model of PAH.

18.2.2 Current iPSC Models of PAH

Our group was the first to publish work on reprogramming patient-derived cells carrying *BMPR2* mutations [13]. Since then, other reports have used iPSC-derived cells to gain insights into PAH.

West et al. [14] used patient-derived iPSCs carrying mutations in *BMPR2* to generate mesenchymal and endothelial-like cells. The authors noted an increase in Wnt signaling in these cells and found this was also the case in adult *BMPR2* mutant fibroblasts and in human tissue. However, although the mesenchymal cells expressed some SMC markers, these cells were unable to model the characteristic hyperproliferative phenotype observed in PASMCs. This highlights the important consideration that iPSC-derived cells must approximate closely enough the relevant adult cell types.

Sa et al. [15] performed RNA-seq on iPSC-derived endothelial cells (iPSC-ECs) and pulmonary artery endothelial cells (PAECs) with and without *BMPR2* mutations and observed that cell adhesion and migration were decreased in cells carrying *BMPR2* mutations compared to controls. This work also showed that *KISS1* was upregulated in *BMPR2* mutant cells compared to wild-type cells.

Gu et al. [16] reiterated the cell adhesion and cell migration defect in iPSC-ECs but went on to look at why not all *BMPR2* mutation carriers develop

PAH. Their approach was to take three different families, in which all individuals carried mutations in *BMPR2*, and then compare the phenotype and transcriptomes of iPSC-ECs of individuals within each family to see if there was a difference between those family members that present with PAH (FPAH) and those that did not (unaffected mutation carriers or UMC). Through this they found that apoptosis was higher in FPAH compared with UMC, while cell adhesion was reduced in both FPAH and UMC. This suggested that genetic modifiers might give UMCs a cell survival advantage. Through transcriptomic analysis, *BIRC3*, a gene implicated in cell survival, was found to be reduced in FPAH compared to UMC. Taken together, the authors concluded that genetic background can influence whether or not an individual will develop PAH. However, as discussed earlier, regardless of the initial instigator (genetic or non-genetic) of PAH, all patients ultimately show a reduction in BMPR2 expression and signaling. Thus, the question of what BMPR2 is doing in disease is fundamental and remained unanswered.

We recently addressed this issue using iPSCs to model arterial ECs and distal PASMCs where we were able to transition cells from a naïve state lacking disease-associated cellular phenotypes to a diseased state, showing that a *BMPR2* mutation *per se* is necessary and sufficient for the establishment of some but not all PAH-associated cellular phenotypes in iPSC-ECs and iPSC-SMCs [21]. Omics analysis of the changes associated with this transition will reveal potentially novel and/or druggable pathways to prevent or reverse PAH disease progression.

18.3   Future Direction and Clinical Implications

Primary future uses of iPSCs include drug screening and the generation of human 3D multi-tissue constructs of the pulmonary system for disease modeling. Protocols to generate endothelial cells (ECs), smooth muscle cells, and pericytes from iPSCs have been established [17, 18], and advanced protocols to generate cells more akin to pulmonary vascular cells are underway. Based on these protocols, functional evaluations in each cell type between normal and disease-carrying subjects can be performed to provide a powerful platform for cell type-specific drug discovery. Considering the importance of cell-cell communication during disease progression, modeling diseases will require using more than one cell type. Although it is possible to co-culture iPSC-derived ECs and perivascular cells [19], the highly specialized and complex nature of the pulmonary vascular bed poses challenges for constructing a 3D pulmonary-specific vasculature. In addition, investigating merely vascular cells might lead us to misinterpret pulmonary vascular disease mechanisms. Although animal models have been widely used to model diseases, they are expensive, time-consuming, and often do not fully recapitulate human pathology. iPSC-derived organ-like tissue, termed 'organoids', might eventually replace animal models [20]. Whilst liver and kidney organoids develop with vasculatures, current lung organoids lack vascular populations [20]. Developing better lung organoids or pulmonary artery-on-a-chip technologies would provide an advanced platform to model pulmonary vascular diseases.

Acknowledgments This research was funded by the British Heart Foundation (BHF) (project grant PG/14/31/30786 and FS/13/51/30636), the Cambridge NIHR Biomedical Research Centre, the Dinosaur Trust, PHA UK, and the Robert McAlpine Foundation. AAR would also like to acknowledge support from the BHF Centre of Regenerative Medicine, Oxford and Cambridge (RM/13/3/30159), the BHF Centre for Research Excellence (RE/13/6/30180), and the BHF IPAH cohort grant (SP/12/12/29836). We apologize to those authors whose work we were unable to cite due to space limitations.

References

1. Humbert M, Morrell NW, Archer SL, Stenmark KR, MacLean MR, Lang IM, et al. Cellular and molecular pathobiology of pulmonary arterial hypertension. J Am Coll Cardiol. 2004;43:13S–24S.
2. Machado RD, Southgate L, Eichstaedt CA, Aldred MA, Austin ED, Best DH, et al. Pulmonary Arterial Hypertension: A Current Perspective on Established and Emerging Molecular Genetic Defects. Hum Mutat. 2015;36(12):1113–27.
3. Ma L, Chung WK. The role of genetics in pulmonary arterial hypertension. J Pathol. 2017;241(2):273–80.
4. Long L, Ormiston ML, Yang X, Southwood M, Gräf S, Machado RD, et al. Selective enhancement of endothelial BMPR-II with BMP9 reverses pulmonary arterial hypertension. Nat Med. 2015;21(7):777–85.
5. Larkin EK, Newman JH, Austin ED, Hemnes AR, Wheeler L, Robbins IM, et al. Longitudinal analysis casts doubt on the presence of genetic anticipation in heritable pulmonary arterial hypertension. Am J Respir Crit Care Med. 2012;186(9):892–6.
6. Ormiston ML, Southgate L, Treacy C, Pepke-Zaba J, Trembath RC, Machado RD, et al. Assessment of a pulmonary origin for blood outgrowth endothelial cells by examination of identical twins harboring a BMPR2 mutation. Am J Respir Crit Care Med. 2013;188(2):258–60.
7. Stenmark KR, Meyrick B, Galie N, Mooi WJ, McMurtry IF. Animal models of pulmonary arterial hypertension: the hope for etiological discovery and pharmacological cure. Am J Physiol Lung Cell Mol Physiol. 2009;297(6):L1013–32.
8. Hurst LA, Dunmore BJ, Long L, Crosby A, Al-Lamki R, Deighton J, et al. TNFα drives pulmonary arterial hypertension by suppressing the BMP type-II receptor and altering NOTCH signalling. Nat Commun. 2017;8:14079.
9. Shi Y, Inoue H, Wu JC, Yamanaka S. Induced pluripotent stem cell technology: a decade of progress. Nat Rev Drug Discov. 2017;16(2):115–30.
10. Ward JP, McMurtry IF. Mechanisms of hypoxic pulmonary vasoconstriction and their roles in pulmonary hypertension: new findings for an old problem. Curr Opin Pharmacol. 2009;9(3):287–96.
11. Yang X, Long L, Southwood M, Rudarakanchana N, Upton PD, Jeffery TK, et al. Dysfunctional Smad signaling contributes to abnormal smooth muscle cell proliferation in familial pulmonary arterial hypertension. Circ Res. 2005;96(10):1053–63.
12. Majesky MW. Developmental basis of vascular smooth muscle diversity. Arterioscler Thromb Vasc Biol. 2007;27(6):1248–58.
13. Geti I, Ormiston ML, Rouhani F, Toshner M, Movassagh M, Nichols J, et al. A practical and efficient cellular substrate for the generation of induced pluripotent stem cells from adults: blood-derived endothelial progenitor cells. Stem Cells Transl Med. 2012;1(12):855–65.
14. West JD, Austin ED, Gaskill C, Marriott S, Baskir R, Bilousova G, et al. Identification of a common Wnt-associated genetic signature across multiple cell types in pulmonary arterial hypertension. Am J Physiol Cell Physiol. 2014;307(5):C415–30.
15. Sa S, Gu M, Chappell J, Shao NY, Ameen M, Elliott KA, et al. Induced Pluripotent Stem Cell Model of Pulmonary Arterial Hypertension Reveals Novel Gene Expression and Patient Specificity. Am J Respir Crit Care Med. 2017;195(7):930–41.

16. Gu M, Shao NY, Sa S, Li D, Termglinchan V, Ameen M, et al. Patient-specific iPSC-derived endothelial cells uncover pathways that protect against pulmonary hypertension in BMPR2 mutation carriers. Cell Stem Cell. 2017;20(4):490–504.e5.
17. Kiskin FN, Chang C-H, Huang CJZ, Kwieder B, Cheung C, Dunmore BJ, Serrano F, Sinha S, Morrell NW, Rana AA. Contributions of mutations and extrinsic factors to cellular phenotypes of pulmonary arterial hypertension revealed by induced pluripotent stem cell modeling. Am J Respir Crit Care Med. 2018;198(2):271–5.
18. Orlova VV, van den Hil FE, Petrus-Reurer S, Drabsch Y, Ten Dijke P, Mummery CL. Generation, expansion and functional analysis of endothelial cells and pericytes derived from human pluripotent stem cells. Nat Protoc. 2014;9(6):1514–31.
19. Cheung C, Bernardo AS, Trotter MW, Pedersen RA, Sinha S. Generation of human vascular smooth muscle subtypes provides insight into embryological origin-dependent disease suscep-tibility. Nat Biotechnol. 2012;30(2):165–73.
20. Heydarkhan-Hagvall S, Helenius G, Johansson BR, Li JY, Mattsson E, Risberg B. Co-culture of endothelial cells and smooth muscle cells affects gene expression of angiogenic factors. J Cell Biochem. 2003;89(6):1250–9.
21. Dye BR, Hill DR, Ferguson MA, Tsai YH, Nagy MS, Dyal R, et al. In vitro generation of human pluripotent stem cell derived lung organoids. Elife. 2015;4. https://doi.org/10.7554/eLife.05098.

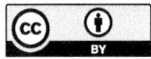

Dysfunction and Restoration of Endothelial Cell Communications in Pulmonary Arterial Hypertension: Therapeutic Implications

19

Christophe Guignabert

Abstract

Impairment of the pulmonary endothelial communications contributes to the development and progression of pulmonary arterial hypertension (PAH). Investigations currently under way are likely to produce novel therapeutic strategies that target pulmonary endothelial dysfunction linked to PAH. This chapter outlines the complex role of the dysfunctional pulmonary endothelium in PAH and its potential value as a target for innovative therapies.

Keywords

Pulmonary hypertension · Pathogenesis · Endothelial dysfunction · Cell-cell communication · Therapeutic target

19.1 Introduction

Pulmonary arterial hypertension (PAH) is a severe and progressive cardiopulmonary disorder characterized by non-specific symptoms (i.e., breathlessness, fatigue, weakness, angina, and syncope) that take years before appearing, usually after the disease is in an advanced stage. In Europe, PAH prevalence and incidence are in the range of 15–60 subjects per million population and 5–10 cases per million per year, respectively. Despite recent progress in the treatment of PAH, most patients still die from the disease or fail to respond adequately to medical therapy with a 5-year survival of 59%. Current treatments can relieve some PAH symptoms and slow the progress of

C. Guignabert (✉)
INSERM UMR_S 999, Hôpital Marie Lannelongue, Le Plessis-Robinson, France

Faculté de Médecine, Université Paris-Sud, Université Paris-Saclay,
Le Kremlin-Bicêtre, France
e-mail: christophe.guignabert@inserm.fr

the disease in some patients, but they have limited impact on the progressive pulmonary vascular remodeling that eventually culminates in right heart failure [1].

Pulmonary endothelial dysfunction is a critical contributor that could be detrimental for the onset and progression of this severe cardiopulmonary disorder [2–4]. Therefore, early diagnosis and better understanding of the mechanisms underlying the altered pulmonary endothelial cell (EC) phenotype and endothelial communications with both resident vascular cells (smooth muscle cells, fibroblasts, myofibroblasts, and pericytes) and inflammatory cells are needed to propose and develop new, more adapted and more powerful therapeutic tools.

19.2 Pulmonary Endothelial Dysfunction and the Pathobiology of PAH

At the interface between bloodstream and lung tissue, the pulmonary ECs play critical roles not only in optimizing gas exchanges but also in the local adaptations of vascular tone, in the maintenance of a thrombosis-free surface, in the control of inflammatory cell adhesion and trafficking, as well as in the maintenance of the vascular wall integrity and for normal angiogenesis. Importantly, they are dynamic and adapt their roles and phenotypes according to the nature of the local milieu (Fig. 19.1). Indeed, the pulmonary ECs are highly metabolically active, sensing and responding to signals from extracellular environments by secreting the correct substance(s) by which it may maintain the vasomotor balance and vascular-tissue homeostasis [4].

As a vital part of the pulmonary vascular wall, alterations of the pulmonary endothelium are now well established to be central role in the pathogenesis of PAH. The main characteristics of pulmonary endothelial alterations or dysfunction in PAH includes, among others, a reduction in the secretion of vasodilator molecules such as prostacyclin (PGI_2) and nitric oxide (NO), and an increase in the potent vasoconstrictor endothelin (ET)-1 [5]. In addition, our group has highlighted that pulmonary ECs from PAH patients exhibit a pro-inflammatory phenotype characterized by an increased

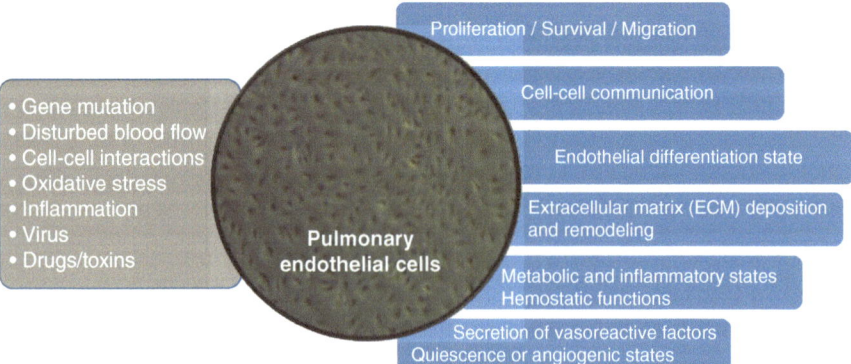

Fig. 19.1 The pulmonary vascular endothelium is a multifunctional organ and is critically involved in modulating vascular tone and structure. Through their capacity to spatially segregate and temporally integrate a diverse range of extracellular signals (in gray), pulmonary ECs adapt their roles and phenotype (in blue) according to the nature of the local milieu

expression of key adhesion molecules (E-selectin, ICAM-1, and VCAM-1) together with an excessive secretion of different inflammatory mediators (such as interleukin (IL)-1α, IL-6, IL-8, IL-12, macrophage migration inhibitory factor (MIF), and CCL2) [6]. Pulmonary ECs from PAH patients also exhibit metabolic alterations including heightened glycolysis [7]. Finally, decreased capacities to form vascular tube in vitro [8] and acquisition of some mesenchymal markers have also been reported [9]. Finally, a pro-proliferative and apoptosis-resistant phenotype has been described [10–12]. Various stimuli such as high glucose, insulin resistance, disturbed blood flow, and oxidative stress can lead to endothelial dysfunction. Therefore, further research is needed to elucidate their specific contribution to the altered pulmonary EC phenotype in PAH.

Importantly, this excessive local secretion of key factors by the dysfunctional pulmonary endothelium in PAH has also been demonstrated to play a critical role in modulating the behavior and functions of adjacent vascular cells (smooth muscle cells, fibroblasts myofibroblasts, and pericytes) and several immune cells that infiltrate the remodeled pulmonary vessels, thereby contributing to the vascular remodeling in PAH [3] (Fig. 19.2). Although considerable progress has been made, the

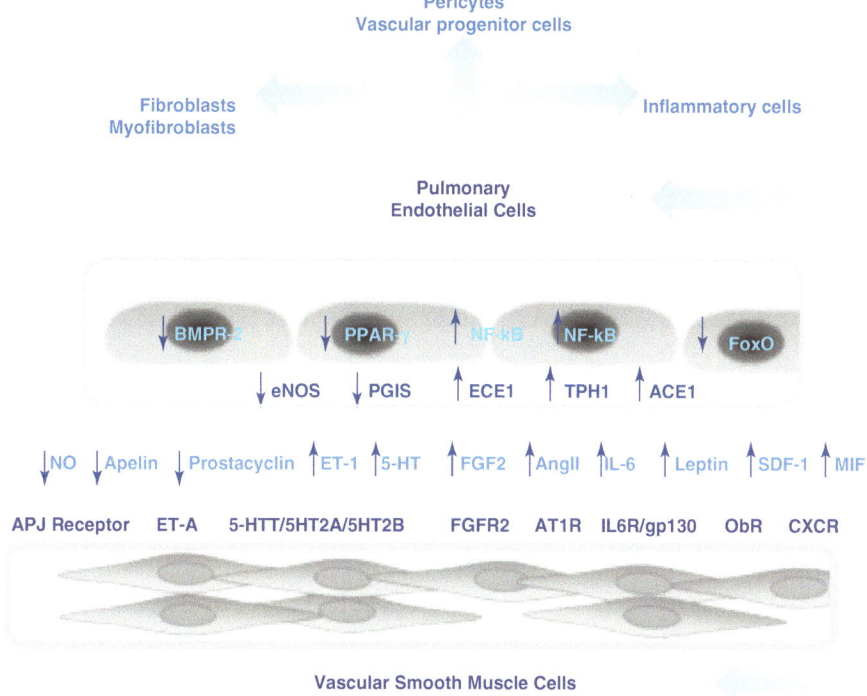

Fig. 19.2 Importance of endothelial miscommunication in PAH. In PAH, the dynamic and unadapted pulmonary vascular remodeling is partly driven by several genetic and environmental factors and also by the presence of different intrinsic abnormalities within the pulmonary ECs that include, among others, a loss and/or dysfunctions of the BMPR-2 signaling, decreased PPAR-γ and FoxO signaling, and constitutive activations of NF-κB and/or PHD2/HIF axes. Consequently, the altered pulmonary ECs create a permissive pericellular/extracellular environment for the progression of the pulmonary vascular remodeling, mainly because they miscommunicate with both resident vascular cells (smooth muscle cells, fibroblasts, myofibroblasts, and pericytes) and inflammatory cells mainly through the secretion of different key molecules

triggers, the mechanisms, and the consequences of dysfunctional pulmonary endothelium in PAH are still not completely understood. A better knowledge of these key aspects would help finding new PAH biomarkers and/or novel therapeutic targets to reverse or even stop the progression of this irreversible vascular remodeling.

19.3 Current Promising Strategies for Restoring Pulmonary Endothelial Dysfunction and Cell-Cell Communications

Below, a few of the most promising therapeutic strategies that target the dysfunctional pulmonary endothelium are underlined.

19.3.1 Restoring the Balance of Vasodilation and Vasoconstriction

In PAH, the discovery of abnormalities affecting the endothelial production and secretion of the three main mediators (NO, PGI2 and ET-1) or defects in their signaling pathways involved in the regulation of pulmonary vasoreactivity has led to the development of currently approved PAH therapies which have drastically improved the quality of life and clinical outcomes in PAH patients. Major therapeutic advances are also leading to the development of new molecules in these three pathways characterized by better pharmaceutical properties, such as longer half-life, increased receptor affinity, prolonged receptor binding, and routes of administration easier to manage. Nevertheless, other vasoreactive mediators are known to be involved and can represent new therapeutic targets, such as RhoA/ROCK inhibitors, anti-serotoninergic drugs, apelin agonists, and inhibitors or blockers of the ACE (angiotensin-converting enzyme)-1/angiotensin (Ang)-II/AT1 receptor, agents that stimulate the ACE2-Ang-(1–7)-Mas pathway [13].

Beyond vasoconstrictors and vasodilators, the recent identification of familial cases of PAH related to heterozygous missense variants in the *KCNK3* gene (encoding TWIK-related acid-sensitive potassium channel (TASK)-1) has revived interest in the concept of channelopathy in PAH [14]. The main challenge is this area is to identify specific small molecules to restore the activity of these ion channels in the dysfunctional pulmonary endothelium in PAH. Undoubtedly, this strategy will have significant impact for future investigations in the field and in other cardiovascular disorders.

19.3.2 Restitution of the Defective BMPR-2 Signaling System

Several notions support that enhancement of the BMPR-2 axis pulmonary vascular cells could offer a novel approach for the treatment of PAH [15, 16]. Consistent with this observation, preliminary data suggested that low-dose of tacrolimus (FK506) is well tolerated and increases BMPR-2 in subsets of PAH patients [17]. Based on these findings, a phase II randomized control trial in PAH has been initiated in stable PAH patients (NCT01647945). Interestingly, promising findings have also been obtained with exogenous BMP9 and ataluren, a drug that induces ribosomal read through of nonsense mutations, and thus may offer the possibility of future therapies [18, 19]. Nevertheless, further studies are needed to validate these hypotheses [20]. Indeed, the low penetrance of the disease among *BMPR2* mutation carriers suggests that additional genetic or environmental factors are required for the development of PAH [15]. In addition, it has been recently shown that the selective BMP9 loss or inhibition does not predispose, but partially prevent or protect against experimental pulmonary hypertension. Therefore, the apparent ambivalent role of the BMP9/BMPR-2 signaling pathway should stimulate work to better understand this feature and the underlying mechanisms.

19.3.3 Targeting Cell Proliferation and Cell accumulation

In PAH, several transcription factors [such as peroxisome proliferator-activated receptor (PPAR-γ), signal transducer and activator of transcription (STAT)-3, HIPPO, FoxO1, and hypoxia-inducible factor (HIF)] and growth factors are known to be overexpressed or overactive in the dysfunctional endothelium [5, 13]. Platelet-derived growth factor (PDGF), fibroblast growth factor (FGF)-2, epidermal growth factor (EGF), vascular endothelial growth factor (VEGF), and nerve growth factor (NGF) are key players in this regard. Furthermore, other factors and signaling may serve as potential target candidates for anti-proliferative strategies in PAH, such as the RhoA/Rho-kinase signaling system, the mammalian target of rapamycin (mTOR) and insulin-like growth factor signaling systems, connective tissue growth factor (CTGF), hepatocyte growth factor (HGF), and placental growth factor (PIGF). However, further studies on their pathogenic roles are important. Although targeting growth factors remains a relevant therapeutic strategy in PAH, a better understanding of tyrosine kinase inhibitor (TKI) properties and characteristics, particularly for lung and heart homeostases, will help designing new drugs that specifically block PAH pathways without severe side effects.

Our group has underlined that the dysfunctional pulmonary endothelium in PAH partly contributes to the excessive pericytic envelope, notably through the overabundance of the endothelial-derived FGF-2 and IL-6 [21]. We also demonstrated that this increase in pulmonary pericyte coverage in PAH could represent a local source of smooth muscle–like cells and actively contributes to the pulmonary vascular remodeling. Pericytes are central regulators of vascular development, stabilization, maturation, and remodeling, modulating EC proliferation, vascular tone and auto-immunity. Although pulmonary pericytes could likely represent a source of promising therapeutic targets in PAH, little is known about the intrinsic characteristics of lung pericytes in PAH and their exact roles in the progression of this irreversible remodeling linked to PAH. Therefore, additional studies are needed.

19.3.4 Restitution of an Adapted Extracellular Matrix (ECM) Remodeling

In PAH, the dynamic and unadapted remodeling of the ECM not only leads to qualitative and quantitative changes that are important to modulate vessel stiffness, but also forms a permissive milieu that profoundly influences cell motility, proliferation, apoptosis, and differentiation. In addition, the excessive release of growth factors and other molecules that are encrypted in the ECM together with the exposure of functionally cryptic sites (i.e., within collagens, fibronectin, laminins, elastin) and the release of ECM fragments also have critical roles in modulating cell behavior and vascular remodeling. Beneficial effects of different strategies that restitute these ECM alterations in PAH have been reported [3].

19.3.5 Targeting Metabolic Changes

Several evidences suggest that a shift in energy production from mitochondrial oxidative phosphorylation to glycolysis is present in pulmonary ECs and contributes to PAH development and progression. In lines with this notion, a recent clinical trial demonstrates that inhibition of pyruvate dehydrogenase kinase (PDK), an inhibitor of the mitochondrial enzyme pyruvate dehydrogenase (PDH, the gatekeeping enzyme of glucose oxidation) improves PAH in the absence of functional variants of *SIRT3* and *UCP2* [22]. Other metabolic pathways and related factors also represent interesting targets for PAH therapy, including modulators of hypoxia-inducible factor (HIF) and the phosphoinositide 3-kinase/protein kinase B/mammalian target of rapamycin (PI3K/Akt/mTOR) pathway, mitochondrial phosphatase and tensin homolog (PTEN)-induced kinase 1 (PINK1), and the HIPPO and p53 signaling pathways. However, a more complete understanding of the overall risk–benefit ratio of these different strategies with long-term follow-up has to be evaluated.

19.3.6 Targeting the Vicious Cycle Between Endothelial Dysfunction and Immune Dysregulation

The interplay between endothelial dysfunction and immune dysregulation warrants future clinical studies of newer biologic agents that can target specific inflammatory pathways [23]. Through the expression of adhesion molecules (ICAM-1, VCAM-1, and E-selectins) and the secretion of various key cytokines and chemokines, the dysfunctional pulmonary endothelium facilitates the infiltration of inflammatory cells in the perivascular area [6, 24]. Remarkably, we demonstrated that the dysfunctional pulmonary endothelium in PAH through its overproduction of leptin inhibits Treg cell function [25]. Consistent with this observation, our group has shown that PAH patients display normal Treg cell count but with an altered function. Interestingly, it is also known that the pulmonary vasculature is sensitive to inflammation and can respond to inflammatory stimuli by abnormal proliferation and/or migration and apoptotic-resistant phenotype. In line with these notions, we recently identified ectopic upregulation of membrane-bound IL-6 receptor (IL6R) on PA-SMCs in PAH patients and in rodent models of pulmonary hypertension and demonstrated its key role for PA-SMC accumulation in vitro and in vivo [26].

19.4   Future Directions and Clinical Implications

In summary, substantial work remains to be done to discover and/or develop a new, better tolerated, and more powerful curative treatment for PAH that combines promotion of vasorelaxation and restoration of endothelial communications. However, important discoveries in the molecular mechanisms contributing to the pulmonary endothelial dysfunction in PAH have been obtained and our knowledge continues to accelerate. Thus, our improved understanding of additional pathways in this condition will presumably lead to the development of novel therapeutic strategies that could specifically target endothelial dysfunction in the near future. A comprehensive estimation and evaluation of risks and benefits, potential ways to circumvent the risk of adverse effects on the adaptative myocardial hypertrophy, and a targeted delivery of these new drugs in a safe and effective manner are still major challenges facing clinical researchers.

Acknowledgments This work was supported by grants from the INSERM, the University of Paris-Sud and the University Paris-Saclay, the Marie Lannelongue Hospital, the ANR (ANR-16-CE17-0014 Tamirah), the FRM (DEQ20150331712), and in part by the DHU TORINO, the AP-HP, *Service de Pneumologie, Centre de Référence de l'Hypertension Pulmonaire Sévère*, the LabEx LERMIT (ANR-10-LABX-0033), the French PAH patient association (HTAP France), and the FRSR-FdS.

References

1. Humbert M, Guignabert C, Bonnet S, Dorfmüller P, Klinger JR, Nicolls MR, Olschewski AJ, Pullamsetti SS, Schermuly RT, Stenmark KR, Rabinovitch M. Pathology and pathobiology of pulmonary hypertension: state of the art and research perspectives. Eur Respir J. 2019;53(1): 1801887. https://doi.org/10.1183/13993003.01887-2018.
2. Guignabert C, Dorfmuller P. Pathology and Pathobiology of Pulmonary Hypertension. Semin Respir Crit Care Med. 2017;38(5):571–84. https://doi.org/10.1055/s-0037-1606214.
3. Guignabert C, Tu L, Girerd B, Ricard N, Huertas A, Montani D, Humbert M. New molecular targets of pulmonary vascular remodeling in pulmonary arterial hypertension: importance of endothelial communication. Chest. 2015;147(2):529–37. https://doi.org/10.1378/chest.14-0862.
4. Huertas A, Guignabert C, Barbera JA, Bartsch P, Bhattacharya J, Bhattacharya S, Bonsignore MR, Dewachter L, Dinh-Xuan AT, Dorfmuller P, Gladwin MT, Humbert M, Kotsimbos T, Vassilakopoulos T, Sanchez O, Savale L, Testa U, Wilkins MR. Pulmonary vascular endothelium: the orchestra conductor in respiratory diseases: Highlights from basic research to therapy. Eur Respir J. 2018;51(4). https://doi.org/10.1183/13993003.00745-2017.
5. Huertas A, Tu L, Guignabert C. New targets for pulmonary arterial hypertension: going beyond the currently targeted three pathways. Curr Opin Pulm Med. 2017;23(5):377–85. https://doi.org/10.1097/MCP.0000000000000404.
6. Le Hiress M, Tu L, Ricard N, Phan C, Thuillet R, Fadel E, Dorfmuller P, Montani D, de Man F, Humbert M, Huertas A, Guignabert C. Proinflammatory signature of the dysfunctional endothelium in pulmonary hypertension. Role of the macrophage migration inhibitory factor/CD74 complex. Am J Respir Crit Care Med. 2015;192(8):983–97. https://doi.org/10.1164/rccm.201402-0322OC.

7. Diebold I, Hennigs JK, Miyagawa K, Li CG, Nickel NP, Kaschwich M, Cao A, Wang L, Reddy S, Chen PI, Nakahira K, Alcazar MA, Hopper RK, Ji L, Feldman BJ, Rabinovitch M. BMPR2 preserves mitochondrial function and DNA during reoxygenation to promote endothelial cell survival and reverse pulmonary hypertension. Cell Metab. 2015;21(4):596–608. https://doi.org/10.1016/j.cmet.2015.03.010.

8. Sa S, Gu M, Chappell J, Shao NY, Ameen M, Elliott KA, Li D, Grubert F, Li CG, Taylor S, Cao A, Ma Y, Fong R, Nguyen L, Wu JC, Snyder MP, Rabinovitch M. Induced pluripotent stem cell model of pulmonary arterial hypertension reveals novel gene expression and patient specificity. Am J Respir Crit Care Med. 2017;195(7):930–41. https://doi.org/10.1164/rccm.201606-1200OC.

9. Ranchoux B, Antigny F, Rucker-Martin C, Hautefort A, Pechoux C, Bogaard HJ, Dorfmuller P, Remy S, Lecerf F, Plante S, Chat S, Fadel E, Houssaini A, Anegon I, Adnot S, Simonneau G, Humbert M, Cohen-Kaminsky S, Perros F. Endothelial-to-mesenchymal transition in pulmonary hypertension. Circulation. 2015;131(11):1006–18. https://doi.org/10.1161/CIRCULATIONAHA.114.008750.

10. Masri FA, Xu W, Comhair SA, Asosingh K, Koo M, Vasanji A, Drazba J, Anand-Apte B, Erzurum SC. Hyperproliferative apoptosis-resistant endothelial cells in idiopathic pulmonary arterial hypertension. Am J Physiol Lung Cell Mol Physiol. 2007;293(3):L548–54. https://doi.org/10.1152/ajplung.00428.2006.

11. Tu L, De Man FS, Girerd B, Huertas A, Chaumais MC, Lecerf F, Francois C, Perros F, Dorfmuller P, Fadel E, Montani D, Eddahibi S, Humbert M, Guignabert C. A critical role for p130Cas in the progression of pulmonary hypertension in humans and rodents. Am J Respir Crit Care Med. 2012;186(7):666–76. https://doi.org/10.1164/rccm.201202-0309OC.

12. Tu L, Dewachter L, Gore B, Fadel E, Dartevelle P, Simonneau G, Humbert M, Eddahibi S, Guignabert C. Autocrine fibroblast growth factor-2 signaling contributes to altered endothelial phenotype in pulmonary hypertension. Am J Respir Cell Mol Biol. 2011;45(2):311–22. https://doi.org/10.1165/rcmb.2010-0317OC.

13. Tu L, Guignabert C. Emerging molecular targets for anti-proliferative strategies in pulmonary arterial hypertension. Handb Exp Pharmacol. 2013;218:409–36. https://doi.org/10.1007/978-3-642-38664-0_17.

14. Ma L, Roman-Campos D, Austin ED, Eyries M, Sampson KS, Soubrier F, Germain M, Tregouet DA, Borczuk A, Rosenzweig EB, Girerd B, Montani D, Humbert M, Loyd JE, Kass RS, Chung WK. A novel channelopathy in pulmonary arterial hypertension. N Engl J Med. 2013;369(4):351–61. https://doi.org/10.1056/NEJMoa1211097.

15. Guignabert C, Bailly S, Humbert M. Restoring BMPRII functions in pulmonary arterial hypertension: opportunities, challenges and limitations. Expert Opin Ther Targets. 2017;21(2):181–90. https://doi.org/10.1080/14728222.2017.1275567.

16. Morrell NW, Bloch DB, ten Dijke P, Goumans MJ, Hata A, Smith J, Yu PB, Bloch KD. Targeting BMP signalling in cardiovascular disease and anaemia. Nat Rev Cardiol. 2016;13(2):106–20. https://doi.org/10.1038/nrcardio.2015.156.

17. Spiekerkoetter E, Sung YK, Sudheendra D, Scott V, Del Rosario P, Bill M, Haddad F, Long-Boyle J, Hedlin H, Zamanian RT. Randomised placebo-controlled safety and tolerability trial of FK506 (tacrolimus) for pulmonary arterial hypertension. Eur Respir J. 2017;50(3). https://doi.org/10.1183/13993003.02449-2016.

18. Drake KM, Dunmore BJ, McNelly LN, Morrell NW, Aldred MA. Correction of nonsense BMPR2 and SMAD9 mutations by ataluren in pulmonary arterial hypertension. Am J Respir Cell Mol Biol. 2013;49(3):403–9. https://doi.org/10.1165/rcmb.2013-0100OC.

19. Long L, Ormiston ML, Yang X, Southwood M, Graf S, Machado RD, Mueller M, Kinzel B, Yung LM, Wilkinson JM, Moore SD, Drake KM, Aldred MA, Yu PB, Upton PD, Morrell NW. Selective enhancement of endothelial BMPR-II with BMP9 reverses pulmonary arterial hypertension. Nat Med. 2015;21(7):777–85. https://doi.org/10.1038/nm.3877.

20. Tu L, Desroches-Castan A, Mallet C, Guyon L, Cumont A, Phan C, Robert F, Thuillet R, Bordenave J, Sekine A, Huertas A, Ritvos O, Savale L, Feige JJ, Humbert M, Bailly S, Guignabert C. Selective BMP-9 Inhibition Partially Protects Against Experimental Pulmonary Hypertension. Circ Res. 2019;124(6):846–55. https://doi.org/10.1161/CIRCRESAHA.118.313356.

21. Ricard N, Tu L, Le Hiress M, Huertas A, Phan C, Thuillet R, Sattler C, Fadel E, Seferian A, Montani D, Dorfmuller P, Humbert M, Guignabert C. Increased pericyte coverage mediated by endothelial-derived fibroblast growth factor-2 and interleukin-6 is a source of smooth muscle-like cells in pulmonary hypertension. Circulation. 2014;129(15):1586–97. https://doi.org/10.1161/CIRCULATIONAHA.113.007469.

22. Michelakis ED, Gurtu V, Webster L, Barnes G, Watson G, Howard L, Cupitt J, Paterson I, Thompson RB, Chow K, O'Regan DP, Zhao L, Wharton J, Kiely DG, Kinnaird A, Boukouris AE, White C, Nagendran J, Freed DH, Wort SJ, Gibbs JSR, Wilkins MR. Inhibition of pyruvate dehydrogenase kinase improves pulmonary arterial hypertension in genetically susceptible patients. Sci Transl Med. 2017;9(413). https://doi.org/10.1126/scitranslmed.aao4583.

23. Huertas A, Perros F, Tu L, Cohen-Kaminsky S, Montani D, Dorfmuller P, Guignabert C, Humbert M. Immune dysregulation and endothelial dysfunction in pulmonary arterial hypertension: a complex interplay. Circulation. 2014;129(12):1332–40. https://doi.org/10.1161/CIRCULATIONAHA.113.004555.

24. Huertas A, Tu L, Thuillet R, Le Hiress M, Phan C, Ricard N, Nadaud S, Fadel E, Humbert M, Guignabert C. Leptin signalling system as a target for pulmonary arterial hypertension therapy. Eur Respir J. 2015;45(4):1066–80. https://doi.org/10.1183/09031936.00193014.

25. Huertas A, Tu L, Gambaryan N, Girerd B, Perros F, Montani D, Fabre D, Fadel E, Eddahibi S, Cohen-Kaminsky S, Guignabert C, Humbert M. Leptin and regulatory T-lymphocytes in idiopathic pulmonary arterial hypertension. Eur Respir J. 2012;40(4):895–904. https://doi.org/10.1183/09031936.00159911.

26. Tamura Y, Phan C, Tu L, Le Hiress M, Thuillet R, Jutant EM, Fadel E, Savale L, Huertas A, Humbert M, Guignabert C (2018) Ectopic upregulation of membrane-bound IL6R drives vascular remodeling in pulmonary arterial hypertension. J Clin Invest 128 (5):1956–1970. https://doi.org/10.1172/JCI96462.

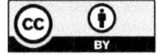

Inflammatory Cytokines in the Pathogenesis of Pulmonary Arterial Hypertension

Yoshikazu Nakaoka, Tadakatsu Inagaki, and Mikiyasu Shirai

Abstract

Interleukin-6 (IL-6) is a multifunctional pro-inflammatory cytokine elevated in the serum of pulmonary arterial hypertension (PAH) patients and can predict the survival of idiopathic (I)PAH patients. Previous animal experiments and clinical human studies indicate that IL-6 is important in the pathogenesis of PAH; however, the molecular mechanisms of IL-6-mediated pathogenesis of PAH have been elusive. We recently identified IL-21 as a novel downstream cytokine of IL-6-signaling in PAH. First, we found that IL-6 blockade by the monoclonal anti-IL-6 receptor antibody, MR16–1, ameliorated hypoxia-induced pulmonary hypertension (HPH) and prevented the hypoxia-induced accumulation of Th17 cells and M2 macrophages in the lungs. Furthermore, the hypoxia-induced upregulation of IL-17 and IL-21, which are primarily produced by Th17 cells, was also ameliorated by IL-6 blockade in mice. Whereas IL-17 blockade with an anti-IL-17 neutralizing antibody had no effect on HPH, IL-21 receptor-deficient mice were resistant to HPH and exhibited no significant accumulation of M2 macrophages in the lungs. Consistently, IL-21 indeed promoted the polarization of primary alveolar macrophages toward the M2 phenotype. Moreover, significantly enhanced expressions of IL-21 and M2 macrophage markers were detected in the lungs of IPAH patients who underwent lung transplantation. Together, the above data suggest that IL-21 promotes PAH through M2 macrophage polarization, downstream of IL-6-signaling. IL-6/Th17/IL-21-signaling axis might be a novel potential target for treating PAH.

Y. Nakaoka (✉) · T. Inagaki
Department of Vascular Physiology, National Cerebral and Cardiovascular Center Research Institute, Suita, Osaka, Japan
e-mail: ynakaoka@ncvc.go.jp

M. Shirai
Department of Advanced Medical Research for Pulmonary Hypertension, National Cerebral and Cardiovascular Center Research Institute, Suita, Osaka, Japan

Keywords
Pulmonary arterial hypertension · Inflammation · Cytokine · Interleukin-6
Interleukin-21

20.1   Background

Pulmonary arterial hypertension (PAH) is a serious disease characterized by arteriopathy in the small- to medium-sized distal pulmonary arteries, which is associated
with arterial muscularization, concentric intimal thickening, and the formation of
plexiform lesions [1, 2]. Inflammation and autoimmunity are currently thought of as
critical factors to the pathogenesis of PAH [3, 4]. Inflammatory cells such as T cells,
B cells, and macrophages infiltrate the plexiform lesions in patients with advanced
PAH. Thus, proinflammatory cytokines produced by these cells may be responsible
for the hyperproliferation of pulmonary artery endothelial cells and pulmonary
artery smooth muscle cells (PASMCs) [5, 6].

Interleukin (IL)-6 is a multifunctional proinflammatory cytokine linked to
numerous autoimmune diseases [7, 8]. Patients with idiopathic (I)PAH exhibit
increased IL-6 serum levels, which correlate with their prognoses [3, 9, 10].
Consistent with these findings, lung-specific IL-6 transgenic mice display spontaneous PH in normoxia and develop greatly exaggerated hypoxia-induced PH (HPH)
[11], whereas IL-6-deficient mice show resistance to HPH [12]. These findings suggest that IL-6 has a significant role in the pathogenesis of PH; however, the downstream target(s) of IL-6 in HPH have been elusive when we started the following
study on the pathogenesis of PH. We recently reported that the IL-6/interleukin-
21(IL-21)-signaling axis played critical roles for the development of HPH in association with M2 macrophage polarization [13]. In this manuscript, we elaborate on
the role of IL-6/IL-21-signaing axis in the pathogenesis of PAH.

20.2   IL-6 in the Pathogenesis of HPH

We examined the effect of hypoxia (10% oxygen) on the expression of *Il-6* mRNA
in the lungs of C57BL/6 mice using quantitative (q)RT-PCR. The *Il-6* mRNA levels
peaked on day 2 and returned to basal levels by day 7 after hypoxia exposure. Next,
we investigated the effect of IL-6 blockade on HPH development by measuring the
right ventricular systolic pressure (RVSP), Fulton's Index (right/[left + septum]
ventricular weight), and the medial wall thickness index, which is estimated by
elastic Van Gieson staining of the pulmonary arterioles. In control antibody-treated
mice, hypoxia exposure for 4 weeks induced significant increases in the RVSP,
Fulton's Index, and medial wall thickness index compared to the values observed
under normoxic conditions. On the other hand, the hypoxia-induced elevation of
these parameters was significantly inhibited by treatment with MR16–1. Similarly,
thickened medial vascular walls were detected in the lung sections of control

antibody-treated mice but not in those of MR16–1-treated mice. These data indicate that IL-6 blockade by MR16–1 effectively prevents HPH.

20.3   IL-21 in the Pathogenesis of HPH

IL-21 is an IL-2 family cytokine produced by activated T cells, including Th17 cells, that regulates immune responses [14]. We found that the *Il-21* mRNA level peaked on day 2, remained elevated until day 14, and returned to the basal levels on day 28 after hypoxia exposure. In addition, hypoxia induced significantly increased numbers of Th17 cells, which produce both IL-17 and IL-21, in the lungs of mice treated with control antibody but not in those treated with MR16–1. These data suggest that IL-6 promotes the accumulation of IL-21-producing Th17 cells in the lungs after hypoxia exposure.

Next, we evaluated the effect of hypoxia on IL-21 receptor (IL-21R) knockout (IL-21RKO) mice [15]. Wild-type (WT) mice exposed to hypoxia for 4 weeks. exhibited significantly increased RVSP, Fulton's Index, and medial wall thickness compared with mice exposed to normoxia. In contrast, the hypoxia-induced elevation of these parameters was significantly inhibited in IL-21RKO mice. Similarly, remodeling of the medial vascular walls following hypoxia exposure in WT mice was also significantly inhibited in the lungs of IL-21RKO mice. These data suggest that IL-21R-deficient mice are resistant to HPH.

Alveolar macrophages have been reported to undergo M2 macrophage polarization in response to hypoxia [16]. We hypothesized that IL-21, which has been reported to be majorly secreted from Th17 cells in mice, might play a role in the hypoxia-induced generation of M2 macrophages in the lung. IL-21 treatment of BALF-isolated alveolar macrophages significantly upregulated the mRNA levels of M2 signature genes, such as *Fizz1*, *Arg1*, and *Cxcl12*, but had no effect on the mRNA levels of M1 signature genes, including *Nos2*, *Il-12β*, and *Tnf-α*, indicating that IL-21 specifically induces the M2 polarization of alveolar macrophages.

We next examined the effect of IL-21R deletion on the hypoxia-induced upregulation of M2 signature genes, including *Fizz1*, *Arg1*, and *Cxcl12*, in the alveolar macrophages isolated from the BALF after exposure to hypoxia for 4 days. All of these genes were significantly upregulated in the alveolar macrophages isolated from WT mice but not in those from IL-21RKO mice. Similarly, Fizz1 protein expression was increased in the lungs of WT mice but not in those of IL-21RKO mice after exposure to hypoxia for 1 week. In contrast, M1 signature gene expression was comparable in the WT and IL-21RKO mice after exposure to hypoxia. Consistent with these findings, the hypoxia-induced generation of M2 macrophages in the lung was significantly inhibited by treatment with an anti-IL-21-neutralizing antibody but not a control antibody. Collectively, these findings suggest that IL-21 is essential for hypoxia-induced M2 macrophage polarization in the lung.

We next examined the effect of IL-21 blockade on the in vivo hypoxia-induced proliferation of PASMCs. Hypoxia exposure significantly increased the number of anti-Ki67 antibody-positive PASMCs in the lungs of WT mice but not in those of

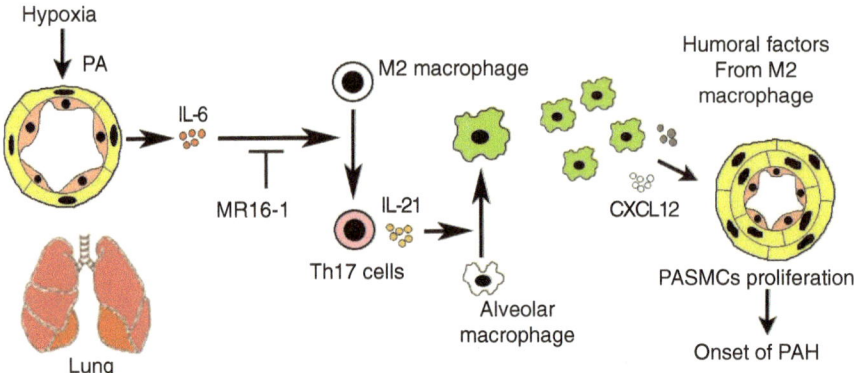

Fig. 20.1 Schematic illustration of the pathogenesis of PAH. IL-6/IL-21-signalling has a central role for the pathogenesis of PAH

IL-21RKO mice. Consistent with this finding, hypoxia exposure significantly increased the number of anti-phospho-Histone H3 antibody-positive PASMCs in the lungs of mice treated with control antibody but not in those treated with the anti-IL-21 neutralizing antibody. Together, these data suggest that IL-21 plays a critical role in the hypoxia-induced proliferation of PASMCs in association with M2 macrophage skewing (Fig. 20.1).

20.4   Increased Expression of IL-21 and M2 Macrophage Markers in the Lungs of IPAH Patients

Immunohistochemical analyses of the lung tissues from IPAH patients undergoing lung transplantation showed an excessive infiltration of IL-21-positive cells in the adventitia, obliterative intimal proliferative lesions, and plexiform lesions of the remodeled pulmonary arteries. In contrast, IL-21-positive cell infiltration was barely detected in the lungs of the control patient. We also observed both Arg1-positive and MRC-1-positive cells in all layers of the remodeled pulmonary arteries and alveolar areas examined in the lungs from IPAH patients but not in the tissue from control patients. Taken together, these findings strongly suggest that IL-6/IL-21-signaling axis is essential for the pathogenesis of human PAH in association with M2 macrophage polarization (Fig. 20.1).

References

1. Pietra GG, Capron F, Stewart S, Leone O, Humbert M, Robbins IM, Reid LM, Tuder RM. Pathologic assessment of vasculopathies in pulmonary hypertension. J Am Coll Cardiol. 2004;43:25S–32S.
2. Rabinovitch M. Molecular pathogenesis of pulmonary arterial hypertension. J Clin Invest. 2012;122:4306–13.
3. Dorfmuller P, Perros F, Balabanian K, Humbert M. Inflammation in pulmonary arterial hypertension. Eur Respir J. 2003;22:358–63.

4. Schermuly RT, Ghofrani HA, Wilkins MR, Grimminger F. Mechanisms of disease: Pulmonary arterial hypertension. Nat Rev Cardiol. 2011;8:443–55.
5. Tuder RM, Groves B, Badesch DB, Voelkel NF. Exuberant endothelial cell growth and elements of inflammation are present in plexiform lesions of pulmonary hypertension. Am J Pathol. 1994;144:275–85.
6. Tuder RM, Voelkel NF. Pulmonary hypertension and inflammation. J Lab Clin Med. 1998;132:16–24.
7. Kishimoto T. Interleukin-6: Discovery of a pleiotropic cytokine. Arthritis Res Ther. 2006;8(Suppl 2):S2.
8. Kishimoto T, Akira S, Taga T. Interleukin-6 and its receptor: A paradigm for cytokines. Science. 1992;258:593–7.
9. Humbert M, Monti G, Brenot F, Sitbon O, Portier A, Grangeot-Keros L, Duroux P, Galanaud P, Simonneau G, Emilie D. Increased interleukin-1 and interleukin-6 serum concentrations in severe primary pulmonary hypertension. Am J Respir Crit Care Med. 1995;151:1628–31.
10. Soon E, Holmes AM, Treacy CM, Doughty NJ, Southgate L, Machado RD, Trembath RC, Jennings S, Barker L, Nicklin P, Walker C, Budd DC, Pepke-Zaba J, Morrell NW. Elevated levels of inflammatory cytokines predict survival in idiopathic and familial pulmonary arterial hypertension. Circulation. 2010;122:920–7.
11. Steiner MK, Syrkina OL, Kolliputi N, Mark EJ, Hales CA, Waxman AB. Interleukin-6 overexpression induces pulmonary hypertension. Circ Res. 2009;104:236–44, 228p following 244.
12. Savale L, Tu L, Rideau D, Izziki M, Maitre B, Adnot S, Eddahibi S. Impact of interleukin-6 on hypoxia-induced pulmonary hypertension and lung inflammation in mice. Respir Res. 2009;10(6).
13. Hashimoto-Kataoka T, Hosen N, Sonobe T, Arita Y, Yasui T, Masaki T, Minami M, Inagaki T, Miyagawa S, Sawa Y, Murakami M, Kumanogoh A, Yamauchi-Takihara K, Okumura M, Kishimoto T, Komuro I, Shirai M, Sakata Y, Nakaoka Y. Interleukin-6/interleukin-21 signaling axis is critical in the pathogenesis of pulmonary arterial hypertension. Proc Natl Acad Sci U S A. 2015;112:E2677–86.
14. Liu SM, King C. Il-21-producing th cells in immunity and autoimmunity. J Immunol. 2013;191:3501–6.
15. Ozaki K, Spolski R, Feng CG, Qi CF, Cheng J, Sher A, Morse HC 3rd, Liu C, Schwartzberg PL, Leonard WJ. A critical role for il-21 in regulating immunoglobulin production. Science. 2002;298:1630–4.
16. Vergadi E, Chang MS, Lee C, Liang OD, Liu X, Fernandez-Gonzalez A, Mitsialis SA, Kourembanas S. Early macrophage recruitment and alternative activation are critical for the later development of hypoxia-induced pulmonary hypertension. Circulation. 2011;123:1986–95.

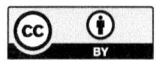

Genotypes and Phenotypes of Chinese Pediatric Patients with Idiopathic and Heritable Pulmonary Arterial Hypertension: Experiences from a Single Center

21

Hong-Sheng Zhang, Qian Liu, Chun-Mei Piao, Yan Zhu, Qiang-Qiang Li, Jie Du, and Hong Gu

Abstract

The aim of this study was to determine the clinical outcomes of gene mutations in Chinese pediatric patients with idiopathic and heritable pulmonary arterial hypertension. We screened gene mutations in 62 pediatric patients who visited Beijing Anzhen Hospital from 2008 September to 2017 August with targeted exome kits containing 22 pulmonary arterial hypertension-related genes. The clinical and hemodynamic characteristics and outcomes of these patients were retrospectively analyzed. In a cohort of 62 patients, a total of 27 gene mutations were identified with 20 mutations

H.-S. Zhang
Department of Pediatrics, Capital Medical University, Beijing, China

Pediatric Cardiology Department, Beijing Anzhen Hospital, Capital Medical University, Beijing, China

Q. Liu
Department of Cardiology, Children's Hospital of Hebei Province, Shijiazhuang, Hebei, China

C.-M. Piao · J. Du
Beijing Anzhen Hospital, The Key Laboratory of Remodeling-Related Cardiovascular Diseases, Capital Medical University, Beijing, China

Beijing Institute of Heart Lung and Blood Vessel Diseases, Beijing, China
e-mail: jiedu@ccmu.edu.cn

Y. Zhu · Q.-Q. Li · H. Gu (✉)
Pediatric Cardiology Department, Beijing Anzhen Hospital, Capital Medical University, Beijing, China

© The Editor(s) (if applicable) and The Author(s) 2020
T. Nakanishi et al. (eds.), *Molecular Mechanism of Congenital Heart Disease and Pulmonary Hypertension*, https://doi.org/10.1007/978-981-15-1185-1_21

in BMPR2, two mutations in ACVRL1, two mutations in KCNK3 and three mutations in NOTCH3. The average age at diagnosis was 77.5 ± 53.8 months. 28 patients (14 mutation carriers) underwent cardiac catherization examinations, with the acute vasodilator testing. Mutation carriers had higher right atrial pressure and tended to have higher pulmonary arterial pressure and pulmonary vascular resistance index than mutation non-carriers. Eight patients responded to acute vasodilator testing and all were mutation non-carriers ($p = 0.002$). The median survival for mutation carriers was 24.0 months. Although similar treatments were employed, mutation carriers had higher mortality rates than mutation non-carriers ($p = 0.036$). The 1-, 2-, 3- year survival rate of mutation non-carriers were 93.6%, 90.0%, and 66.9%, respectively, while for mutation carriers, the proportion were 79.8%, 49.9%, and 33.3%. In conclusion, early gene screening for pediatric patients with idiopathic pulmonary arterial hypertension and heritable pulmonary arterial hypertension is recommended, and more aggressive treatment for mutation carriers is advisable.

Keywords
Mutation · hemodynamics · mortality

21.1 Introduction

Pulmonary arterial hypertension (PAH) is a progressive pulmonary vessel disease, which can ultimately lead to progressive right-sided heart failure and premature death [1]. Idiopathic pulmonary arterial hypertension (IPAH) is a sporadic form of PAH, which occurs without family aggregation or known etiology [2], while heritable pulmonary arterial hypertension (HPAH) occurs in a familial aggregate. Without adequate treatment, these patients' condition deteriorates rapidly with a median survival time of 2.8 years in adults and 10 months in children [3, 4]. Despite recent advances in management and improvement of prognosis, the pathophysiology of IPAH is not yet explained in detail.

Genetic studies showed that gene mutations in some members of the transforming growth factor-β (TGF-β) pathway were associated with heritable PAH, including bone morphogenetic protein receptor type II (BMPR2), activin receptor-like kinase 1 (ALK1), endoglin (ENG) and SMAD family [5–8]. Mutations in ALK1 and ENG are thought to be linked to hereditary hemorrhagic telangiectasia (HHT), an autosomal dominant genetic disorder typically characterized by small arteriovenous malformations [9, 10]. With the development of gene detection technology, more additional gene mutations were found out to be the disease-causing genes, including KNCK3 (potassium two pore domain channel subfamily K member 3), CAV1 (Caveolin 1), NOTCH3, BMPR1B (bone morphogenetic protein receptor, type 1B), EDN1 (endothelin 1), TBX4 (T-box 4), TRPC6 (transient receptor potential cation channel, subfamily C, member 6), TOPBP1 (topoisomerase (DNA) II binding protein 1), and SERPINE1 (serpin family E member 1) [7, 8, 11]. IPAH and HPAH were seen more commonly in pediatric patients [12, 13], indicating more genetic factors participate in the pathogenesis of pediatric PAH.

In addition to the effect on the pathogenicity of PAH, gene mutations have previously been linked to worse clinical outcomes in adult patients [14, 15]. An international multi-center research revealed that patients with childhood IPAH or HPAH with BMPR2 or ACVRL1 mutation have poorer clinical outcomes than mutation non-carriers [16]. However, the study sample was relatively small, and data addressing the relationship of gene mutations with clinical outcomes of pediatric patients is scarce till now.

In this study, we applied a targeted capture exome sequence to investigate the genetic etiology of Chinese pediatric patients with IPAH and HPAH. We aimed to assess the prevalence of gene mutations in this group of patients and to assess the relationship between genotypes and phenotypes.

21.2 Methods

21.3 Selection of Patients

Sixty-two pediatric patients with IPAH and HPAH who visited Beijing Anzhen Hospital from 2008 September to 2017 August were included in the study. PAH was defined as a mean pulmonary arterial pressure (MPAP) ≥ 25 mmHg with a pulmonary artery wedge pressure ≤ 15 mmHg and pulmonary vascular resistance >3 Wood units by cardiac catheterization [1]. Acute vasodilator testing was performed during cardiac catheterization and a positive response was defined according to current guidelines as a decrease in MPAP of at least 10 to <40 mmHg with a stable cardiac output [17]. Clinical, functional, and hemodynamic characteristics of patients were collected at the time of diagnosis and during the follow-up period. The study procedures were approved by the Research Ethics Committee of Beijing Anzhen Hospital. All patients gave informed consent in accordance with local ethical guidelines.

21.4 Genetic Studies

Genomic DNA was isolated using QIAamp Blood Midi kit (Qiagen). Libraries were prepared according to the Illumina standard protocol. Exon and exon–intron junction sequences of 22 candidate genes (ACVRL1, AGTR2, ANGPT1, BMPR2, BMPR1A, BMPR1B, ENG, NOS3, HTR2B, KCNA5, KCNQ1, SLC6A4, SMAD1, SMAD2, SMAD3, SMAD4, SMAD5, SMAD6, SMAD7, TGFB1, TRPC6, THBS1) were enriched using a GenCap custom enrichment kit (My-Genostics). The enriched libraries were sequenced on an Illumina Hi Seq 2000 sequencer for paired reads of 100 bp in length.

21.5 Statistical Analysis

Qualitative variables were expressed as frequency and percentage and mean ± standard deviation and median [interquartile range] for quantitative variables. We compared clinical and hemodynamic characteristics between mutation carriers and non-carriers by one-way analysis of variance or the median test for continuous measures and the chi-square test for categorical measures. The Kaplan-Meier survival curve and the Log-rank test were used to assess the difference in survival rates between two groups. A p-value less than 0.05 was considered to indicate statistical significance. All analyses were performed with the Statistical Package for Social Sciences for Windows (SPSS, Chicago, IL) version 19.0.

21.6   Results

21.6.1 Clinical Characteristics

Sixty-two unrelated childhood IPAH or HPAH probands, 26 (41.9%) female, were included in this study. The average age at diagnosis was 77.5 ± 53.8 months. The median interval from onset of symptoms to diagnosis was 4 months (1~48 months). Twenty-eight (45.2%) patients were presented with markedly decreased cardiac function (NYHA class III–IV). The average plasma BNP concentration was 1198.8 ± 2239.9 pg/mL. Of 62 children evaluated, 20 (32.3%) carried BMPR2 mutations, and 2 (3.2%) carried ALK1 mutations; 2 (3.2%) carried KCNK3 mutations and 3 (4.8%) carried NOTCH3 mutation. Patients were divided into two groups based on the presence or absence of gene mutations, and clinical and hemodynamic characteristics were compared (details in Table 21.1). Twenty-eight patients, half of them mutation carriers, underwent cardiac catherization examinations, with acute vasodilator testing (details in Table 21.2). Mutation non-carriers had lower right atrial pressure than mutation carriers ($p = 0.016$). Mutation carriers tended to have higher pulmonary arterial pressure and higher pulmonary vascular resistance index than mutation non-carriers although the differences were not statistically significant. Eight patients responded to acute vasodilator challenge testing; all were mutation non-carriers ($p = 0.002$).

Table 21.1 Clinical characteristics of patients at diagnosis

Variables	Mutation carriers ($n = 27$)	Mutation non-carriers ($n = 35$)	p-value
Female (%)	8 (29.6)	18 (51.4)	0.120
Age at diagnosis, months	80.7 ± 49.8	77.5 ± 53.6	0.992
NYHA function class			0.921
I–II	15	19	
III–IV	12	16	
BNP, pg/mL	953.0 ± 1874.7	1358 ± 2487.8	0.502
TBIL, μmol/L	13.3 ± 5.7	16.0 ± 9.4	0.220
DBIL, μmol/L	3.3 ± 1.5	4.0 ± 2.5	0.214
UA, μmol/L	421.2 ± 173.0	424.7 ± 159.3	0.940

NYHA New York Heart Association, *BNP* brain natriuretic peptide, *TBIL* total bilirubin, *DBIL* direct bilirubin, *UA* uric acid

Table 21.2 Hemodynamic characteristics of patients at diagnosis

Variables	Mutation carriers, $n = 14$	Mutation non-carriers, $n = 14$	p-value
PASP, mmHg	100.1 ± 22.9	83.8 ± 33.4	0.144
PADP, mmHg	59.8 ± 14.0	45.7 ± 22.0	0.054
MPAP, mmHg	74.5 ± 16.2	59.1 ± 23.3	0.052
RAP, mmHg	10.5 ± 4.1	7.2 ± 2.0	0.016
PVRI, WU·m²	20.3 ± 11.1	14.1 ± 9.5	0.130
CI, l/min/m²	3.3 ± 1.3	3.9 ± 1.1	0.669
SvO₂, %	59.3 ± 11.3	67.2 ± 6.6	0.564
AVT (%)	0 (0)	8 (57.1)	0.002

PASP pulmonary artery systolic pressure, *PADP* pulmonary artery diastolic pressure, *MPAP* mean pulmonary arterial pressure, *RAP* right atrial pressure, *PVRI* pulmonary vascular resistance index, *WU* Wood units, *CI* cardiac index, *SvO₂* mixed venous oxygen saturation, *AVT* acute pulmonary vasodilatation test

Table 21.3 Targeted drugs' protocols of patients

Protocols	All, $n = 56$	Carriers, $n = 24$	Non-carriers, $n = 32$
Monotherapy (%)	29 (51.8)	10 (41.7)	19 (59.4)
Bosentan	21	8	13
Sildenafil	2	0	2
Tadalafil	4	0	4
Beraprost sodium	2	0	2
Dual therapy (%)	23 (41.1)	11 (45.8)	12 (37.5)
Bosentan and sildenafil	5	3	2
Bosentan and tadalafil	10	2	8
Bosentan and beraprost sodium	3	3	0
Ambrisentan and sildenafil	1	1	0
Ambrisentan and tadalafil	1	1	0
Macitentan and sildenafil	1	1	0
Sildenafil and beraprost sodium	1	0	1
Vardenafil and beraprost sodium	1	0	1
Triple therapy (%)	4 (7.1)	3 (12.5)	1 (3.1)
Bosentan, sildenafil, and iloprost	2	2	0
Bosentan, tadalafil, and beraprost sodium	1	0	1
Bosentan, beraprost sodium, and treprostinil	1	1	0

21.6.2 Targeted Drug Therapy

Fifty-six patients received PAH-targeted treatment. The utilization of targeted drugs is listed in Table 21.3. Endothelin-receptor antagonists were the medications most commonly used. The percentage of patients who received monotherapy, dual therapy, and triple therapy were 41.7%, 45.8%, and 12.5% in mutation carriers and 59.4%, 37.5%, and 3.1% in mutation non-carriers, respectively. No differences were found between mutation carriers and mutation non-carriers.

21.6.3 Outcome of Patients

The median duration of follow-up was 20.5 months (0–108 months). One patient underwent lung transplantation at the age of 16, after 4 years of targeted drug therapy. Eleven out of 20 BMPR2 mutation carriers, both of the 2 ALK1 mutation carriers, 1 of 2 KCNK3 mutation carriers, and 9 of 39 mutation non-carriers died during the follow-up period. The median survival for mutation carriers was 24.0 months. The 1-, 2-, 3-year survival of mutation non-carriers were 93.6%, 80.0%, and 66.9%, respectively, while for mutation non-carriers, the proportions were 79.8%, 49.9%, and 33.3% (see Fig. 21.1), respectively. The clinical characteristics between the death group and survival group

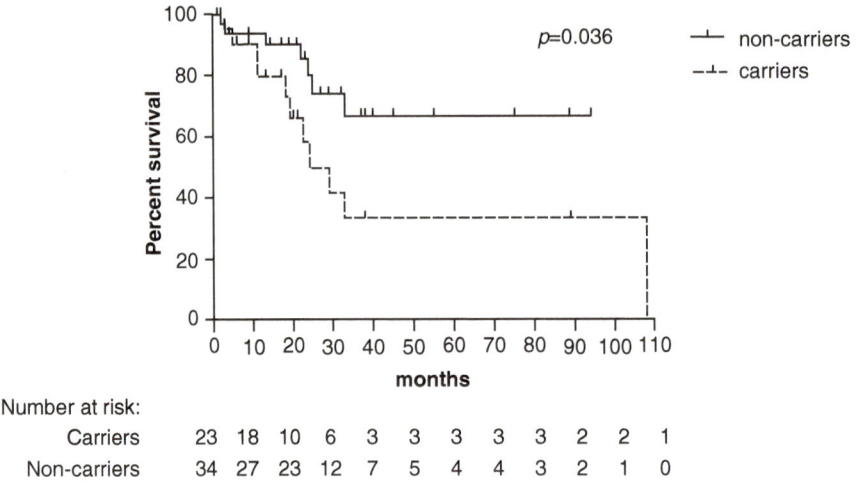

Fig. 21.1 Survival rate of mutation carriers and non-carriers with IPAH/HPAH

Table 21.4 Characteristics of dead and surviving patients

Variables	Deaths, $n = 23$	Survivors, $n = 34$	p-value
Female (%)	7 (30.4)	18 (52.9)	
Age, months	69.9 ± 57.6	87.9 ± 50.0	0.227
NYHA function class			0.849
I-II	15	23	
III-IV	8	11	
Gene mutation, (%)	14 (60.9)	11 (32.4)	0.033
BNP, pg/ml	1763.9 ± 3179.5	920.1 ± 1367.5	0.195
PASP, mmHg	97.2 ± 13.4	89.1 ± 37.2	0.496
PADP, mmHg	58.2 ± 10.0	50.0 ± 23.6	0.292
MPAP, mmHg	75.4 ± 10.3	63.3 ± 26.3	0.277
RAP, mmHg	11.9 ± 3.8	6.9 ± 2.1	0.000
PVRI, WU·m²	22.8 ± 11.5	14.0 ± 9.5	0.044
CI, L/min/m²	2.9 ± 1.2	4.0 ± 1.1	0.032
SvO₂, %	64.5 ± 12.5	70.8 ± 6.2	0.098

NYHA New York Heart Association, *BNP* brain natriuretic peptide, *PASP* pulmonary artery systolic pressure, *PADP* pulmonary artery diastolic pressure, *MPAP* mean pulmonary arterial pressure, *RAP* right atrial pressure, *PVRI* pulmonary vascular resistance index, *CI* cardiac index, *SvO₂* mixed venous oxygen saturation

were compared (for details, see Table 21.4). The results showed that dead patients had higher RAP, PVRI, and lower cardiac index than the survival group. The mutation of PAH-related genes is the main risk factor of death (OR = 6.418, 95% CI 1.393, 27.123).

21.7 Discussion

In this study, we retrospectively analyzed the clinical outcomes of gene mutations in Chinese pediatric patients with idiopathic and heritable pulmonary arterial hypertension. Gene mutations are important causes of PAH. The BMPR2 gene encodes a transmembrane serine/threonine kinase receptor of the bone morphogenetic protein (BMP) pathway, which is involved in the regulation of growth and apoptosis of pulmonary smooth muscle cells and pulmonary endothelial cells [18]. Hundreds of BMPR2 mutations have been identified in 70% of familial PAH patients and up to 40% of IPAH cases [12, 19]. In our study, BMPR2 was also the most often mutation—accounting for 32.3% of all the patients.

Mutations in ALK1 are identified as the major cause of HHT [15]. Neither of the two patients with ALK1 mutations in our study met the diagnostic criteria for HHT. As clinical manifestations of HHT develop with increasing age, the majority of ALK1 mutation carriers might not have clinical evidence of HHT during childhood [15]. Both of the two patients carrying ALK1 mutations died during the follow-up period, suggesting it a rapidly progressing type. A larger sample size is needed for the assessment of ALK1 on phenotype of these patients.

The KCNK3 gene encodes for an outward K+ channel and is a member of two-pore-domain K+ channels (K2P) [20]. KCNK3 inhibition participates extensively in the whole spectrum of PAH pathomechanism from vasoconstriction and vascular cell proliferation to PAH-associated chronic inflammation [21]. NOTCH3 is a transmembrane receptor protein that participates in the modulation of cell proliferation, differentiation, apoptosis, and migration [22]. Compared with that of BMPR2 and ALK1, the research on KCNK3 and NOTCH3 is relatively less. The relationship between these gene mutations and clinical phenotypes needs further verification.

Previous studies on adult patients have suggested that mutation carriers present PAH approximately 10 years earlier than noncarriers, with more compromised hemodynamic status and worse prognosis [14]. Similar results were also obtained from studies on pediatric patients with IPAH and HPAH [16, 23]. In our study, two groups of patients were similar in gender and age, while mutation carriers tended to have higher pulmonary arterial pressure and pulmonary arterial resistance index than mutation non-carriers although the difference was not statistically significant. Moreover, mutation carriers had higher right atrial pressure compared with mutation non-carriers, indicating right heart burden of mutation carriers higher than mutation non-carriers. Similar with the results of previous research, our study showed that pediatric patients with PAH-related gene mutations responded poorly to acute vasodilator testing. No differences were found between two groups in WHO function class and blood biochemical index. As the clinical symptoms of IPAH were atypical, the majority of patients came to our center until obvious symptoms of right heart failure occurred and, thus, blood biochemical index and heart function indexes at baseline could not be used to assess the whole progression of the disease.

Targeted drugs have benefited the patients with pulmonary hypertension [24, 25]. Targeted drugs were approved in China from 2000s: bosentan in 2005, followed by iloprost, inhaled, in 2007, ambrisentan in 2012, treprostinil in 2014, and tadalafil in 2015. Endothelin receptor antagonists were the most commonly used targeted drugs in our patients, followed by phosphodiesterase inhibitors. More than 90% of our patients accepted monotherapy or dual therapy in spite of the relatively serious condition. Treatment options were usually made according to the status of the patients, as well as their financial situation. As the only available intravenous prostanoid, the application of treprostinil was limited due to the price and side effects of subcutaneous catheterization.

Our results indicated that the prognosis of pediatric patients with IPAH and HPAH was poor in China. The 3-year survival rate of patients with gene mutations was only 33.3%, with a median survival time of 24 months, even in the modern targeted drugs era. More effort is needed to explore the pathophysiological mechanisms of IPAH and HPAH as well as more effective treatments.

In conclusion, pediatric patients with IPAH and HPAH had worse outcomes when gene mutations exist. Early gene screening for pediatric patients with IPAH and HPAH is recommended, and more aggressive treatment for mutation carriers is advisable.

Acknowledgments We are grateful to the patients and their families whose generosity and cooperation have made this study possible.

Conflicting Interests: The authors declare that there is no conflict of interest.

Funding: This work was supported by the National Natural Science Foundation of China (81570442).

Author Contributions: Hong Gu and Jie Du conceived and designed the research; Hong-sheng Zhang performed all the research. Hong-sheng Zhang wrote the main manuscript text. Qian Liu and Qiang-qiang Li analyzed data; Yan Zhu prepared tables and the figure; Hong-sheng Zhang and Chun-mei Piao edited and revised the manuscript. All authors reviewed the manuscript.

References

1. Galiè N, Humbert M, Vachiery JL, et al. ESC/ERS guidelines for the diagnosis and treatment of pulmonary hypertension. Kardiol Pol. 2016;73(12):1127.
2. Loyd JE, Atkinson JB, Pietra GG, Virmani R, Newman JH. Heterogeneity of pathologic lesions in familial primary pulmonary hypertension. Am Rev Respir Dis. 1988;138(4):952–7.
3. Runo JR, Loyd JE, hypertension P p. Lancet. 2003;361(9368):1533–44.
4. Barst RJ, Maislin G, Fishman AP. Vasodilator therapy for primary pulmonary hypertension in children. Circulation. 1999;99(9):1197–208.
5. International PPHC, Lane KB, Machado RD, et al. Heterozygous germline mutations in BMPR2, encoding a TGF-beta receptor, cause familial primary pulmonary hypertension. Nat Genet. 2000;26(1):81–4.
6. Machado RD, Pauciulo MW, Thomson JR, et al. BMPR2 haploinsufficiency as the inherited molecular mechanism for primary pulmonary hypertension. Am J Hum Genet. 2001;68(1):92–102.
7. Elliott CG. Genetics of pulmonary arterial hypertension. Clin Chest Med. 2013;34(4):651–63.
8. Garcia-Rivas G, Jerjes-Sanchez C, Rodriguez D, Garcia-Pelaez J, Trevino VA. Systematic review of genetic mutations in pulmonary arterial hypertension. BMC Med Genet. 2017;18(1):82.
9. McAllister KA, Grogg KM, Johnson DW, et al. Endoglin, a TGF-beta binding protein of endothelial cells, is the gene for hereditary haemorrhagic telangiectasia type 1. Nat Genet. 1994;8(4):345–51.

10. Johnson DW, Berg JN, Baldwin MA, et al. Mutations in the activin receptor-like kinase 1 gene in hereditary haemorrhagic telangiectasia type 2. Nat Genet. 1996;13(2):189–95.
11. Girerd B, Lau E, Montani D, Humbert M. Genetics of pulmonary hypertension in the clinic. Curr Opin Pulm Med. 2017;23(5):386–91.
12. Hansmann G, Hoeper MM. Registries for paediatric pulmonary hypertension. Eur Respir J. 2013;42(3):580–3.
13. Berger RM, Beghetti M, Humpl T, et al. Clinical features of paediatric pulmonary hypertension: a registry study. Lancet. 2012;379(9815):537–46.
14. Sztrymf B, Coulet F, Girerd B, et al. Clinical outcomes of pulmonary arterial hypertension in carriers of BMPR2 mutation. Am J Respir Crit Care Med. 2008;177(12):1377–83.
15. Girerd B, Montani D, Coulet F, et al. Clinical outcomes of pulmonary arterial hypertension in patients carrying an ACVRL1 (ALK1) mutation. Am J Respir Crit Care Med. 2010;181(8):851–61.
16. Chida A, Shintani M, Yagi H, et al. Outcomes of childhood pulmonary arterial hypertension in BMPR2 and ALK1 mutation carriers. Am J Cardiol. 2012;110(4):586–93.
17. Sitbon O, Humbert M, Jais X, et al. Long-term response to calcium channel blockers in idiopathic pulmonary arterial hypertension. Circulation. 2005;111(23):3105–11.
18. van der Bruggen CE, Happe CM, Dorfmuller P, et al. Bone morphogenetic protein receptor Type 2 mutation in pulmonary arterial hypertension: a view on the right ventricle. Circulation. 2016;133(18):1747–60.
19. Soubrier F, Chung WK, Machado R, et al. Genetics and genomics of pulmonary arterial hypertension. J Am Coll Cardiol. 2013;62(25 Suppl):D13–21.
20. Ma L, Roman-Campos D, Austin ED, et al. A novel channelopathy in pulmonary arterial hypertension. N Engl J Med. 2013;369(4):351–61.
21. Antigny F, Hautefort A, Meloche J, et al. Potassium Channel Subfamily K Member 3 (KCNK3) contributes to the development of pulmonary arterial hypertension clinical perspective. Circulation. 2016;133(14):1371–85.
22. Li X, Zhang X, Leathers R, et al. Notch3 signaling promotes the development of pulmonary arterial hypertension. Nat Med. 2009;15(11):1289–97.
23. Rosenzweig EB, Morse JH, Knowles JA, et al. Clinical implications of determining BMPR2 mutation status in a large cohort of children and adults with pulmonary arterial hypertension. J Heart Lung Transplant. 2008;27(6):668–74.
24. Zhang R, Dai LZ, Xie WP, et al. Survival of Chinese patients with pulmonary arterial hypertension in the modern treatment era. Chest. 2011;140(2):301–9.
25. Rival G, Lacasse Y, Martin S, Bonnet S, Provencher S. Effect of pulmonary arterial hypertension-specific therapies on health-related quality of life: a systematic review. Chest. 2014;146(3):686–708.

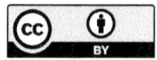

Fundamental Insight into Pulmonary Vascular Disease: Perspectives from Pediatric PAH in Japan

22

Yoshihide Mitani and Hirofumi Sawada

Abstract

In Japan, we have a unique experience with pulmonary arterial hypertension (PAH): mandatory electrocardiography (ECG) screening in apparently healthy school children and lung biopsy study in infants with congenital heart disease and atypical PAH. Our recent nationwide survey demonstrated that the school ECG screening in Japan detects a substantial pediatric IPAH population that is associated with already established PH but without apparent right heart failure; early treatment in PAH patients was associated with better outcomes. Our lung biopsy study in small infants with atypical CHD-PAH in a single institute showed that microscopic respiratory disease was associated with the development of severe PH, which is unexplained by CHD but is reversible in acute vasodilator testing. We presented some experimental data supporting the benefit in initiating early treatment in PAH and targeting at-risk population from the perinatal period.

Keywords

Pulmonary hypertension · Electrocardiogram · Lung biopsy · Lifelong cardiology · Congenital heart disease

Pulmonary arterial hypertension (PAH) is a progressive and fatal disorder characterized by occlusive vascular disease (PVD), including intimal hyperplasia and plexiform lesions in small pulmonary arteries. Since PAH still remains an incurable disease, it is required to explore the pathobiological mechanisms, which may confer new therapeutic targets and strategies. In Japan, we have a unique experience with

Y. Mitani (✉) · H. Sawada
Department of Pediatrics, Mie University Graduate School of Medicine, Tsu, Mie, Japan
e-mail: ymitani@clin.medic.mie-u.ac.jp

PAH: mandatory electrocardiography (ECG) screening in apparently healthy school children and lung biopsy study in infants with congenital heart disease and atypical PAH. In this presentation, recent clinical and experimental data are presented on the basis of lessons from PAH in Japan.

22.1 Early Detection and Early Treatment of PAH: Mechanistic Insights

For the early detection of cardiovascular diseases, a school ECG screening has been executed for all the first graders in elementary, middle and high schools in Japan. Our recent nationwide survey demonstrated that the school ECG screening in Japan detects a substantial pediatric IPAH population that is associated with already established PH but without apparent right heart failure; early treatment in PAH patients was associated with better outcomes. In exploring the pathobiological basis of these findings, experimental studies using a human PAH-like rat model produced by Sugen/hypoxia (SuHx) treatment were performed. Animal studies showed that early but not late treatment reversed occlusive PVD, which was associated with increased apoptosis and suppressed anti-apoptotic molecule survin expression in α-SMA cells in the intima. Further studies using SuHx models and human samples showed α-SMA cells in the intima were immature SMC-like cells although the origin of such cells remains to be explored; microarray analysis indicated distinct gene expression profiles in the early treatment.

22.2 Pathological Basis of Atypical CHD-PAH: Clinical and Mechanistic Implications

Some patients with Eisenmenger syndrome experience no obvious heart failure due to systemic pulmonary shunting in infancy, which is unexplained. Although a complex interplay of epithelial-endothelial cells is required for lung morphogenesis, its clinical relevance is unclear. Our lung biopsy study in small infants with atypical CHD-PAH showed that microscopic respiratory disease was associated with the development of severe PH, which is unexplained by CHD but is reversible in acute vasodilator testing. Such lung disease could be related to high functional PVR in infancy and late irreversible PAH unless CHD is timely repaired.

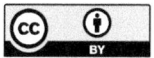

Risk Stratification in Paediatric Pulmonary Arterial Hypertension

23

Shahin Moledina

Abstract

Risk stratification can be defined as clinical assessment and investigation with the purpose of determining a person's risk of suffering a particular outcome and thereby guiding the need for preventative intervention (*McGraw-Hill Concise Dictionary of Modern Medicine* 2002). The need for risk stratification comes from the realisation that although the presence of pulmonary arterial hypertension significantly impairs survival, the degree of impairment can vary across the population of patients by as much as an order of magnitude.

Furthermore the understanding that therapies aimed at palliating symptoms and prolonging life has negative consequences both for the patients by way of side effects and society by way of costs and should therefore be targeted at those for whom potential benefit outweighs harm.

Keywords

Prognosis · Paediatric · Pulmonary hypertension

23.1 Why Risk Stratify?

Current drug therapies for pulmonary hypertension are licensed based on randomised control trials primarily demonstrating improvement in exercise intolerance. Currently there are five main therapy classes which may be used in combination, resulting in potentially numerous permutations of therapy. However, with polypharmacy comes a potential

S. Moledina (✉)

United Kingdom National Paediatric Pulmonary Hypertension Service, Great Ormond Street Hospital, London, UK

e-mail: Shahin.moledina@gosh.nhs.uk

© The Editor(s) (if applicable) and The Author(s) 2020

T. Nakanishi et al. (eds.), *Molecular Mechanism of Congenital Heart Disease and Pulmonary Hypertension*, https://doi.org/10.1007/978-981-15-1185-1_23

177

for increased disease burden and side effects. Data from our own centre (unpublished) shows that the number of therapies a patient is receiving negatively impacts health-related quality of life scores even when adjusting for other measures of disease severity. Tools to identify those patients at highest risk of adverse outcome in whom to offer more aggressive therapy are therefore increasingly important. The same is true for interventional procedures used to treat pulmonary hypertension such as balloon atrial septostomy or reverse Potts procedure. Each has a significant procedural mortality between 5 and 15% which must be balanced against the potential for significant palliation. They therefore should be targeted at those patients who are most likely to benefit.

Finally, cadaveric lung transplantation is a special case where risk stratification is exceedingly important. Lung transplantation especially for younger patients in whom the potential donor pool is restricted, by size and therefore availability, requires anticipation of prognosis. At the time of listing, for a young child in the United Kingdom, for example, might expect to wait a median of 12 months before a suitable matched graft is available. Therefore, if one enters the transplant waiting list too late there is a chance that the patient will succumb to their disease prior to transplantation [1]. Conversely, transplantation itself carries both immediate and longer-term morbidity. The procedure risk is between 5 and 10%, and the median survival is approximately 10 years. Therefore, listing a patient too early in the disease course will serve to impair the outcome and will result in harm.

23.2   Multidimensional Risk Stratification

Risk stratification is borne from the observation of discernible differences between patients who experience an early adverse outcome and those who enjoy better longer-term results. These differences span a number of domains and are not always congruous. For example, a patient with very severe vascular disease may have mild symptoms or a patient with mildly increased vascular resistance at assessment may have a particularly aggressive form of disease with rapid progression in vascular disease. Therefore, we proposed a multidimensional assessment of patients to guide risk stratification but also to allow a full understanding of the patient for more holistic treatment and to further understanding of the disease.

23.3   Factors to Consider in Multidimensional Risk Stratification of children with Pulmonary Arterial Hypertension

The paradigm of pulmonary arterial hypertension is of vascular remodelling resulting in progressive vascular obstruction and therefore the haemodynamic sequelae of the disease. These processes are thought to result from a combination of inherent susceptibility combined with vascular injury. It is therefore natural to consider the cause of pulmonary hypertension in a particular patient to inform the likely progression of the vascular disease. Since the core of the disease is vascular remodelling, measures of vascular structure and function are also considered important in gauging disease severity and risk. Data however indicate that whilst vascular disease is the source of the problem in pulmonary hypertension, outcome is largely mediated by its impact on cardiac function. Finally, as with any chronic disease, the body employs different compensatory mechanisms and therefore a downstream indicator of severity and risk would be the impact of the disease on the patient as a whole.

23.4   Cause of Pulmonary Hypertension

It is well known that different aetiologies of pulmonary arterial hypertension have different survival rates [2]. Patients with Eisenmenger syndrome have better survival in most registries than those with idiopathic or postoperative disease. It is likely that patients who develop pulmonary vascular disease despite minimal vascular injury may have more aggressive disease progression compared to those where vascular disease develops only after considerable insult to the vasculature. A prime example of this is the BMPR2 mutation. It has now been demonstrated that patients harbouring a BMPR2 mutation have poorer survival than those with idiopathic pulmonary arterial hypertension without this mutation [3].

23.5   Vascular Burden

Since vascular remodelling is central to the disease, measures of remodelling may aid risk stratification. Vascular disease at the microscopic level is difficult to study in patients due to access to tissue, and histology is not routinely performed. Functional cellular assays acting as biomarkers of vascular disease burden have not been well validated and are not in routine clinical use; however, they do represent exciting potential for further research. The classical way of assessing burden of disease in the vasculature in totality is to measure its impact on haemodynamics and, in particular, on pulmonary vascular resistance. As a vessel lumen obstructs the resistance will increase resulting in an aggregate assessment of vascular disease. The ability of pulmonary vascular resistance to predict outcome understandably has been assessed in numerous studies with varying results. A meta-analysis of these data demonstrates a significant association between pulmonary vascular resistance index (PVRI) and outcome with a 32% increased risk of adverse event for every 10 $WU.m^2$ increase in PVRI [4]. Since the pulmonary vasculature experiences pulsatile blood flow the degree of vascular remodelling cannot be described solely in terms of resistance. The other components of vascular load are total arterial compliance and wave reflection. Wave reflection has not been studied; however, arterial compliance has been investigated to some extent and does predict mortality with the total arterial compliance falling with increased vascular disease. In a number of small studies, pulmonary arterial compliance is seen to be as good as, or better, at predicting outcome than pulmonary vascular resistance. The reason for this is unclear. Finally assessing the acute response of the vascular bed to vasodilators is important. In this procedure, patients undergo acute testing of the pulmonary vaso-dilator, typically inhaled nitric oxide to assess the degree to which the vascular bed will respond by dilating. It is estimated that patients who respond to acute vasodila-tor testing have about a quarter to a third the risk of patients who do not respond to acute vasodilator testing [4].

As well as assessment of haemodynamics, one can image the vasculature itself with three-dimensional imaging techniques such as computed tomography. In one study CT angiograms from patients with varying degrees of pulmonary hyperten-sion were segmented to look at the complexity of the overall branching structure as a measure of vascular remodelling. In the pilot study, vascular branching complex-ity correlated both with functional class and pulmonary vascular resistance index but most importantly predicted survival [5].

23.6   Ventricular Function

Many of the effects of vascular disease are mediated via its impact on right ventricu-lar function resulting in the observation that patients with very advanced disease, but preserved ventricular function often has a lower symptom burden and better outcome than those with more modest vascular disease but more severe ventricular dysfunction. Ventricular function can be assessed in aggregate during haemody-namic testing by considering total cardiac index which informs prognosis (hazard ratio of 0.66 per 1 L/min/m^2 increase). Pump failure may also be assessed by mea-suring right atrial pressure RAP, and this is a robust prognostic indicator with hazard ratio of 1.12 per 1 mmHg increase in RAP. NT-proBNP has been used in various forms of heart failure as a circulating biomarker of ventricular wall stress and dys-function. Tested in a number of small paediatric studies, this measure also informs prognosis and can be used for risk stratification. One advantage to this measure is that it can be performed in a serial fashion.

Finally the gold standard for measuring cardiac function is cardiac MRI. This can now be performed even for the youngest of children. One study of 100 children undergoing cardiac MRI found a number of measures which are prognostic. These include measures of right ventricular dilatation, severity of tricuspid regurgitation and right ventricular mass; however, the most robust measure in predicting outcome was right ventricular ejection fraction [6].

23.7   Impact on the Patient

The most common symptom experienced by patients with pulmonary hypertension is exertional dyspnoea and exercise limitation with nearly 80% of patients experi-encing this [7]. Exercise limitation may be measured by 6-min walking distance; however, numerous studies have failed to demonstrate this as a useful prognostic indicator. A more objective measure of exercise tolerance can be obtained by car-diopulmonary exercise testing, and in an unpublished study from our centre both peak oxygen consumption peak O_2 and ventilatory efficiency slope (VE/VCO$_2$)

were highly prognostic. Perhaps the best way of determining the impact on a patient's ability to function as a result of that disease is to ask them in a structured fashion. This can be scored as in the WHO functional class assessing severity of symptoms. Despite its crude appearance as a subjective score, functional class has been demonstrated consistently to inform prognosis and is a very robust measure. Other ways of assessing impact on patient is to use a structured quality of life questionnaire to score measures of quality of life in different domains. A study from our centre using the PedQL questionnaire has demonstrated good correlation between physical domain of the questionnaire and prognosis.

Finally, children are in the unique position of growing and developing. Chronic diseases impact on this growth and development and therefore measures of growth may be considered as an aggregate measure of the impact on the disease on the patient's biology as a whole. Children with pulmonary hypertension have been shown to have growth failure, and their severity of the growth failure also predicts outcome [7].

23.8   Summary

Whilst there is no cure for paediatric pulmonary arterial hypertension at present, treatments have advanced and with more treatment options comes complexity in decision making leading to a need to stratify risk. Numerous markers of adverse outcome have been described across the breadths of domains; however, we believe a multidimensional assessment considering causation, vascular disease burden, cardiac function and overall impact on patient will lead to more accurate risk stratification, promote holistic care of patients and provide deeper insight into disease mechanisms which can later be exploited to therapeutic advantage. Such assessments should be a dynamic process.

References

1. Lammers AE, Burch M, Benden C, et al. Lung transplantation in children with idiopathic pulmonary arterial hypertension. Pediatr Pulmonol. 2010;45(3):263–9.
2. Haworth SG, Hislop AA. Treatment and survival in children with pulmonary arterial hypertension: the UK Pulmonary Hypertension Service for Children 2001-2006. Heart. 2009;95(4):312–7.
3. Evans JD, Girerd B, Montani D, et al. BMPR2 mutations and survival in pulmonary arterial hypertension: an individual participant data meta-analysis. Lancet Respir Med. 2016;4(2):129–37.
4. Ploegstra MJ, Zijlstra WM, Douwes JM, et al. Prognostic factors in pediatric pulmonary arterial hypertension: A systematic review and meta-analysis. Int J Cardiol. 2015;184:198–207.
5. Moledina S, de Bruyn A, Schievano S, et al. Fractal branching quantifies vascular changes and predicts survival in pulmonary hypertension: a proof of principle study. Heart. 2011;97(15):1245–9.
6. Moledina S, Pandya B, Bartsota M, et al. Prognostic significance of cardiac magnetic resonance imaging in children with pulmonary hypertension. Circ Cardiovasc Imaging. 2013;6(3):407–14.
7. Moledina S, Hislop AA, Foster H, et al. Childhood idiopathic pulmonary arterial hypertension: a national cohort study. Heart. 2010;96(17):1401–6.

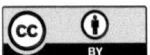

The Adaptive Right Ventricle in Eisenmenger Syndrome: Potential Therapeutic Targets for Pulmonary Hypertension?

24

Rebecca Johnson Kameny, Sanjeev A. Datar, Jason Boehme, and Jeffrey R. Fineman

Abstract

Pulmonary hypertension (PH) is a rare disease with significant mortality despite targeted therapies. Among patients with PH, both survival and functional class are more closely correlated with right ventricular (RV) function than with the degree of pulmonary artery pressure elevation or pulmonary vascular resistance. Unfortunately, the RV is usually exquisitely sensitive to increases in afterload associated with PH, and progressive RV failure is the typical clinical course among most patients over time. However, in the subset of PH patients with congenital heart disease and Eisenmenger syndrome, survival is prolonged and RV function is preserved compared to patients with primary PH. This functional superiority may be due to a persistent RV fetal phenotype as patients continue to have a biventricular hypertrophy pattern which mimics fetal cardiac morphology. We have utilized an ovine model of congenital heart disease to demonstrate superior RV function following acute afterload stimulus—a unique RV Anrep effect. Further, we have shown shared gene expression patterns in the fetal and CHD model RV. In the future, understanding the underlying mechanisms of RV adaptation in CHD and PH may yield novel therapeutic strategies for all patients with pulmonary hypertension.

Keywords

Eisenmenger syndrome · Pulmonary hypertension · Right ventricle

R. J. Kameny · S. A. Datar · J. Boehme
Department of Pediatrics, University of California, San Francisco, San Francisco, CA, USA

J. R. Fineman (✉)
Department of Pediatrics, University of California, San Francisco, San Francisco, CA, USA

Cardiovascular Research Institute, University of California, San Francisco,
San Francisco, CA, USA
e-mail: jeff.fineman@ucsf.edu

24.1   Introduction

Pulmonary arterial hypertension (PAH) is a rare but devastating disease that carries a significant burden of morbidity and mortality. Most investigations have focused on mechanisms that underlie abnormal pulmonary vascular reactivity and remodeling, which have led to the development of new therapies and improved survival. Similarly, much of the clinical evaluation of patients with PAH is based upon assessments of pulmonary arterial pressure and pulmonary vascular resistance. However, mortality is due to right ventricular (RV) failure, and there is growing recognition that indices of RV function in patients with PAH—including right atrial pressure and cardiac index—are correlated most closely with not only survival but also functional class [1, 2]. Interestingly, patients with PAH associated with CHD have better functional capacity and survival than patients with other forms of PAH despite equivalent pulmonary artery pressures and advanced pulmonary arteriopathy [3]. However, the mechanisms that might account for this difference are unknown and have been the subject of limited investigation. Among patients with primary PH, there is considerable variability in indices of RV function (cardiac output and right atrial pressure) relative to pulmonary artery pressure elevation. There is a subpopulation of patients who retain an adaptive phenotype with concentric hypertrophy and preserved mechanical efficiency; accordingly, these patients have improved survival compared to patients with a "maladaptive" RV phenotype [4]. A better understanding of preserved RV function in these patients might lead to novel therapeutic targets.

24.2   Improved Survival in Eisenmenger Syndrome

For decades, there has been a consistently observed survival advantage among patients with Eisenmenger syndrome compared to those with idiopathic PH or PH secondary to other causes [5]. Despite equivalent elevations in PA pressure and pulmonary vascular resistance compared with patients with IPAH, these patients have lower right atrial pressures and higher cardiac output. Moreover, at a similar level of PAP elevation, patients with ES have superior echocardiographic features of RV function [6]. Two major mechanisms for this observed survival benefit have been theorized. The presence of a communication at either the atrial or ventricular level (or both) allows right-to-left shunting of blood—a "pop-off"—preserving left-sided output during right ventricular failure. Another intriguing potential factor is persistence of a fetal RV phenotype due to the presence at birth of an unrestrictive post-tricuspid valve left-to-right shunt that applies systemic-level afterload to the RV. In this situation, the RV does not undergo the deconditioning that normally occurs as pulmonary vascular resistance decreases after birth and, thereby, may be better suited to function against an increasing afterload as pulmonary hemodynamics worsen [5, 7]. Interestingly, a recent multicenter study of predictive factors of survival in patients with ES found that those with pre-tricuspid lesions had worse survival [8]. These data support the hypothesis that RV remodeling in the setting of high afterload associated with post-tricuspid CHD lesions confers additional benefit beyond right-to-left unloading through an intracardiac shunt.

24.3   Preserved Fetal Morphology in Eisenmenger Syndrome

During fetal life, the right ventricle is the dominant ventricle, responsible for approximately two-thirds of combined cardiac output [9]. Commensurate with this function, the right and left ventricles are equally hypertrophied in fetal life; in normal physiology, RV hypertrophy regresses postnatally as the RV remodels into a highly efficient, compliant chamber which pumps a full cardiac output to the low resistance pulmonary vascular bed with approximately 1/5 the energy expenditure of the left ventricle. In patients with post-tricuspid lesions, the RV is continually exposed to high afterload and regression from fetal characteristics is attenuated or absent. Hopkins and Waggoner compared morphologic characteristics of 50 patients with Eisenmenger syndrome, infants with unrestrictive VSDs, and fetuses with normal anatomy; they found a consistent linear relationship between LV and RV wall thickness among these groups (Fig. 24.1) [10]. Furthermore, among patients with Eisenmenger syndrome, those with post-tricuspid (as opposed to

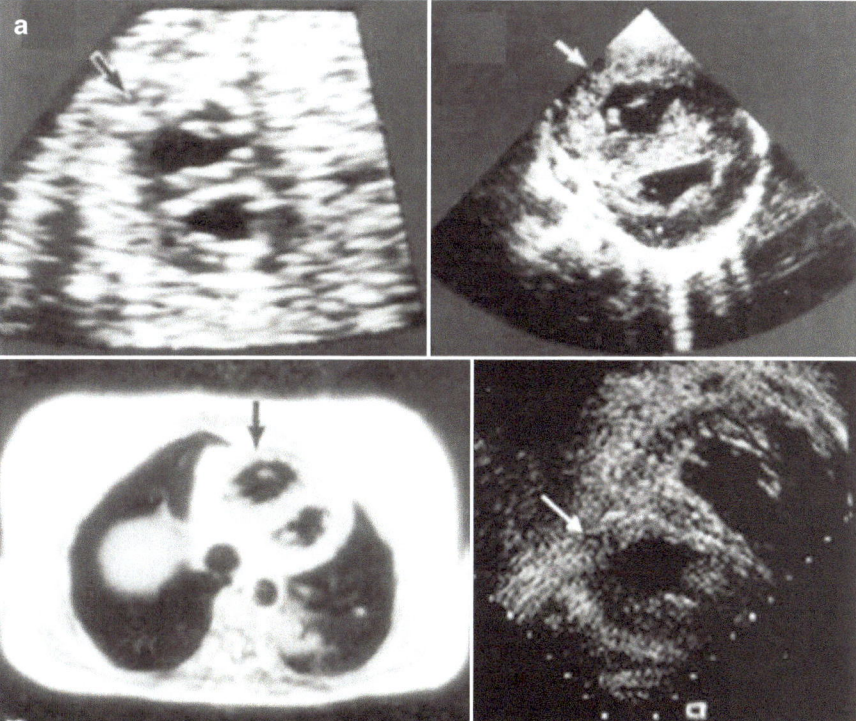

Fig. 24.1 Preserved fetal biventricular hypertrophy in patients with Eisenmenger syndrome (ES). Adapted from Hopkins and Waggoner. Severe pulmonary hypertension without right ventricular failure: the unique hearts of patients with Eisenmenger syndrome. *AJC* 2002. Reproduced with permission. (**a**) **Cardiac imaging** *top left*, normal 20-week fetal echo; *top right*, echo of 26-year old with truncus arteriosus and ES; bottom left, magnetic resonance imaging of 41-year old with patent ductus arteriosus and ES, 77-year old with perimembranous ventricular septal defect and ES. (**b**) **Wall thickness**. Linear Regression of LV and RV wall thickness in structurally normal fetal hearts, infants with unrestrictive ventricular septal defects, and adolescents and adults with unrestrictive post-tricuspid lesions and ES

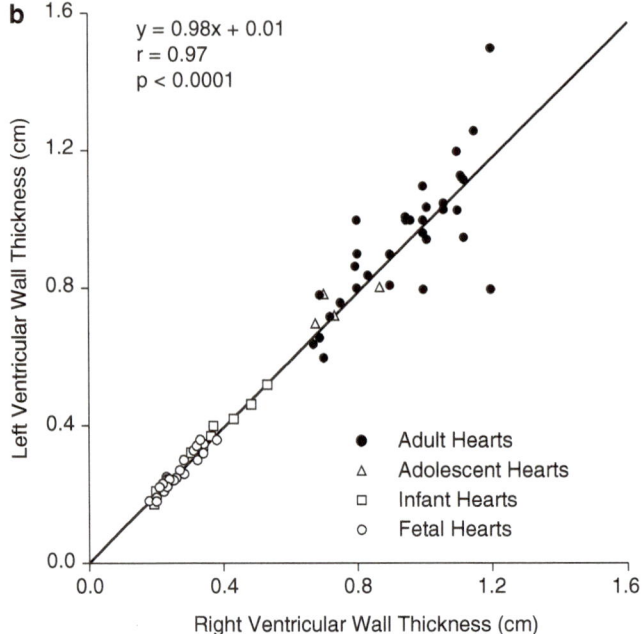

Fig. 24.1 (continued)

pre-tricuspid) lesions have better RV function and survival [11]. These findings suggest that post-tricuspid CHD lesions allow for continued postnatal exposure of the RV to systemic-level afterload, prevent the typical regression of RV hypertrophy postnatally, and condition the RV to respond to later increases in afterload associated with PH.

24.4   Fetal Phenotype in Ovine CHD Model

Our laboratory has a well-established, clinical relevant model of CHD utilizing a large, fetally implanted aortopulmonary shunt, which continually exposes the RV to systemic level afterload during the perinatal transition and beyond (Fig. 24.2a) [12]. As a consequence of this hemodynamic stimulus, the RV in the juvenile shunt lamb is significantly hypertrophied compared to the control (Fig. 24.2b) [13]. In this CHD model, the RV of shunt lambs has many gene expression similarities with the RV of fetal lambs, including in α- and β-myosin heavy chain expression [13] and nitric oxide synthase expression and activity [14]. Further, we have utilized RNA sequencing to compare RV gene expression among fetal and juvenile shunt and control lambs. Eighty-two percent of genes that were differentially expressed in fetal RV tissue (compared to control) were also upregulated in shunt RV tissue (unpublished data). When subjected to gene ontology analysis, these 142 shared differentially expressed genes enrich a total of 25 biological pathways, including those associated with ECM remodeling, negative regulation of cellular proliferation, and cardiovascular system development—all pathways which might contribute to the observed adaptive RV phenotype.

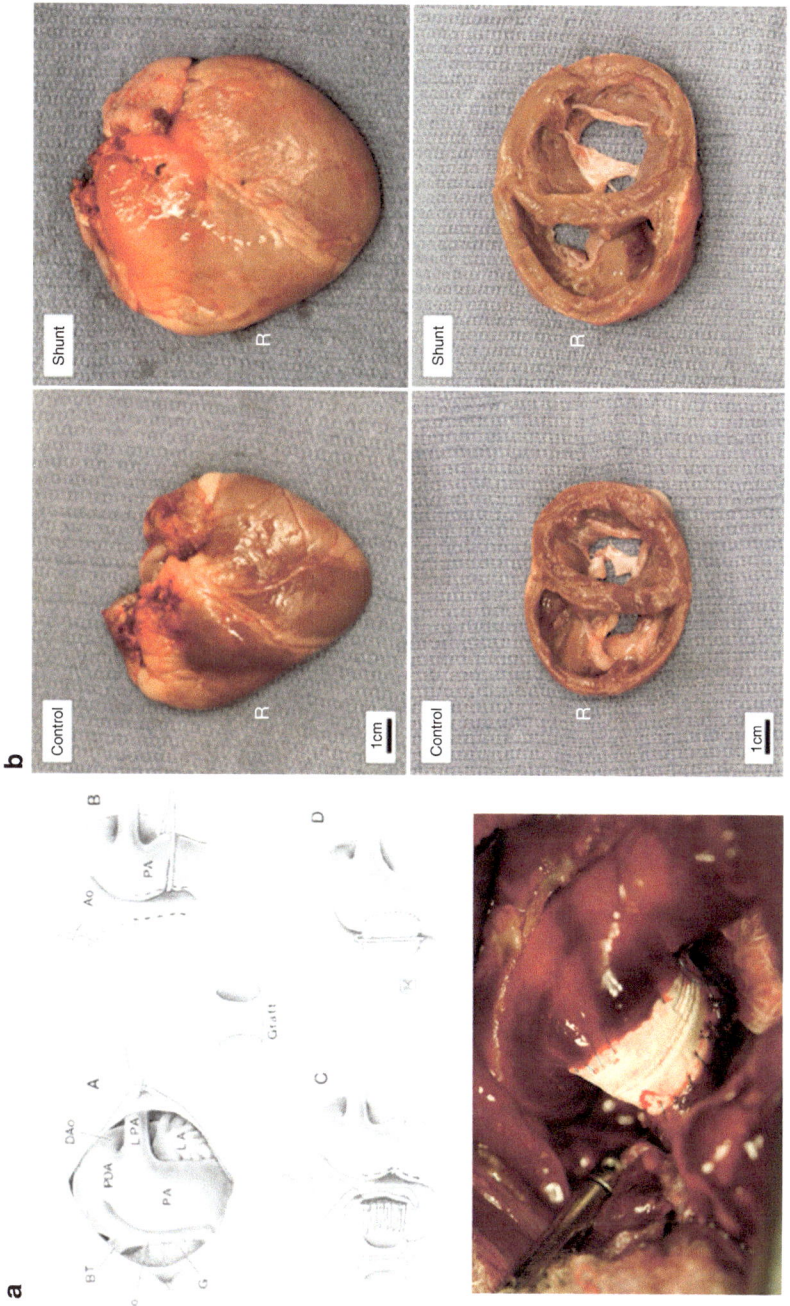

Fig. 24.2 Ovine model of congenital heart disease (CHD) with biventricular hypertrophy. (**a**) Cartoon drawing and in situ image of fetally implated aortopulmonary shunt. (**b**) *Top panel*, whole heart; *bottom panel*, cut section of juvenile control and shunt hearts, in all images, RV indicated with "R"

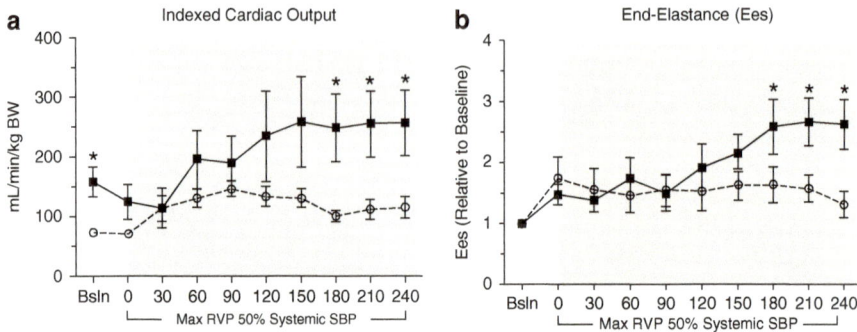

Fig. 24.3 Superior RV performance in ovine CHD model with acute RV afterload stimulus. Following 4 h of acute pulmonary artery banding to 50% of systemic pressure, (**a**) shunt lambs demonstrated continued superior cardiac index compared to controls and (**b**) shunt lambs increased RV contractility (Ees) by 2.5-fold baseline

24.5 The Adaptive RV Response to Acute Afterload—RV Anrep Effect

In our model of CHD with chronic left-to-right shunting, we demonstrated that the RV of shunt lambs has an adaptive response compared to control RV when challenged with an acute afterload increase (imposed by pulmonary artery banding) with increased contractility and preservation of mechanical efficiency and ventricular-vascular coupling (Fig. 24.3). Our observation of a sustained increase in contractility in the shunt RV following afterload challenge is evidence of a novel Anrep effect, the second slow increase in contractility in response to myocyte stretch. Previously, this critical physiologic mechanism had only been observed in the left ventricle (LV) as the normal RV is exquisitely sensitive to increased afterload. Furthermore, after pulmonary artery banding, the RV in shunted animals had preserved ventricular-vascular coupling and ventricular efficiency relative to controls [13]. These adaptive physiologic responses to acutely increased afterload in shunted lambs may correlate with the response in patients with CHD and PH.

24.6 Potential Mechanisms of RV Anrep Effect

Having established this novel Anrep effect, we next sought to understand potential underlying mechanisms. We first examined nitric oxide signaling as increased cardiac NO signaling has a variety of paracrine and autocrine effects which ultimately maximize cardiac function including improved excitation-contraction coupling, which is crucial for the Anrep effect [15]. We found a

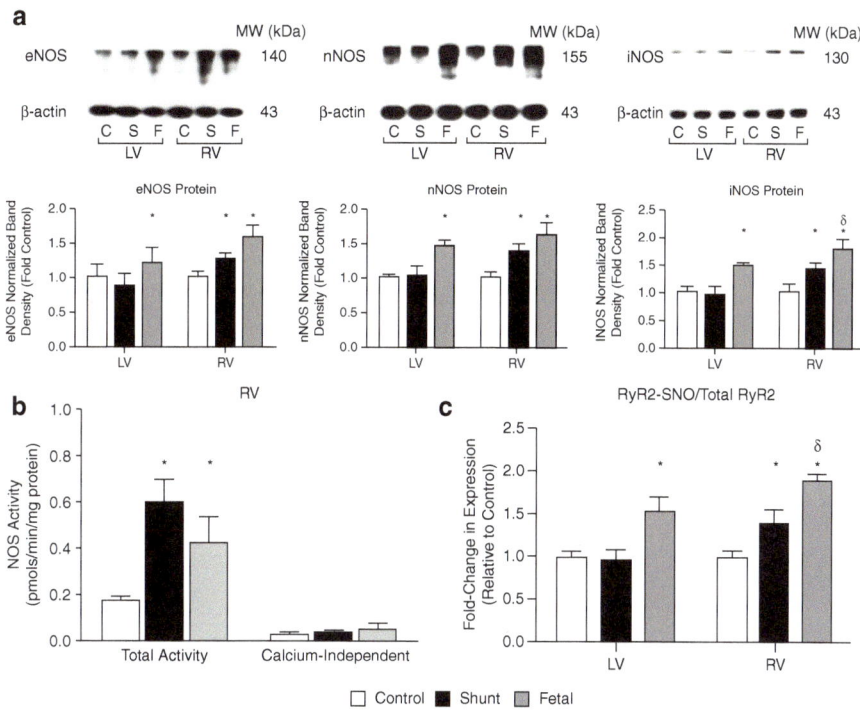

Fig. 24.4 RV nitric oxide signaling in ovine CHD model. (**a**) Increased expression of all nitric oxide synthase isoforms (eNOS, nNOS, and iNOS) in shunt and fetal RV. (**b**) Increased NOS activity in shunt and fetal RV, and (**c**) increased post-translational nitrosylation of ryanodine receptor 2 (RyR2) in shunt and fetal RV. Nitrosylation of RyR2 predisposes the open confirmation with resultant increased intracellular calcium and increased contractility

distinct shunt RV phenotype with consistently increased NOS expression, activity, and association of important cofactors for NOS activation; this distinct pattern was consistent in the RV of fetal and shunt but not control lambs (Fig. 24.4).

We next examined non-coding microRNA expression patterns as potential modulators of multiple pathways of gene expression [16]. We found important differences in miRNA expression in our adaptive RVH model compared human and animal maladaptive RVH with significant overlap in the fetus. Next, we investigated downstream effects of miR-199b and miR-29a expression as they relate to NFAT-calcineurin mediated cardiac hypertrophy and fibrosis. Alterations in miR-199b and miR-29a and downstream effects are shown in Fig. 24.5 [17]. These changes yield valuable insight into one of the potential mechanisms behind adaptive RV hypertrophy seen in our model of ovine CHD.

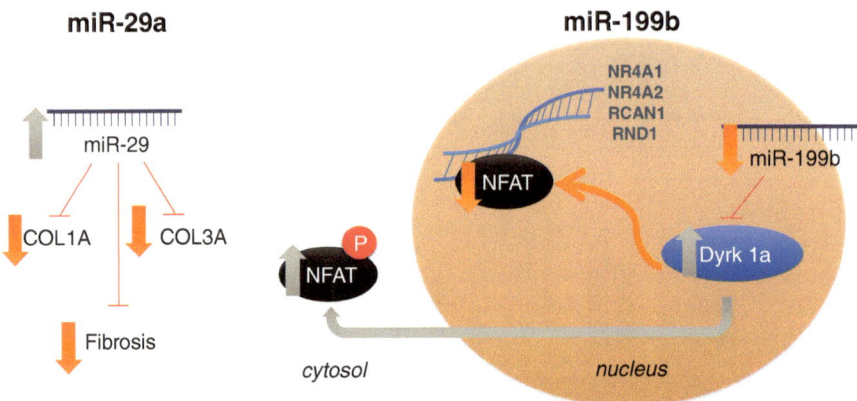

Fig. 24.5 miR 29 and 199b effects. Cartoon of downstream effects of observed changes in miR expression in shunt and fetal RV tissue. Increased miR-29 leads to decreased collagen 1 and 3 expression and decreased fibrosis. Decreased miR199b expression leads to increased Dyrk1a expression, which promotes NFAT phosphorylation and inhibits NFAT translocation to nucleus and transcription of NFAT/calcineurin-dependent heart failure gene program

24.7 Future Directions and Clinical Implications

Preserved RV function among patients with Eisenmenger Syndrome remains a clinical observation without a clearly identified pathophysiologic mechanism. Although a preserved RV fetal phenotype in these ES patients seems a logical conclusion based on both cardiovascular development and preliminary animal data, this hypothesis remains unproven. As the mechanisms for preserved RV function in these circumstances is better defined, the next step will be targeting of these pathways in all patients with preserved RV function in the hopes of improving the survival and functional status of these patients.

Ackowledgments This research was supported by grants from the National Institutes of Health (HL61284 to J.R.F. and 5T32HD049303-07 to J.R.F. and R.J.K.) and American Heart Association (14FTF19670001 to R.J.K.).

References

1. Voelkel NF, Quaife RA, Leinwand LA, et al. Right ventricular function and failure: report of a National Heart, Lung, and Blood Institute working group on cellular and molecular mechanisms of right heart failure. Circulation. 2006;114:1883–91. https://doi.org/10.1161/CIRCULATIONAHA.106.632208.
2. Roche SL, Redington AN. The failing right ventricle in congenital heart disease. Can J Cardiol. 2013;29:768–78. https://doi.org/10.1016/j.cjca.2013.04.018.

3. Hopkins WE, Ochoa LL, Richardson GW, Trulock EP. Comparison of the hemodynamics and survival of adults with severe primary pulmonary hypertension or Eisenmenger syndrome. J Heart Lung Transplant. 1996;15:100–5.
4. Simon MA, Deible C, Mathier MA, et al. Phenotyping the right ventricle in patients with pulmonary hypertension. Clin Transl Sci. 2009;2:294–9. https://doi.org/10.1111/j.1752-8062.2009.00134.x.
5. Hopkins WE. The remarkable right ventricle of patients with Eisenmenger syndrome. Coron Artery Dis. 2005;16:19–25.
6. Giusca S, Popa E, Amzulescu MS, et al. Is right ventricular remodeling in pulmonary hypertension dependent on etiology? An echocardiographic study. Echocardiography. 2016;33:546–54. https://doi.org/10.1111/echo.13112.
7. Hopkins WE. Right ventricular performance in congenital heart disease: a physiologic and pathophysiologic perspective. Cardiol Clin. 2012;30:205–18. https://doi.org/10.1016/j.ccl.2012.03.006.
8. Kempny A, Hjortshøj CS, Gu H, et al. Predictors of death in contemporary adult patients with Eisenmenger syndrome: a multicenter study. Circulation. 2017;135:1432–40. https://doi.org/10.1161/CIRCULATIONAHA.116.023033.
9. Rudolph AM. Circulatory adjustments after birth: effects on ventricular septal defect. Br Heart J. 1971;33(Suppl):32–4.
10. Hopkins WE, Waggoner AD. Severe pulmonary hypertension without right ventricular failure: the unique hearts of patients with Eisenmenger syndrome. Am J Cardiol. 2002;89:34–8.
11. Alonso-Gonzalez R, Lopez-Guarch CJ, Subirana-Domenech MT, et al. Pulmonary hypertension and congenital heart disease: an insight from the REHAP National Registry. Int J Cardiol. 2015;184:717–23. https://doi.org/10.1016/j.ijcard.2015.02.031.
12. Reddy VM, Meyrick B, Wong J, et al. In utero placement of aortopulmonary shunts. A model of postnatal pulmonary hypertension with increased pulmonary blood flow in lambs. Circulation. 1995;92:606–13.
13. Johnson RC, Datar SA, Oishi PE, et al. Adaptive right ventricular performance in response to acutely increased afterload in a lamb model of congenital heart disease: evidence for enhanced Anrep effect. Am J Physiol Heart Circ Physiol. 2014;306(8):H1222–30.
14. Kameny RJ, He Y, Morris C, et al. Right ventricular nitric oxide signaling in an ovine model of congenital heart disease: a preserved fetal phenotype. Am J Physiol Heart Circ Physiol. 2015;309:H157–65. https://doi.org/10.1152/ajpheart.00103.2015.
15. Balligand JL, Feron O, Dessy C. eNOS activation by physical forces: from short-term regulation of contraction to chronic remodeling of cardiovascular tissues. Physiol Rev. 2009;89:481–534. https://doi.org/10.1152/physrev.00042.2007.
16. Latronico MVG, Condorelli G. MicroRNAs and cardiac pathology. Nat Rev Cardiol. 2009;6:419–29. https://doi.org/10.1038/nrcardio.2009.56.
17. Kameny RJ, He Y, Zhu T, et al. Analysis of the microRNA signature driving adaptive right ventricular hypertrophy in an ovine model of congenital heart disease. Am J Physiol Heart Circ Physiol. 2018;315:H847–54. https://doi.org/10.1152/ajpheart.00057.2018.

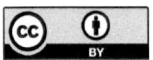

Impaired Right Coronary Vasodilator Function in Pulmonary Hypertensive Rats Assessed by In Vivo Synchrotron Microangiography

25

Tadakatsu Inagaki, Hirotsugu Tsuchimochi,
James T. Pearson, Daryl O. Schwenke, Keiji Umetani,
Mikiyasu Shirai, and Yoshikazu Nakaoka

Keywords

Coronary microangiography · Synchrotron radiation · Right heart failure · Endothelial dysfunction

Pulmonary hypertension (PH) causes cardiac hypertrophy in the right ventricle (RV) and eventually leads to RV failure due to persistently elevated afterload. Considerable clinical and experimental animal studies have shown that abnormalities of endothelial function represent a hallmark of heart failure. However, the relationships between right coronary endothelial dysfunction and the development of heart failure remain to be fully established especially in the right heart. Synchrotron

T. Inagaki · Y. Nakaoka (✉)
Department of Vascular Physiology, National Cerebral and Cardiovascular Center,
Osaka, Japan
e-mail: ynakaoka@ncvc.go.jp

H. Tsuchimochi · J. T. Pearson
Department of Cardiac Physiology, National Cerebral and Cardiovascular Center,
Osaka, Japan

D. O. Schwenke
Department of Physiology, University of Otago, Dunedin, New Zealand

K. Umetani
Japan Synchrotron Radiation Research Institute, Sayo-gun, Hyogo, Japan

M. Shirai
Department of Advanced Medical Research for Pulmonary Hypertension, National Cerebral and Cardiovascular Center, Osaka, Japan

© The Editor(s) (if applicable) and The Author(s) 2020
T. Nakanishi et al. (eds.), *Molecular Mechanism of Congenital Heart Disease and Pulmonary Hypertension*, https://doi.org/10.1007/978-981-15-1185-1_25

radiation (SR) microangiography has provided the temporal and spatial resolution required to visualize microvessels of various organs in vivo [1]. Therefore, in this study, we aimed to validate a new approach for the in vivo assessment of endothelial coronary function of the rat right heart using SR microangiography.

Imaging of the right coronary circulation was performed under pentobarbital anesthesia with monochromatic SR at 33.2 keV for producing maximal absorption contrast of the iodine contrast agent in the vascular lumen (Fig. 25.1a). ImageJ (ver. 1.41, NIH, Bethesda, MD) was used to identify coronary vessels and determine their caliber. Vessels were labeled and classified according to branching orders from first-order main segment (Fig. 25.1b). The visible vessel internal diameter (ID) of each vessel was determined from a single field of view for all cine sequences. The ID of each vessel was averaged over at least ten consecutive frames [2].

The figure shows a typical imaging pattern of right coronary arteries from the aortic root to the third or fourth branching. It was possible to observe an arteriole with a diameter of about 50 μm (Fig. 25.1c). The ID of the first, second, and third

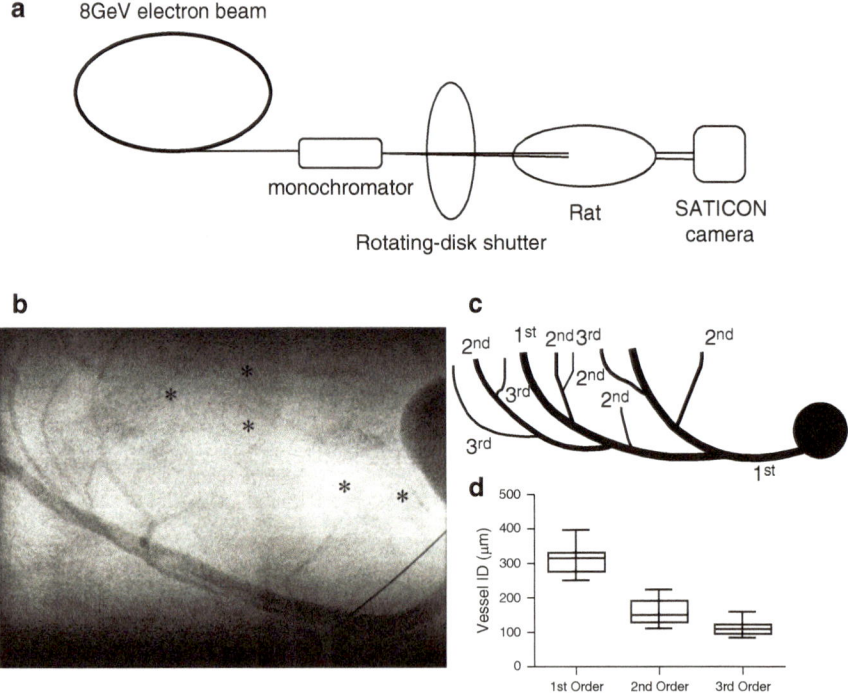

Fig. 25.1 SR microangiography for assessing vascular function in a rat. Schematic of SR microangiography for the rat right coronary artery using SPring-8 facilities (**a**). Typical SR angiogram image of the right coronary vasculature (**b**). Schematic of right coronary arteries in lateral view depicting the coronary branching nomenclature used in this study (**c**). Range of vessel size at each of the branching generations of right coronary circulation in the normal rat (**d**). Asterisks indicate ~50 μm vessels not included in (**d**)

branches were 312.7 ± 15.4, 159.3 ± 12.4, and 113.1 ± 7.5 µm, respectively (Fig. 25.1d). The present investigation demonstrates the ability to clearly visualize the right coronary circulation of the closed-chest anesthetized rat using SR micro-angiography. The use of SR microangiography provides a powerful tool for assessing coronary hemodynamics in unprecedented detail in PH models. Ultimately, future studies using SR microangiography will provide important new insights into the pathophysiology of right heart failure.

Acknowledgments Experiments were performed at the Japan Synchrotron Radiation Research Institute (SPrimg-8, BL28B2, Proposals 2014B1801 and 2015A1868). This work was supported by JSPS KAKENHI JP25860184 to T.I.

References

1. Shirai M, et al. Synchrotron radiation imaging for advancing our understanding of cardiovascular function. Circ Res. 2013;112:209–21.
2. Jenkins MJ, et al. Dynamic synchrotron imaging of diabetic rat coronary microcirculation in vivo. Arterioscler Thromb Vasc Biol. 2012;32:370–7.

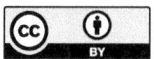

Relationship Between Mutations in *ENG* and *ALK1* Genes and the Affected Organs in Hereditary Hemorrhagic Telangiectasia

26

Toru Iwasa, Osamu Yamada, Hiroko Morisaki, Takayuki Morisaki, Ken-ichi Kurosaki, and Isao Shiraishi

Keywords

Hereditary hemorrhagic telangiectasia · Genetic analysis · Arteriovenous fistula

Hereditary hemorrhagic telangiectasia (HHT) is a hereditary disorder that causes refractory nasal bleeding, arteriovenous malformations in the lung (pulmonary arteriovenous fistula: PAVF), central nervous system (CNS-AVF), and liver (hepatic AVF). HHT is caused by genetic abnormalities in endoglin (*ENG*), ACVRL1 (*ALK1*), and other rare genes (e.g., *SMAD4*). The relationship between these gene mutations and the affected organs remains unclear.

We performed genetic analysis from whole blood of 464 suspected HHT patients or HHT carriers from April 2005 to November 2015 in 35 hospitals and found 264

T. Iwasa (✉) · K.-i. Kurosaki · I. Shiraishi
Department of Pediatric Cardiology, National Cerebral and Cardiovascular Center, Osaka, Japan
e-mail: tiwasa@ncvc.go.jp

O. Yamada
Department of Pediatric Cardiology, National Cerebral and Cardiovascular Center, Osaka, Japan

Department of Pathology, National Cerebral and Cardiovascular Center, Osaka, Japan

H. Morisaki
Department of Biochemistry, Research Institute of National Cerebral and Cardiovascular Center, Osaka, Japan

Department of Medical Genetics, The Sakakibara Heart Institute, Tokyo, Japan

T. Morisaki
Department of Biochemistry, Research Institute of National Cerebral and Cardiovascular Center, Osaka, Japan

patients positive for mutation in *ENG*, *ALK1*, and *SMAD4* genes. Of these 264 positive results, we excluded 68 patients who were sporadic, non-familial cases and performed proband gene analysis. We also excluded 107 non-symptomatic mutation carriers and leaving a total of 89 patients with AVFs.

To clarify the relationship between gene mutations and the affected organs, we assessed the mutations and clinical presentation of these 89 patients. We found 25 mutations in the *ENG* gene from 68 patients and 8 mutations in the *ALK1* gene from 21 patients. We then grouped patient AVF presentation (PAVF, CNS-AVF and hepatic AVF) according to the genetic mutation (Table 26.1).

Among patients with mutations in *ENG*, 19/25 (79%) mutations and 46/68 (69%) of patients presented with the same affected organ pattern. PAVFs were tending to

Table 26.1 Gene mutation and affected organs

Gene	Mutation	N	Type	PAVF	CNS-AVF	HAVF
ENG	Met368Thr	4	Missense	All(+)	ALL(−)	NA
ENG	Cly331Ser	6	Missense	All(+)	NA	NA
ENG	IVS3 ds G-C +1	3	Splicing	All(+)	ALL(−)	NA
ENG	Leu162Pro	2	Missense	All(+)	NA	NA
ENG	Skipping of ex.2	2	Splicing	All(+)	NA	NA
ENG	Ala229Profs	2	Frame shift	All(+)	ALL(−)	NA
ENG	Gln505Ter	2	Nonsense	All(+)	ALL(−)	NA
ENG	Leu107Cysfs	2	Frame shift	All(+)	NA	NA
ENG	Gln145Ter	3	Nonsense	All(+)	NA	NA
ENG	Leu194Pro198del5	2	Missense	All(+)	NA	NA
ENG	Glu276IlefsX57	2	Frame shift	All(+)	All(+)	NA
ENG	(Novel1)	2	Frame shift	All(+)	ALL(−)	NA
ENG	(Novel2)	2	Missense	All(+)	ALL(−)	NA
ENG	(Novel3)	2	Splicing	All(+)	NA	NA
ENG	Arg93Ter	2	Nonsense	All(+)	NA	NA
ENG	Arg339GlyfsX22	2	Frame shift	All(+)	ALL(−)	NA
ENG	Glu563Lysfs	2	Frame shift	All(+)	NA	NA
ENG	Leu506Pro	2	Missense	All(+)	NA	NA
ENG	IVS7−1G>A	2	Splicing	All(+)	ALL(−)	NA
ENG	IVS3+1G>A	2	Splicing	Hetero	Hetero	NA
ENG	IVS6 ds T-A +2	4	Splicing	All(+)	Hetero	NA
ENG	Ex.3-8 del	4	Exon del.	All(+)	Hetero	NA
ENG	Cys412Thr	3	Missense	Hetero	All(+)	NA
ENG	IVS8 ds G-A −1	7	Splicing	Hetero	Hetero	Hetero
ENG	(Novel4)	2	Splicing	Hetero	Hetero	NA
ALK1	Arg479Ter	5	Nonsense	All(+)	ALL(−)	All(+)
ALK1	IVS6ds insAA+4_5	3	Splicing	All(+)	NA	NA
ALK1	Pro424Leu	2	Missense	ALL(−)	NA	All(+)
ALK1	Arg200Gly	2	Missense	All(+)	ALL(−)	All(+)
ALK1	Gln118Ter	2	Nonsense	NA	ALL(−)	All(+)
ALK1	IVS5-3C>G	2	Splicing	All(+)	NA	NA
ALK1	Arg484Gln	3	Missense	NA	ALL(−)	Hetero
ALK1	Asp437Gly	2	Missense	ALL(−)	ALL(−)	Hetero

PAVF pulmonary arterio-venous fistula, *CNS-AVF* central nervous system arterio-venous fistula, *HAVF* hepatic arterio-venous fistula, *NA* not assessed
Novel1-Novel4 gene: novel gene mutations

be the same. Hepatic AVFs were rarely described in patient profiles so we were unable to evaluate hepatic AVF presentation patterns in mutated *ENG* patients.

In patients with mutations in *ALK1*, 8/10 (80%) mutations, 16/21 (76%) patients presented with the same affected organ pattern. For example, all five patients with the Arg479X mutation presented with the same affected organ pattern.

Previous reports have suggested that patients with mutations in *ENG* frequently have PAVFs. In contrast, patients with mutations in *ALK1* frequently have hepatic AVFs and gastrointestinal telangiectasias but rarely have CNS-AVFs [1–3]. However, previous reports have not discussed similarity and combination of AVF patterns for each mutation.

In our analysis, approximately 70–80% of HHT patients with a previously detected genetic mutation presented with the same AVF pattern. Our result emphasizes the importance of genetic testing in HHT even if the patient had already been diagnosed according to other clinical findings.

References

1. Letteboer TG, Mager JJ, Snider RJ, et al. Genotype-phenotype relationship in hereditary haemorrhagic telangiectasia. J Med Genet. 2006;43(4):371–3.
2. Arthur H, Geisthoff U, Gossage JR, et al. Executive summary of the 11th HHT international scientific conference. Angiogenesis. 2015;18:511–24.
3. Komiyama M, Ishiguro T, Yamada O, et al. Hereditary hemorrhagic telangiectasia in Japanese patients. J Hum Genet. 2013;59:37–41.

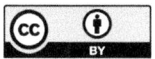

A Genetic Analysis for Patients with Pulmonary Arterial Hypertension

27

Yu Yoshida, Keiko Uchida, Kazuki Kodo, Yoshiyuki Furutani, Toshio Nakanishi, and Hiroyuki Yamagishi

Keywords

T-box · TBX4 · Pulmonary hypertension · Genetic analysis

Pulmonary arterial hypertension (PAH) is a lethal disease [1]. Although mutations in *BMPR2* and other genes have been reported, the genetic causes in large numbers of patients, especially with sporadic PAH, remain unknown. In 2013, Kerstjens-Frederikse et al. first reported *TBX4* mutations in patients with PAH [2]. TBX4 is an essential transcription factor for the development of the hindlimbs and lungs [3]. In European countries, the frequency of *TBX4* mutation was reported as 2.4–4.1% in adult-onset PAH [2, 4] and as 7.5–30% in child-onset PAH [2, 5] (Fig. 27.1). However, its frequency in Asian patients with PAH has yet to be studied.

In our genetic analysis for patients with PAH, at least nine sequence variants in exons and six sequence variants in flanking introns of *TBX4* were found. The allele frequencies of variants in the Japanese population are under investigation. The detected variants will be validated using the following web databases: UCSC genome browser (https://genome-asia.ucsc.edu), Ensembl (http://www.ensembl.org), PolyPhen-2 (http://genetics.bwh.harvard.edu/pph2), SIFT (http://sift.jcvi.org), Human Splicing Finder (http://umd.be/HSF3), and Protein Data Bank Japan (https://

Y. Yoshida · K. Uchida · K. Kodo
Department of Pediatrics, Keio University School of Medicine, Shinjuku, Tokyo, Japan

Y. Furutani · T. Nakanishi
Department of Pediatric Cardiology, Tokyo Women's Medical University, Tokyo, Japan
e-mail: nakanishi.toshio@twmu.ac.jp

H. Yamagishi (✉)
Division of Pediatric Cardiology, Department of Pediatrics,
Keio University School of Medicine, Tokyo, Japan
e-mail: hyamag@keio.jp

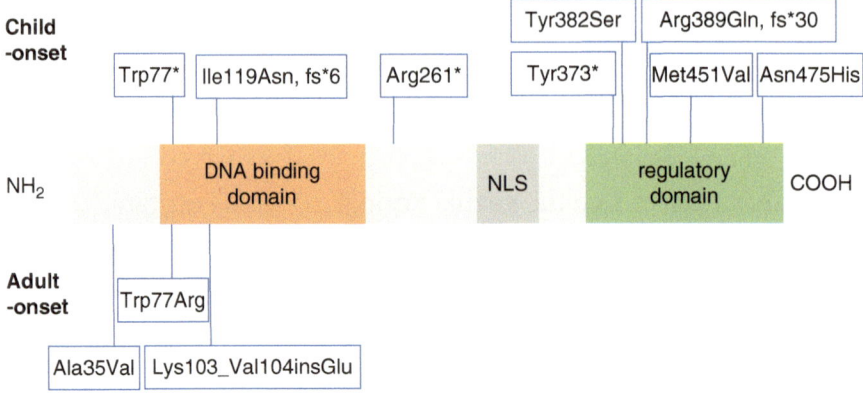

Fig. 27.1 Summary of the position of the previously reported variants in TBX4. Upper labels indicate variants with child-onset PAH; lower labels indicate variants with adult-onset PAH. *NLS* nuclear localization signal

pdbj.org) for their functional significance. We are further attempting to establish the experimental system of functional analysis for the identified variants of *TBX4* using cell culture with luciferase, immunoprecipitation, and immunohistochemistry assays in order to elucidate the molecular mechanism underlying PAH resulting from *TBX4* mutations.

This study suggests that *TBX4* may be a prevalent genetic cause of PAH not only in Caucasians but also within Japanese/Asian populations. Our ongoing studies would soon reveal the functional relevance and genotype–phenotype correlations in patients with PAH associated with *TBX4* mutations.

References

1. Chin K, Torres F, Rubin LJ. Idiopathic and heritable pulmonary hypertension: introduction to pathophysiology and clinical aspects. In: Peacock AJ, Naeije R, Rubin LJ, editors. Pulmonary circulation: diseases and their treatment. 3rd ed. London: Hodder Arnold; 2012. p. 207–11.
2. Kerstjens-Frederikse WS, Bongers EM, Roofthooft MT, et al. TBX4 mutations (small patella syndrome) are associated with childhood-onset pulmonary arterial hypertension. J Med Genet. 2013;50:500–6.
3. Papaioannou VE. The T-box gene family: emerging roles in development, stem cells and cancer. Development. 2014;141:3819–33.
4. Navas P, Tenorio J, Quezada CA, et al. Molecular analysis of BMPR2, TBX4, and KCNK3 and genotype-phenotype correlations in Spanish patients and families with idiopathic and hereditary pulmonary arterial hypertension. Rev Esp Cardiol. 2016;69:1011–9.
5. Levy M, Eyries M, Szezepanski I, et al. Genetic analyses in a cohort of children with pulmonary hypertension. Eur Respir J. 2016;48:1118–26.

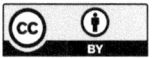

Evaluation and Visualization of the Right Ventricle Using Three-Dimensional Echocardiography

28

Yui Ito, Yusaku Kamiya, Azuma Ikari,
and Katsuaki Toyoshima

Keywords
Pulmonary hypertension · Three-dimensional echocardiography · Right ventricular
function

As neonatal right ventricular (RV) function undergoes transition from fetal to neonatal circulation, evaluation of the neonatal right ventricle is important. We analyzed the RV function of three infants with persistent pulmonary hypertension of the newborn (PPHN) using three-dimensional transthoracic echocardiography (3D echo) and herein report the results.

Patient 1 was a boy born at 40 weeks (weight, 3284 g; Apgar score (Ap), 7/8) with neonatal asphyxia, meconium aspiration syndrome, and PPHN. His oxygen saturation increased with inhaled nitric oxide (iNO) therapy; 3D echo was performed 6 and 12 h after iNO therapy.

Patient 2 was a girl born at 41 weeks (weight, 3010 g; Ap, 1/6) with neonatal asphyxia, neonatal pneumonia, and PPHN. She underwent iNO therapy and improved; 3D echo was performed before and after iNO therapy.

Patient 3 was a boy with congenital cystic adenomatoid malformation and hydrops fetalis. He was born by cesarean section at 35 weeks with uncontrollable pleural fluid and ascites. His pulmonary hypertension (PH) and respiratory condition did not improve even after thoracentesis, lobectomy, and sildenafil. He died 27 h after birth. Echocardiography was performed after lobectomy.

In each case, we performed 3D echo with an EPIQ system and X7-2 transducer (Philips Healthcare, Amsterdam, Netherlands) and analyzed the images with a TomTec system (TomTec Imaging Systems, Unterschleißheim, Germany) (Fig. 28.1). 3D data were acquired in a full-volume data set from the four-chamber

Y. Ito (✉) · Y. Kamiya · A. Ikari · K. Toyoshima
Neonatology, Kanagawa Children's Medical Center, Yokohama, Kanagawa, Japan

© The Editor(s) (if applicable) and The Author(s) 2020
T. Nakanishi et al. (eds.), *Molecular Mechanism of Congenital Heart Disease
and Pulmonary Hypertension*, https://doi.org/10.1007/978-981-15-1185-1_28

Fig. 28.1 3D RV image by a TomTec System

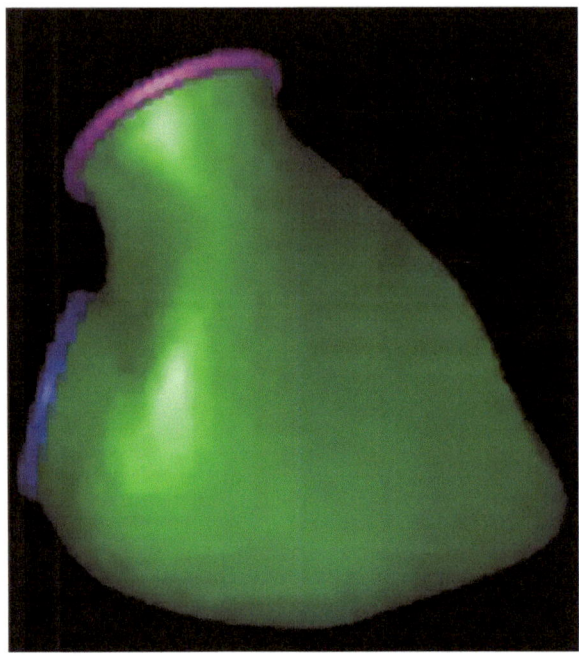

CASE1

	iNO 6h	iNO 12h
RVEDV (ml)	5.7	5.7
RVSV (ml)	1.6	2.3
RVEF (%)	28	40

CASE2

	Before iNO	After iNO
RVEDV (ml)	5.1	4.9
RVSV (ml)	1.4	1.9
RVEF (%)	28	39

CASE3

		CPAM
RVEDV (ml)		4.8
RVSV (ml)		3.5
RVEF (%)		27

Fig. 28.2 Data of RVEDV, RVSV, RVEF in Cases 1–3

apical view. The frame rate was 50 Hz. In Patient 1, the right ventricular end-diastolic volume (RVEDV) was the same (5.7 ml) at 6 and 12 h after starting iNO therapy; however, the right ventricular stroke volume (RVSV) and right ventricular ejection fraction (RVEF) increased from 1.6 to 2.3 ml and from 28% to 40%, respectively. In Patient 2, the RVEDV slightly decreased from 5.1 to 4.9 ml before and after iNO therapy. The RVSV and RVEF increased from 1.4 to 1.9 ml and from 28% to 39%, respectively. In Patient 3, the RVEDV was 4.7 ml, RVSV was 3.5 ml, and RVEF was 27% (Fig. 28.2).

The RVEF increased in Patients 1 and 2 following the improvement of PH and remained low in Patient 3. This may suggest that RVEF is significantly correlated with PH. Murata et al. [1] reported that RVEF measured by 3D echo could help to noninvasively predict the clinical outcomes of PH. Thus, 3D echo data might be useful for evaluating patients' cardiac condition and choosing treatment.

Reference

1. Murata M. Prognostic value of three-dimensional echocardiographic right ventricular ejection fraction in patients with pulmonary arterial hypertension. Oncotarget. 2016;7(52):86781–90. https://doi.org/10.18632/oncotarget.13505.

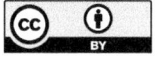

Pulmonary Hypertension Associated with Postoperative Tetralogy of Fallot

29

Jun Yasuhara and Hiroyuki Yamagishi

Keywords

Pulmonary artery · Major aortopulmonary collateral artery · Percutaneous pulmonary angioplasty · Pulmonary vascular bed · Segmental pulmonary hypertension

Pulmonary hypertension (PH) is a frequent complication in patients with congenital heart disease (CHD), before or after cardiac surgery. According to the recent clinical classification, PH associated with CHD is categorized into subclasses depending on the pathogenesis: (1) Eisenmenger syndrome, (2) left-to-right shunts, (3) PH with coincidental CHD, and (4) postoperative PH [1]. Postoperative PH means that CHD was repaired, but PH either persists immediately after surgery or recurs/develops months or years after surgery, in the absence of significant postoperative hemodynamic lesions. The anatomical features are varied and the clinical phenotype is often aggressive [2–4].

We encountered many patients with PH associated with postoperative tetralogy of Fallot (TOF), especially those with major aortopulmonary collateral arteries (MAPCAs). The etiology of PH associated with TOF with or without MAPCAs is uncertain. During cardiovascular development, MAPCAs are formed to supply blood flow to the lungs through remnants of inter-segmental arteries (ISAs) as a result of abnormal regression of the sixth pharyngeal arch arteries (PAA) in the embryonic stages (Fig. 29.1). Maldevelopment of the sixth PAA also leads to

J. Yasuhara
Department of Pediatrics, Keio University School of Medicine, Shinjuku, Tokyo, Japan

H. Yamagishi (✉)
Division of Pediatric Cardiology, Department of Pediatrics,
Keio University School of Medicine, Tokyo, Japan
e-mail: hyamag@keio.jp

T. Nakanishi et al. (eds.), *Molecular Mechanism of Congenital Heart Disease and Pulmonary Hypertension*, https://doi.org/10.1007/978-981-15-1185-1_29

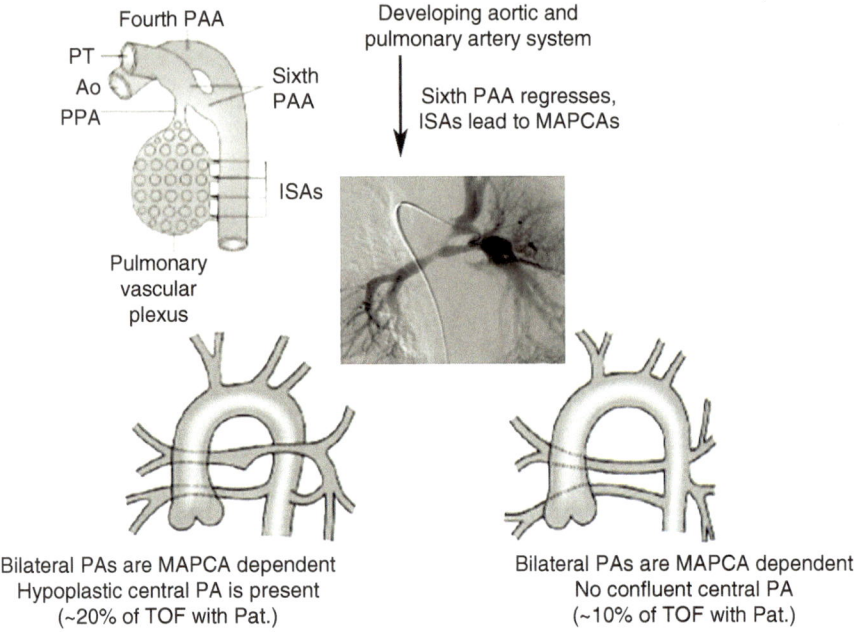

Fig. 29.1 Development of the aortic and pulmonary artery system, and the genesis of major aorto-pulmonary collateral arteries (MAPCAs). MAPCAs are formed to supply blood flow to the lungs through remnants of inter-segmental arteries (ISAs). Types of pulmonary blood supply in tetralogy of Fallot (TOF) with pulmonary atresia (Pat.) are illustrated with approximate frequencies. Pulmonary angiography of the patient is also shown. *Ao* aorta, *PA* pulmonary artery, *PAA* pharyngeal arch artery, *PPA* peripheral pulmonary artery, *PT* pulmonary trunk

hypoplasia or aplasia of the ductus arteriosus and peripheral pulmonary artery (PPA). The postoperative TOF, especially with MAPCAs, was implicated in hypoplasia of the lungs and pulmonary vasculature, thrombosis, and/or previously large systemic-to-pulmonary shunts. MAPCAs are connected to hypoplastic or segmentally unequal pulmonary vascular beds and branches, resulting in arborization abnormalities as observed in the pulmonary angiography (Fig. 29.1) [5]. We, therefore, speculate that inadequate pulmonary vascular beds due to segmentally unequal pulmonary blood flow, vascular spasm in the area of alveolar hypoventilation, and/or residual peripheral pulmonary stenosis (PPS) may result in high pulmonary blood pressure in postoperative TOF with MAPCAs. The hemodynamic and clinical presentations of patients with PH associated with postoperative TOF and MAPCAs are sometimes similar to those in Eisenmenger syndrome.

To better recognize the PH associated with TOF, especially with MAPCAs, the updated subclass as "segmental PH associated with CHD" should be important. Our clinical experience suggests that PH-targeted therapy may be effective for some of such patients, especially combined with percutaneous pulmonary angioplasty for the repair of residual PPS.

References

1. Simonneau G, Gatzoulis MA, Adatia I, et al. Updated clinical classification of pulmonary hypertension. J Am Coll Cardiol. 2013;62(25 Suppl):D34–41. https://doi.org/10.1016/j.jacc.2013.10.029.
2. Ivy DD, Abman SH, Barst RJ, et al. Pediatric pulmonary hypertension. J Am Coll Cardiol. 2013;62(25 Suppl):D117–26. https://doi.org/10.1016/j.jacc.2013.10.028.
3. D'Alto M, Mahadevan VS. Pulmonary arterial hypertension associated with congenital heart disease. Eur Respir Rev. 2012;21(126):328–37. https://doi.org/10.1183/09059180.00004712.
4. Marelli AJ, Mackie AS, Ionescu-Ittu R, et al. Congenital heart disease in the general population: changing prevalence and age distribution. Circulation. 2007;115(2):163–72.
5. Yasuhara J, Yamagishi H. Pulmonary arterial hypertension associated with tetralogy of Fallot. Int Heart J. 2015;56:S17–21. https://doi.org/10.1536/ihj.14-351.

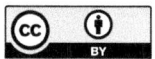

Microscopic Lung Airway Abnormality and Pulmonary Vascular Disease Associated with Congenital Systemic-to-Pulmonary Shunt

30

Hirofumi Sawada, Yoshihide Mitani, Hiroyuki Ohashi, Shoichiro Otsuki, Noriko Yodoya, Hidetoshi Hayakawa, Hironori Oshita, Jane C. Kabwe, Takeshi Konuma, Kyoko Imanaka-Yoshida, Hideto Shimpo, Kazuo Maruyama, and Masahiro Hirayama

Keywords

Pulmonary hypertension · Congenital heart disease · Lung biopsy · Pulmonary vascular disease

Links between impaired lung development/growth and pulmonary hypertension (PH) have been demonstrated in infants with bronchopulmonary dysplasia or congenital diaphragmatic hernia. Experimental studies also suggest that a complex interplay of epithelial-endothelial cells is required for normal pre/postnatal lung

H. Sawada (✉)
Departments of Pediatrics, Mie University School of Medicine, Tsu, Mie, Japan

Department of Anesthesiology and Critical Care Medicine, Mie University School of Medicine, Tsu, Mie, Japan
e-mail: hsawada@clin.medic.mie-u.ac.jp

Y. Mitani · H. Ohashi · S. Otsuki · N. Yodoya · H. Hayakawa · H. Oshita · M. Hirayama
Departments of Pediatrics, Mie University School of Medicine, Tsu, Mie, Japan

J. C. Kabwe · K. Maruyama
Department of Anesthesiology and Critical Care Medicine, Mie University School of Medicine, Tsu, Mie, Japan

T. Konuma · H. Shimpo
Department of Thoracic and Cardiovascular Surgery, Mie University School of Medicine, Tsu, Mie, Japan

K. Imanaka-Yoshida
Department of Pathology, Mie University School of Medicine, Tsu, Mie, Japan

© The Editor(s) (if applicable) and The Author(s) 2020
T. Nakanishi et al. (eds.), *Molecular Mechanism of Congenital Heart Disease and Pulmonary Hypertension*, https://doi.org/10.1007/978-981-15-1185-1_30

morphogenesis [1]. In this chapter, we focus on the role of lung development/growth abnormality in the development of pulmonary vascular disease (PVD) associated with congenital heart defect (CHD).

Children with large systemic-to-pulmonary shunt typically exhibit symptoms of heart failure in early infancy (tachypnea, failure to thrive), have PH with increased pulmonary blood flow and do not develop irreversible PVD if closure of defect is performed before 9 months to 2 years of age [2]. In general, the patient's age and type of lesion contribute to the risk of developing irreversible PVD. Conditions with pressure overload and high flow, such as large ventricular septal defect or patent ductus arteriosus, are likely to cause PVD earlier than low-pressure, high-flow lesions (pre-tricuspid shunt such as atrial septal defect). However, we sometimes encounter children with "atypical" PH which is associated with CHD but unexplained by the type or magnitude of coexisting CHD (e.g., pre-tricuspid shunt or small post-tricuspid shunt with severe PH and elevated pulmonary vascular resistance [PVR]; large post-tricuspid shunt lacking symptom of heart failure due to high PVR sustained from neonatal period.

Our recent observation suggests that microscopic airway abnormality caused by genetic or pre/postnatal conditions may be associated with PVD in infants with "atypical" PH.

References

1. Abman SH. Bronchopulmonary dysplasia: "a vascular hypothesis". Am J Respir Crit Care Med. 2001;164:1755–6.
2. Rabinovitch M, Keane JF, Norwood WI, et al. Vascular structure in lung tissue obtained at biopsy correlated with pulmonary hemodynamic findings after repair of congenital heart defects. Circulation. 1984;69:655–67.

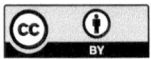

Respiratory Syncytial Virus Infection in Infants with Heart and Lung Diseases

Hiroyuki Yamagishi

Abstract

Respiratory syncytial virus (RSV) is a major causative agent of respiratory infection in infants because of its affinity for bronchial and alveolar epithelial cells. Serious and sometimes fatal RSV infection may develop in premature infants as well as infants with chronic lung disease and congenital heart disease (CHD). In infants with CHD, the addition of RSV infection to the underlying respiratory pathology resulting from increase or decrease in pulmonary blood flow may cause significant problems such as serious symptoms, increases in hospitalization rate, postponement of elective heart surgery, or death. Strict infection control measures with administration of anti-RSV antibody are essential in the management of infants with heart and lung diseases.

31.1 Clinical Characteristics of RSV Infection

Respiratory syncytial virus (RSV) accounts for more than 30% of hospitalizations of children under 3 years of age due to respiratory infection [1]. RSV infection typically develops acute upper respiratory tract inflammation associated with watery nasal discharge, cough, and fever. Although RSV infection causes only mild or moderate upper respiratory tract inflammation in most adults and older children, serious RSV infection may develop in babies and young infants who often experience acute bronchiolitis and pneumonia associated with expiratory wheezing and tachypnea. Serious and sometimes fatal RSV infection may develop in infants with

H. Yamagishi (✉)

Division of Pediatric Cardiology, Department of Pediatrics,
Keio University School of Medicine, Tokyo, Japan
e-mail: hyamag@keio.jp

underlying conditions such as a history of premature birth, chronic lung disease (CLD), and congenital heart disease (CHD).

31.2 Impact of RSV Infection on CHD

RSV infection in infants with CHD is of particular significance in the following respects:

1. Severe RSV infection may develop in infants with CHD [2, 3].
   (a) The rate of hospitalization due to RSV infection is higher in infants with CHD than in those without CHD.
   (b) The use of ICU care and ventilation for the treatment of RSV infection is more common in infants with CHD than in those without CHD.
   (c) Mortality due to RSV infection is higher in infants with CHD than in those without CHD.
2. The prognosis of surgical treatment for CHD (open heart surgery) is poor when surgery is performed before complete recovery from RSV infection [4].

31.3 Respiratory Pathophysiology and Severe RSV Infection in Infants with CHD

CHD is classified into two main classes: left-to-right shunt lesion associated with congestive heart failure and right-to-left shunt lesion associated with cyanosis. In both types of CHD, infants typically have the respiratory pathophysiological changes which may predispose to severe RSV infection [5].

Normal respiratory function in normal infants features sufficient tidal volume, pulmonary compliance, and airway resistance. It is known that RSV infection decreases alveolar liquid clearance and pulmonary compliance by injuring alveolar epithelial cells and inducing inflammatory edema of tissues surrounding the peripheral pulmonary arteries. Bronchiolitis due to RSV infection causes airway obstruction with increase in airway resistance as well. These changes result in decrease in tidal volume and increase in imbalance of ventilation and blood flow (V/Q mismatch), which promote hypoxemia and hypercapnia.

In cases of CHD with a left-to-right shunt such as ventricular septal defect and patent ductus arteriosus, increases in pulmonary capillary wedge pressure and left atrial pressure due to the increase in pulmonary blood flow are observed, and pulmonary hypertension may occur in some cases. Due to the presence of extravasation of fluid resulting from increased blood flow and pressure in the pulmonary vessels, the excessive fluid leaking into interstitial tissues tends to flow into the alveoli. In cases of significant pulmonary congestion, decrease in pulmonary compliance and increase in airway resistance due to compression of the airways by surrounding dilated vessels may occur, resulting in increase in respiratory rate. When children with such underlying conditions contract RSV infection, alveolar liquid compliance and lung compliance will be further decreased, and airway resistance will rapidly increase. As a result, lung tissue swelling and pulmonary edema may develop with decrease in functional residual capacity and rapid deterioration of V/Q mismatch, and severe respiratory signs/symptoms may occur. RSV infection may become particularly serious in children with pulmonary hypertension, who must thus be monitored carefully.

On the other hand, in cases of CHD with right-to-left shunt and decrease in pulmonary blood flow such as the tetralogy of Fallot, cyanosis and hypoxemia are constantly present. Due to the small lung volume and underdevelopment of airways resulting from low pulmonary blood flow, peripheral airway resistance is high and lung compliance is low in such patients. Although this type of CHD is not frequently associated with pulmonary edema, unlike CHD with increased pulmonary blood flow, RSV infection accelerates the increase in airway resistance and decrease in pulmonary compliance with significant deterioration of cyanosis and hypoxemia and development of severe respiratory signs and symptoms.

In cases of complex heart disease such as complete transposition of the great arteries and hypoplastic left heart syndrome, which are characterized by increase in pulmonary blood flow and hypoxemia, mixtures of the above-described pathophysiological conditions are present, and RSV infection induces clinical deterioration.

31.4 Prevention of RSV Infection in Infants with CHD

To date, no specific treatment for RSV infection has been established. Therefore, prevention of RSV infection is essential in the management of infants with CHD.

In our hospital, infants and young children ≤3 years of age are usually hospitalized in the infant ward (a large room) with full nursing service. In the infant ward, standard infection control procedures including hand washing when entering and leaving the ward, hand disinfection before and after examining each patient, wearing a gown specific to each patient, and use of a stethoscope specific to each patient are strictly adhered to. Since many children hospitalized in the infant ward have CHD and/or CLD and are at high risk for severe RSV infection, all children to be hospitalized in the infant ward are subjected to a rapid RSV antigen test in the ambulatory setting on the day of hospitalization during RSV infection is prevalent. Children with a positive test for RSV antigen are not allowed to enter the infant ward and are hospitalized in a private room or referred to other hospitals. The first step to preventing RSV infection in infants with CHD is preventing sources of infection from entering the infant ward.

When signs/symptoms of respiratory infection develop in patients hospitalized in the infant ward especially during the period of prevalent RSV infection, they are subjected to a rapid RSV antigen test to detect RSV infection as early as possible. Children with mild RSV infection (a positive RSV antigen test) who do not require ventilation or intensive care are transferred to private rooms with prior consent while children with severe RSV infection requiring ventilation and/or intensive care, who are difficult to care for in private rooms, enter the infant ICU with the following measures taken to avoid transmission of RSV infection. Each infected child's bed is surrounded by portable partitions with metal frames and transparent plastic panels to separate the child from others and avoid droplet infection in the crowded infant ward, which features small distances between beds. In addition, a hand washer and a specific door to the infant ward are used only by healthcare professionals and visitors who care for children with RSV infection to ensure separation of them in the infant ward. Children with RSV infection are attended only by designated nurses who do not attend other children.

Education of staff members is essential to ensuring appropriate infection control measures. In the CDC's guidelines, education of hospital staff is rated as Category IA [6]. In our hospital, an infection control section regularly provides "pediatric infection control seminars" by pediatric infection specialists in order to increase awareness of infection control.

31.5   The Use of Palivizumab in Infants with CHD

A humanized monoclonal antibody specific to RSV (palivizumab, Synagis®) was developed and released. Palivizumab is an antibody specific to the antigenic region of the F protein of RSV, neutralizes the infectivity of RSV, inhibits amplification and growth of RSV, and thereby prevents the onset of severe lower respiratory tract disease.

From 1998 to 2002, a multicenter clinical study of palivizumab in CHD patients was conducted in Europe and the United States. A total of 1, 287 children were randomized and allocated to a palivizumab group (639 children) or placebo group (648 children). The rate of hospitalization due to RSV infection was decreased by 45% in the palivizumab group (9.7% in the placebo group vs. 5.3% in the palivizumab group; $p = 0.03$) [7]. Palivizumab was administered intramuscularly at a dose of 15 mg/kg body weight every month throughout the RSV season.

In October 2005, palivizumab was approved for infants with CHD by the National Health Insurance in Japan, and Japanese guidelines for the use of palivizumab in infants with CHD was prepared [8]. Since palivizumab does not affect the efficacy of vaccinations, treatment with it can be continued without changing vaccination schedules. Even if RSV infection develops during treatment with palivizumab, palivizumab should continue to be administered thereafter during the RSV season since reinfection with RSV causing serious disease may occur during the same season.

31.6   Conclusions and Future Perspectives

Cox et al. noted that "conventional infection control measures failed to prevent spread of RSV infection, and palivizumab could prevent occurrence of nosocomial RSV infections" [9]. We believe that performance of standard infection control measures considering the mode of transmission of RSV and education of hospital staff are important steps in preventing RSV infection in children with CHD. Efforts to detect sources of infection as early as possible and use of preventive treatment with palivizumab are also essential.

It has been generally accepted that palivizumab should be administered from September–October to March–April in Japan. However, a child with a positive RSV antigen test is recently often observed in May, July, and August. Duration of palivizumab treatment should thus be modified based on the prevalence of RSV infection in the relevant geographical area and trends in the incidence of RSV infection in each year. It is preferable that serum palivizumab concentration be high enough to ensure prevention of RSV infection. Physicians should also consider whether to perform additional administration of palivizumab after surgery using cardiopulmonary bypass, which is known to decrease serum palivizumab concentration. Although no serious adverse events related to treatment with palivizumab have been reported, monitoring should be continued to ensure the safety of palivizumab treatment in each year.

References

1. Kaneko M, Watanabe J, Kuwahara M, et al. Impact of respiratory syncytial virus infection as a cause of lower respiratory tract infection in children younger than 3 years of age in Japan. J Infect. 2002;44:240–3.
2. Boyce TG, Mellen BG, Mitchel EF Jr, et al. Rates of hospitalization for respiratory syncytial virus infection among children in Medicaid. J Pediatr. 2000;137:865–70.
3. Navas L, Wang E, de Carvalho V, Robinson J. Pediatric Investigators Collaborative Network on Infections in Canada; Improved outcome of respiratory syncytial virus infection in a high-risk hospitalized population of Canadian children. J Pediatr. 1992;121:348–54.
4. Khongphatthanayothin A, Wong PC, Samara Y, et al. Impact of respiratory syncytial virus infection on surgery for congenital heart disease: postoperative course and outcome. Crit Care Med. 1999;27:1974–81.
5. MacDonald NE, et al. Respiratory syncytial viral infection in infants with congenital heart disease. N Engl J Med. 1982;307:397–400.
6. Greenough A. Respiratory syncytial virus infection; clinical features, management, and prophylaxis. Curr Opin Pulm Med. 2002;8:214–7.
7. Feltes TF, Cabalka AK, Meissner HC, et al. Palivizumab prophylaxis reduces hospitalization due to respiratory syncytial virus in young children with hemodynamically significant congenital heart disease. J Pediatr. 2003;143:532–40.
8. Nakazawa M, Saji T, Ichida F, et al. Guideline for the use of palivizumab in infants and young children with congenital heart disease. Pediatr Int. 2006;48:190–3.
9. Cox RA, Rao P, Brandon-Cox C, et al. The use of palivizumab monoclonal antibody to control an outbreak of nosocomial respiratory syncytial virus infection in a special care baby unit. J Hosp Infect. 2001;48:186–92.

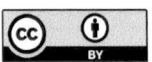

Part III

Ductus Arteriosus:
Bridge Over Troubled Vessels

Perspective for Part III

32

Toshio Nakanishi

The ductus arteriosus (DA) is open before birth and normally closes after birth. The unique anatomy and normal and abnormal behavior of the DA are discussed by Gittenberger, Shelton, and Sterren in this chapter.

The DA sometimes closes before birth or does not close after birth; both situations cause problems. Normally only 10–20% of right ventricular output goes to the lung and the rest goes to the aorta though DA during fetal life. If the DA closes before birth, right ventricular afterload increases because the right ventricle has to eject blood to the lung, which has high pulmonary arterial resistance. Early closure of the DA may result in right ventricular hypertrophy and somehow left ventricular dilatation [1].

If the DA does not close after birth, left (aorta) to right (pulmonary artery) shunt occurs, resulting in patent DA. In congenital heart diseases with severe outflow stenosis or atresia to the pulmonary artery, pulmonary circulation is dependent on the DA from the aorta. In hypoplastic left heart syndrome, systemic circulation is dependent on the DA from the pulmonary artery. Thus, the DA is clinically an important bridge over troubled vessels.

The precise mechanisms for the DA closure after birth remain unclear. The trigger for the DA closure is most likely O_2, but how O_2 causes DA closure has not been clarified. We [2] reported that ATP-sensitive K channel (KATP) might be an O_2 sensor, which causes DA closure based on in vitro experiments. Momma et al. also report in this symposium that inhibition of KATP results in closure of DA in in vivo experiments. The group of Archer, however, reported that voltage-dependent K channels (Kv) might be an O_2 sensor [3, 4]. They suggest that Kv channels close in the DA, resulting in DA closure, and open in the pulmonary artery, resulting in pulmonary artery dilation, in response to O_2 and reactive oxygen species produced in mitochondria.

T. Nakanishi (✉)

Department of Pediatric Cardiology, Tokyo Women's Medical University, Tokyo, Japan
e-mail: nakanishi.toshio@twmu.ac.jp

In addition to O_2, prostaglandin E plays an important role in opening DA before birth and closure of DA after birth. Prostaglandin E concentration in the neonatal blood decreases after birth, facilitating DA closure. Furthermore, Yokoyama et al. [5, 6] have shown that prostaglandin E and its receptor EP4 promote neointimal formation during fetal life and inhibit elastic fiber formation, preparing DA closure after birth.

The DA is such an important and interesting vessel. Further investigation of the O_2 sensor in the DA is necessary because the O_2 sensor is biologically important not only in the DA but also in other vessels such as the pulmonary artery. Basic research regarding arterial elastogenesis could be expanded to the aorta in which the elastic fiber is disrupted in some patients with tetralogy of Fallot [7].

References

1. Momma K, Takao A. Right ventricular concentric hypertrophy and left ventricular dilatation by ductal constriction in fetal rats. Circ Res. 1989;64:1137–46.
2. Nakanishi T, Gu H, Hagiwara N, Momma K. Mechanisms of oxygen-induced contraction of ductus arteriosus isolated from the fetal rabbit. Circ Res 1993;72(6):1218–1228.
3. Tristani-Firouzi M, Reeve HL, Tolarova S, Weir EK, Archer SL. Oxygen-induced constriction of rabbit ductus arteriosus occurs via inhibition of a 4-aminopyridine-, voltage-sensitive potassium channel. J Clin Invest. 1996;98:1959–65.
4. Kajimoto H, Hashimoto K, Bonnet SN, Haromy A, Harry G, Moudgil R, Nakanishi T, Rebeyka I, Thébaud B, Michelakis ED, Archer SL. Oxygen activates the Rho/Rho-kinase pathway and induces RhoB and ROCK-1 expression in human and rabbit ductus arteriosus by increasing mitochondria-derived reactive oxygen species: a newly recognized mechanism for sustaining ductal constriction. Circulation 2007;115(13):1777–1788.
5. Yokoyama U, Minamisawa S, Quan H, Ghatak S, Akaike T, Segi-Nishida E, Iwasaki S, Iwamoto M, Misra S, Tamura K, Hori H, Yokota S, Toole BP, Sugimoto Y, Ishikawa Y. Chronic activation of the prostaglandin receptor EP4 promotes hyaluronan-mediated neointimal formation in the ductus arteriosus. J Clin Invest 2006;116(11):3026–3034.
6. Yokoyama U, Minamisawa S, Shioda A, Ishiwata R, Jin MH, Masuda M, Asou T, Sugimoto Y, Aoki H, Nakamura T, Ishikawa Y. Prostaglandin E2 inhibits elastogenesis in the ductus arteriosus via EP4 signaling. Circulation 2014;129(4):487–496.
7. Niwa K, Perloff JK, Bhuta SM, Laks H, Drinkwater DC, Child JS, Miner PD. Structural abnormalities of great arterial walls in congenital heart disease: light and electron microscopic analyses. Circulation 2001;103(3):393–400.

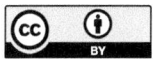

The Ductus Arteriosus, a Vascular Outsider, in Relation to the Pulmonary Circulation

33

Adriana C. Gittenberger-de Groot, Arno A. W. Roest,
Regina Bökenkamp, Monique R. M. Jongbloed,
Margot M. Bartelings, Marco C. DeRuiter,
and Robert E. Poelmann

Abstract

The muscular ductus arteriosus (DA) has many unique characteristics setting it apart from the adjoining elastic arteries. Preparation for neonatal closure takes place in utero with the development of intimal thickening. Ductus-specific gene and protein expression patterns were demonstrated during this process. We postulated that the closing process, with increased expression of progerin, might reflect aspects of premature ageing. Persistent patency of the DA, can be congenitally or immaturity based. During embryonic development the sixth pharyngeal arch arteries are the last to develop. In avian embryos this arch is divided into a proximal (part of the future pulmonary artery) and a distal part (on the left side the origin of the DA). The consequence is that the pulmonary arteries have a double vascular contribution being a proximal sixth arch artery component and

A. C. Gittenberger-de Groot (✉)
Department of Cardiology, Leiden University Medical Center, Leiden, The Netherlands
e-mail: acgitten@lumc.nl

A. A. W. Roest · R. Bökenkamp
Department of Pediatrics, Leiden University Medical Center, Leiden, The Netherlands

M. R. M. Jongbloed
Department of Cardiology, Leiden University Medical Center, Leiden, The Netherlands

Department of Anatomy and Embryology, Leiden University Medical Center, Leiden, The Netherlands

M. M. Bartelings · M. C. DeRuiter
Department of Anatomy and Embryology, Leiden University Medical Center, Leiden, The Netherlands

R. E. Poelmann
Department of Cardiology, Leiden University Medical Center, Leiden, The Netherlands

Department of Animal Sciences and Health, Leiden University, Leiden, The Netherlands

a distal true pulmonary artery segment. We have conclusive evidence that this is not encountered in the human embryo. Both sixth arch arteries and the right and left pulmonary arteries connect separately and at distinct locations to the pulmonary trunk side of the aortic sac. The insertion of the wall of the DA between the proximal and distal part of the left pulmonary artery, referred to as pulmonary coarctation, constitutes a congenital malformation and not a remnant of what is encountered during normal development. This configuration is found almost exclusively in combination with pulmonary atresia leading to neonatal interruption of the proximal left pulmonary artery with consequences for surgical or intervention repair.

Keywords
Vascular development · Patent ductus arteriosus · Persistent ductus arteriosus · Congenital heart disease · Pulmonary atresia · Pulmonary ductal coarctation · Juxtaductal pulmonary coarctation

33.1   The Normal Closing Ductus Arteriosus

The DA is a functional shunt before birth, directing oxygen-rich blood to the systemic circulation, bypassing the pulmonary circulation. Perinatally, the DA shows a physiological contraction followed by anatomical closure after birth. Eventually the closed DA is remodeled into a fibrous strand, the ligamentum arteriosum [1]. The characteristics of the muscular DA are reflected in its histological make-up, setting it apart from the elastic adjoining arteries [2]. Around 17 weeks of human gestation there is the start of formation of typical intimal thickenings (cushions). The first indication is the subendothelial appearance of hyaluronic acid and detachment of the endothelium [3]. The process of hyaluronic acid production continues during ductal maturation and even after birth [4]. In the second half of gestation the maturation process progresses and marked intimal thickenings develop containing media-derived synthetic smooth muscle cells and fine elastin fibers [5]. Accompanying the first physiological contractions the DA develops degeneration of the inner media, showing apoptosis and extracellular matrix filled mucoid lakes [5]. A recent study shows that this process is accompanied by a different lamin A/C to progerin balance. Progerin, an indicator of vascular ageing, is increased in the mature DA [6]. This observation has lead us to postulate that a process akin to premature ageing might accompany postnatal ductal closure [6]. In Fig. 33.1, schematic and correlating histological features of the DA are presented.

More advanced methodology has allowed to shift focus to the unique gene and protein profiles of the DA. The data derive from DNA microarray profiling [7], transcriptional profiles [8] and gene profiling after single-cell microcapture isolation [9]. These studies unravel pieces of the puzzle underlying DA closure and maturation. Results show that the important relaxing factor, PGE2, inhibits elastogenesis, clarifying the muscular nature of the DA [10]. Furthermore the endothelin receptor EP4 promotes hyaluronic acid–induced intimal thickening [4].

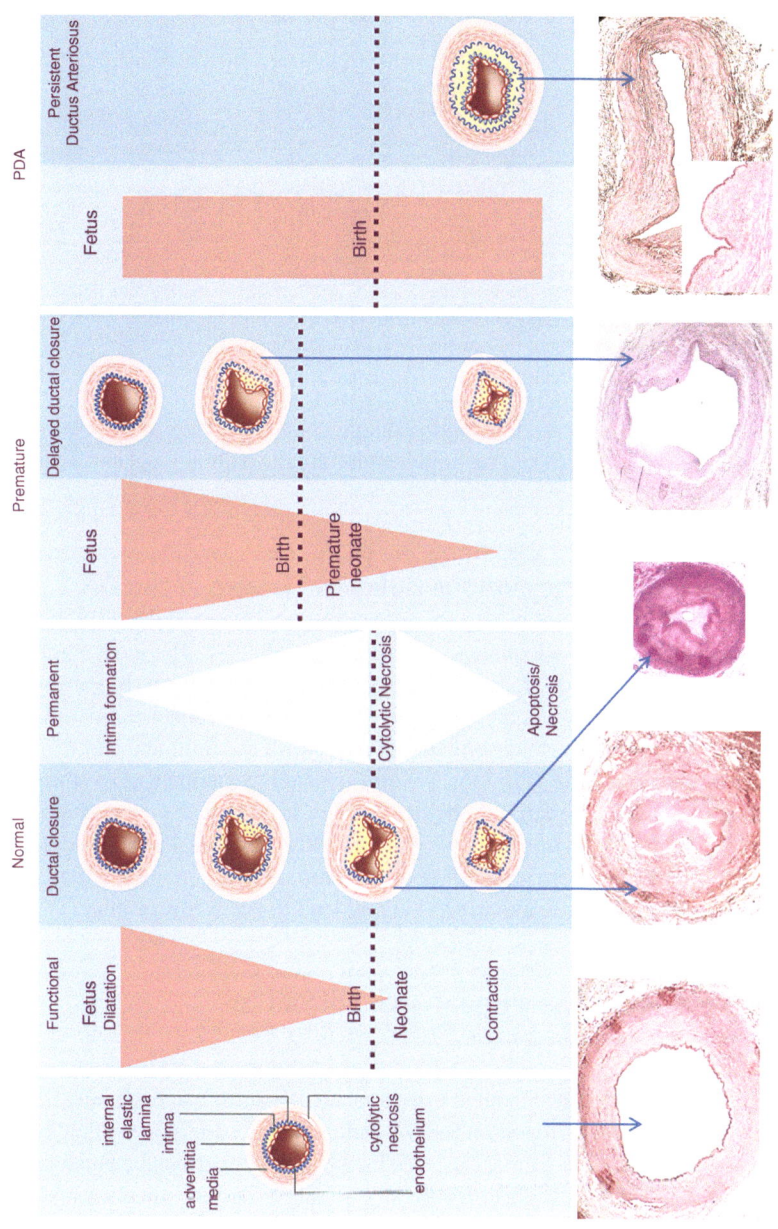

Fig. 33.1 Schematic presentation of normal closure, delayed closure and persistent patency of the ductus arteriosus with corresponding histology and histopathology (Modified after [1])

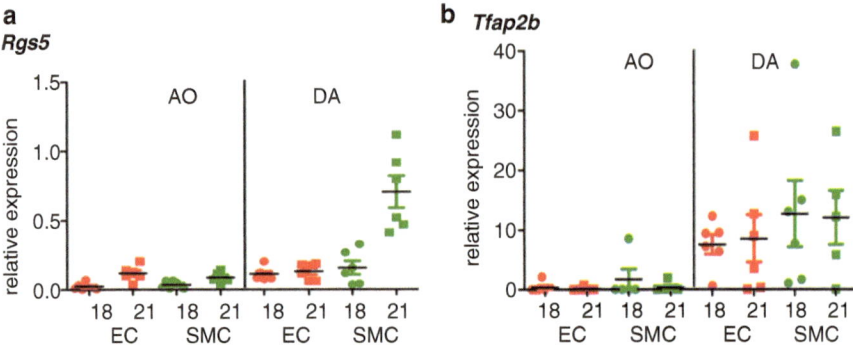

Fig. 33.2 Relative gene expression levels of Rgs5 and Tfap2B after microarray and quantitative RT-PCR, showing the differences between endothelial cells (EC: red) and smooth muscle cells (SMC: green) in aorta (Ao) and ductus arteriosus (DA) (Modified after [9])

With increased information, showing the distinct characteristics of smooth muscle and endothelial cells (Fig. 33.2) we gain insight into the pathological and delayed DA closure.

33.2 Persistent Patency Versus Delayed Closure of the DA

Several causes lead to a non-adequate to non-closure of the DA. The most common cause is delayed closure after premature birth because of immaturity of the ductal wall [5]. A different cause for ductal patency is a structural wall abnormality inhibiting anatomical closing. We have described that a DA with an additional and marked subendothelial elastic lamina (Fig. 33.1) is not capable of permanent anatomical closure [2]. As this anomaly can only be detected by histology, it poses a problem to differentiate it clinically from delayed closure. Very little is known about the genetic or environmental background of persistent DA. A few genes have been discovered like the TFAP2B gene mutation [11] that lead to persistent patency.

33.3 Normal Sixth Pharyngeal Arch Formation and Connections to the Surrounding Arteries

During development, pharyngeal arch arteries connect the aortic sac bilaterally to the dorsal aortae. The sixth arch, important for DA and pulmonary artery formation, has a separate status [12]. In various animal species it has been described that the putative left and right pulmonary arteries connect end to side to the sixth pharyngeal arch artery [13]. We have shown in quail embryos that this connection results from ingrowth of the pulmonary sprout into the sixth arch artery opposed to an outgrowth towards the lung mesenchyme [12]. This implies that the proximal part of the sixth arch artery forms the proximal part of the left pulmonary artery while the distal end develops the

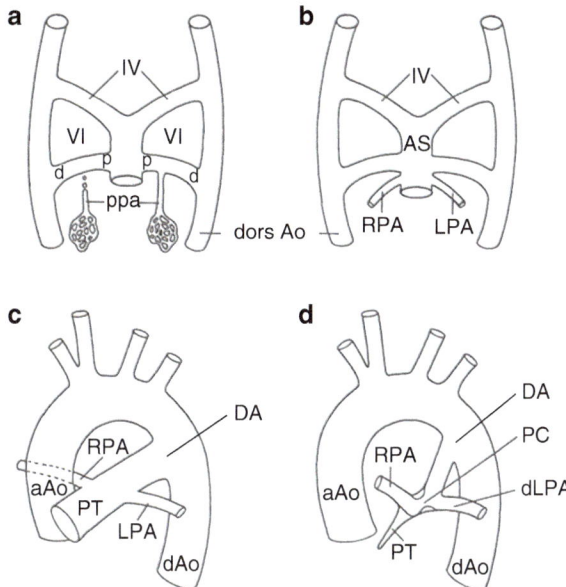

Fig. 33.3 (**a**) Schematic configuration of end-to-side ingrowth of pulmonary sprout (ppa) between the proximal (p) and distal (d) part of the sixth arch artery (VI). (**b**) Situation as encountered in a 6 week human embryo with right (RPA) and left (LPA) arteries connecting to the aortic sac (AS). (**c**) Normal neonatal situation with distinct connections of RPA, LPA and ductus arteriosus (DA) to the pulmonary trunk (PT). (**d**) Pulmonary coarctation (PC) in a case of pulmonary atresia. Ascending aorta (aAo), descending aorta (dAo), fourth arch artery (IV)

characteristic DA structure. This necessitates a major remodeling process to achieve the mature situation in the human fetus and neonate in which the DA and left and right pulmonary arteries have a distinct connection site with the pulmonary trunk (Fig. 33.3). Investigation of human embryos, before 6 weeks of age, revealed that the ingrowth of the pulmonary arteries together with the proximal part of the sixth arch is incorporated into the pulmonary side of the aortic sac. Thus the distal part of the left-sided sixth pharyngeal artery develops into the left-sided DA. The distal right-sided sixth arch disappears together with the distal part of the right-sided dorsal aorta early in development by selective apoptosis [14]. These observations in the human embryo are relevant for understanding some forms of congenital heart disease and related complications.

33.4   Pulmonary Coarctation (PC) and Proximal Left Pulmonary Artery Interruption

DA problems can exist in right heart congenital heart disease with narrowing to atresia of the right ventricular outflow tract and hypoplasia of the pulmonary trunk. The most extreme is complete absence of the DA with the question whether a sixth arch artery ever developed. The VEGF120/120 mouse revealed that with increase of mild pulmonary stenosis towards complete atresia the DA became hypoplastic to atretic. In the most severe cases major aorto-pulmonary collateral arteries (MAPCAs) developed [15]. We published data on a set of human neonatal specimens with various degrees of pulmonary stenosis and atresia that had developed a PC [16]. We assumed that this anomaly mimicked the aortic coarctation in which DA tissue extends within the inner circumference of the aortic arch in which the roof of the coarctation always consisted of elastic aorta tissue (Fig. 33.2). More recent observations showed that PDC could lead to a complete obstruction of the proximal left pulmonary artery. DA tissue was, however, not only observed on the inside lining of the pulmonary artery but could completely encircle the lumen [17], being thus interposed between the proximal and distal part of the left pulmonary artery. Progressive narrowing by DA tissue could result in left pulmonary artery interruption. We concluded that a more left lateral insertion of the DA into the left pulmonary artery is not a normal position but a congenital anomaly. Reversed hemodynamics through the DA might play a secondary role as cause for PC.

33.5 Future Directions and Clinical Implications

- Is PC exclusively linked to anomalies with pulmonary atresia or can it also be associated with less severe obstructions of the right ventricular outflow tract and pulmonary valve?
- Is there a link to the 22q11 deletion syndrome and thus to mutations within the second heart field and its interaction with neural crest cells?
- A clinical implication of the complete encircling of the DA tissue of the left pulmonary artery is that by surgical restoration of the left pulmonary artery it should be aimed to completely excise the DA tissue or completely stent the DA-infested region.

References

1. Bökenkamp R, DeRuiter MC, VanMunsteren C, et al. Insights into the pathogenesis and genetic background of patency of the ductus arteriosus. Neonatology. 2010;98:6. https://doi.org/10.1159/000262481.
2. Gittenberger-de Groot AC. Persistent ductus arteriosus: most probably a primary congenital malformation. Br Heart J. 1977;39:610–8.
3. De Reeder EG, Girard N, Poelmann RE, et al. Hyaluronic acid accumulation and endothelial cell detachment in intimal thickening of the vessel wall; the normal and genetically defective ductus arteriosus. Am J Pathol. 1988;132:574–85.
4. Yokoyama U, Minamisawa S, Quan H, et al. Chronic activation of the prostaglandin receptor EP4 promotes hyaluronan-mediated neointimal formation in the ductus arteriosus. J Clin Invest. 2006;116:3026–34.
5. Gittenberger-de Groot AC, van Ertbruggen I, Moulaert AJ, et al. The ductus arteriosus in the preterm infant: histologic and clinical observations. J Pediatr. 1980;96:88–93.

6. Bökenkamp R, Raz V, Lie-Venema A, et al. Differential temporal and spatial progerin expression during closure of the ductus arteriosus in neonates. PLoS One. 2011;6:e23975. https://doi.org/10.1371/journal.pone.0023975.
7. Jin MH, Yokoyama U, Sato Y, et al. DNA microarray profiling identified a new role of growth hormone in vascular remodeling of rat ductus arteriosus. J Physiol Sci. 2011;61:167. https://doi.org/10.1007/s12576-011-0133-3.
8. Liu NM, Yokota T, Maekawa S, et al. Transcription profiles of endothelial cells in the rat ductus arteriosus during a perinatal period. PLoS One. 2013;8:e73685. https://doi.org/10.1371/journal.pone.0073685.
9. Bökenkamp R, van Brempt R, VanMunsteren JC, et al. Dlx1 and Rgs5 in the ductus arteriosus: vessel-specific genes identified by transcriptional profiling of laser-capture microdissected endothelial and smooth muscle cells. PLoS One. 2014;9:e86892. https://doi.org/10.1371/journal.pone.0086892.
10. Yokoyama U, Minamisawa S, Shioda A, et al. Prostaglandin E2 inhibits elastogenesis in the ductus arteriosus via EP4 signaling. Circulation. 2014;129:487. https://doi.org/10.1161/CIRCULATIONAHA.113.004726.
11. Ivey KN, Sutcliffe D, Richardson J, et al. Transcriptional regulation during development of the ductus arteriosus. Circ Res. 2008;103:388. https://doi.org/10.1161/CIRCRESAHA.108.180661.
12. DeRuiter MC, Gittenberger-de Groot AC, Poelmann RE, et al. Development of the pharyngeal arch system related to the pulmonary and bronchial vessels in the avian embryo. With a concept on systemic-pulmonary collateral artery formation. Circulation. 1993;87:1306–19.
13. Bergwerff M, DeRuiter MC, Gittenberger-de Groot AC. Comparative anatomy and ontogeny of the ductus arteriosus, a vascular outsider. Anat Embryol. 1999;200:559–71.
14. Molin DGM, DeRuiter MC, Wisse LJ, et al. Altered apoptosis pattern during pharyngeal arch artery remodelling is associated with aortic arch malformations in Tgf beta 2 knock-out mice. Cardiovasc Res. 2002;56:312–22.
15. Rammeloo LA, DeRuiter MC, van den Akker NM, et al. Development of major aorto-pulmonary collateral arteries in vegf120/120 isoform mouse embryos with tetralogy of Fallot. Pediatr Cardiol. 2015;36:89. https://doi.org/10.1007/s00246-014-0969-4.
16. Elzenga NJ, Gittenberger-de Groot AC. The ductus arteriosus and stenoses of the pulmonary arteries in pulmonary atresia. Int J Cardiol. 1986;11(2):195–208. https://doi.org/10.1016/0167-5273(86)90179-8.
17. Waldman JD, Karp RB, Gittenberger-de Groot AC, et al. Spontaneous acquisition of discontinuous pulmonary arteries. Ann Thorac Surg. 1996;62:161–8.

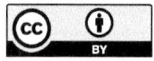

Molecular, Genetic, and Pharmacological Modulation of the Ductus Arteriosus: K$_{ATP}$ Channels as Novel Drug Targets

34

Elaine L. Shelton and Jerod S. Denton

Abstract

Maintaining fetal patency and facilitating neonatal closure of the ductus arteriosus are complex processes that involve nuanced developmental programing and a precise balance of perinatal vasodilators and constrictors. Work over the past 40 years has identified "master regulators" of ductus tone, namely oxygen, prostaglandins, and nitric oxide signaling. Yet, prolonged neonatal patency of the ductus remains a significant clinical problem with limited therapeutic options. Understanding the molecular and genetic underpinnings of normal ductus function and PDA pathophysiology will facilitate the development of new therapeutic strategies to regulate ductus tone.

Keywords

Ductus arteriosus · PDA · K$_{ATP}$ channel

E. L. Shelton (✉)

Department of Pediatrics, Monroe Carell Jr. Children's Hospital at Vanderbilt and Vanderbilt University Medical Center, Nashville, TN, USA

Department of Pharmacology, Vanderbilt University School of Medicine, Nashville, TN, USA
e-mail: Elaine.L.Shelton@vanderbilt.edu

J. S. Denton
Department of Pharmacology, Vanderbilt University School of Medicine, Nashville, TN, USA

Department of Anesthesiology, Vanderbilt University Medical Center, Nashville, TN, USA

34.1   Introduction

The ductus arteriosus (DA) is an essential fetal vessel connecting the main pulmonary artery and aorta. In utero, high pulmonary vascular resistance coupled with relatively low systemic resistance promotes right-to-left blood flow through the DA, allowing blood oxygenated by the placenta to bypass the developing lungs [1, 2]. Soon after birth, the DA must close in order to facilitate proper perfusion of the newly inflated lungs, a process normally complete by 12–48 h in full-term neonates.

In some cases, the DA fails to close after birth, a condition termed patent ductus arteriosus (PDA). PDA is a common congenital heart defect, occurring in up to 80% of premature infants weighing <1000 g [3]. Several comorbidities including neurodevelopmental impairment, intraventricular hemorrhage, pulmonary hemorrhage, respiratory distress syndrome, bronchopulmonary dysplasia, necrotizing enterocolitis, and spontaneous intestinal perforation have been attributed to or associated with prolonged patency of the DA [4]. In contrast, keeping the DA open to preserve pulmonary or systemic circulation is essential in certain cardiovascular conditions where blood flow to the lungs or body is disrupted [5]. Unfortunately, there are surprisingly few therapies currently available to promote DA closure or maintain vessel patency. Pharmacology-based therapeutics are non-specific and relatively inefficient. While surgical ligation, catheter-based closure, and stent implantation are effective alternatives, these mechanical approaches come with their own risks and are sometimes limited by the anatomical size constraints of extremely premature newborns [6].

34.2   Molecular Regulation of the DA

The fetal DA has intrinsic tone and requires factors to maintain its patency in utero (summarized in Table 34.1) [2, 7, 8]. While nitric oxide (NO) and prostaglandin E_2 (PGE_2) are typically considered the primary mediators of DA dilation, other factors clearly play a role. Potassium (K^+) channels are well-characterized

Table 34.1 Molecular regulators of DA tone

Promote DA patency	Promote DA constriction
Blood flow	Oxygen
Nitric oxide (cGMP/PKG)	Endothelin 1
Prostaglandin E2 (cAMP/PKA)	8-iso-PGF2α
Adenosine (cAMP)	Reactive oxygen species (H_2O_2)
Atrial naturetic peptide (cGMP)	TRPM3
Voltage-gated K^+ channels: Kv1.2, Kv1.5, Kv2.1	Angiotensin II
Large-conductance voltage-dependent and calcium-activated	RhoA/B, Rock1/2
(BK_{Ca}) channels	Bradykinin
ATP-gated K^+ (K_{ATP}) channels	Acetylcholine, norepinephrine

DA dilators. Voltage-gated K^+ channels, large-conductance voltage-dependent and calcium-activated K^+ (BK_{Ca}) channels, and ATP-gated K^+ (K_{ATP}) channels are all specifically enriched in the DA compared to other vascular beds [9]. K_{ATP} channels are hetero-octameric complexes of pore-forming inward rectifier K^+ channel subunits (Kir6.1 or Kir6.2) and regulatory sulfonylurea receptor subunits (SUR1, SUR2a, or SUR2b) [10]. Different combinations of these subunits are expressed in a tissue-specific manner and exhibit different pharmacological properties, thereby making them attractive targets for DA-specific therapies. This notion is supported by animal studies demonstrating that activating or inhibiting K_{ATP} channels directly modulates DA tone [11, 12].

While nitric oxide (NO) and prostaglandin E_2 (PGE_2) are typically considered the primary mediators of DA dilation, other factors clearly play a role. Potassium (K^+) channels are well-characterized DA dilators. Voltage-gated K^+ channels, large-conductance voltage-dependent and calcium-activated K^+ (BK_{Ca}) channels, and ATP-gated K^+ (K_{ATP}) channels are all specifically enriched in the DA compared to other vascular beds [9]. K_{ATP} channels are hetero-octameric complexes of pore-forming inward rectifier K^+ channel subunits (Kir6.1 or Kir6.2) and regulatory sulfonylurea receptor subunits (SUR1, SUR2a, or SUR2b) [10]. Different combinations of these subunits are expressed in a tissue specific manner and exhibit different pharmacological properties, thereby making them attractive targets for DA-specific therapies. This notion is supported by animal studies demonstrating that activating or inhibiting K_{ATP} channels directly modulates DA tone [11, 12].

At birth, the DA constricts in response to a sharp increase in oxygen (O_2) tension coupled with a loss of vasodilators. Several mechanisms have been proposed to explain the DA's unique ability to sense and respond to O_2. These include cytochrome P450-mediated induction of endothelin 1 and production of "constrictor" isoprostanes (8-iso-$PGF2\alpha$), and mitochondrial-mediated reactive oxygen species inhibition of Kv1.5 and Kv2.1 [8]. O_2 can also inhibit K_{ATP} channels resulting in membrane depolarization, activation of voltage-dependent calcium (Ca^{2+}) channels, and increased intracellular Ca^{2+} accumulation [12]. Other factors known to regulate DA contraction are listed in Table 34.1 [2, 6–8]. While it is clear that multiple mechanisms are involved, all pathways eventually converge on Ca^{2+}-mediated phosphorylation of myosin light chain, leading to actin/myosin interaction and ultimately DA smooth muscle cell contraction [2, 8].

34.3 Genetic Regulation of the DA

While occurring most often in the setting of prematurity, twin studies gave the first indication that PDA has a genetic component [6]. Several mouse models of PDA have been created and are summarized in Table 34.2 [6–8]. Not surprisingly, many of these models result from disruption of genes involved in smooth muscle function or prostaglandin signaling.

Syndromes featuring PDA (Table 34.2) can also be informative regarding genetic regulation of DA development and function [6, 13]. For instance, clinically

Table 34.2 Genetic regulators of DA tone

Mouse models of PDA	Human syndromes	Non-syndromic SNPs
Smooth muscle related:	Char (TFAP2B)	*Increased risk of PDA*:
Tfap2b$^{-/-}$	Mowat-Wilson (SMADIP1)	TFAP2B (rs987237)
Myocd$^{-/-}$	Loeys-Dietz (TGFBR1/2)	TRAF1 (rs1056567)
Myh11$^{-/-}$	Noonan (PTPN11)	AGTR1 (rs5186)
Prostaglandin pathway:	Holt-Oram (TBX5)	*Decreased risk of PDA*:
Ptgs2$^{-/-}$	Rubinstein-Taybi (CREBP)	PTGIS (rs493694,
Ptgs1/Ptgs2 double$^{-/-}$	DiGeorge (TBX1)	rs693649)
EP4$^{-/-}$	Periventricular heterotopia	ESR1 (rs2234693)
Sloco2a1$^{-/-}$	(FLNA)	IFN-γ (rs2430561)
Hpdg$^{-/-}$	Cantu (ABCC9, KCNJ8)	
Others:		
Notch2$^{-/-}$		
Notch2/Notch3 double$^{-/-}$		
Jag1$^{-/-}$		
Brg1$^{-/-}$		
Bmp9$^{-/-}$ with loss of		
Bmp10		
Nfe2$^{-/-}$		
Itga2b$^{-/-}$		

significant PDA occurs in 50% of patients with Cantu syndrome, a condition caused by gain-of-function mutations in K_{ATP} channel genes, *KCNJ8* and *ABCC9*, which encode the vascular-specific K_{ATP} channel subtype Kir6.1/SUR2B. In these cases, PDA is resistant to indomethacin therapy and often requires surgical ligation to achieve closure [14].

While only 10% of PDA cases are associated with chromosomal abnormalities [7], identifying single-nucleotide polymorphisms (SNPs) associated with non-syndromic PDA may be more informative regarding the more common sporadic cases of PDA (Table 34.2). Variants in *TFAP2β*, TRAF1 (TNF receptor-associated factor 1), and *AGTR1* (Angiotensin II type 1 receptor) were associated with an increased risk of PDA while SNPs in *PTGIS* (prostaglandin I2 synthase), *ESR1* (estrogen receptor-α), and *IFN-γ* (interferon-γ) were found to be protective [6]. Unfortunately, replicating many of these findings in other cohorts has proved difficult to this point [15].

34.4   Pharmacological Regulation of the DA

Only three drugs are currently available to treat PDA (indomethacin, ibuprofen, and acetaminophen). All are non-selective cyclooxygenase inhibitors that suppress prostaglandin signaling. Alternately, infusion of prostaglandin E_1 (PGE_1) is the only pharmacologic option used to maintain DA patency in cases of ductus-dependent congenital heart defects. None of these therapies specifically target the DA, leading to off-target effects on other vascular beds. Furthermore, indomethacin and ibuprofen have been associated with spontaneous intestinal perforation and necrotizing

Table 34.3 Pharmacological regulators of DA tone

Maternal drugs	Neonatal drugs
Increased risk of PDA:	*Dilates DA*:
Tocolytics (indomethacin, nifedipine, magnesium sulfate)	PGE_1
	Gentamicin
ACE inhibitors	PDE inhibitors (milrinone, amrinone,
Antihistamines	sildenafil)
Anticonvulsants (valproic acid, phenytoin)	Cimetidine
Amphetamines	Heparin
Alcohol	Diazoxide
Cause fetal DA constriction:	*Constricts DA*:
NSAIDs	NSAIDs
SSRIs antidepressants (sertraline, fluoxetine)	Caffeine
Polyphenols	K_{ATP} inhibitors (glibenclamide)
Betamethasone	

enterocolitis while PGE_1 has been associated with apnea, fever, and other physiologic disturbances [16, 17].

The fetal DA can also be affected by drugs administered to pregnant women (summarized in Table 34.3). Use of tocolytics, ACE inhibitors, antihistamines, anticonvulsants, amphetamines, and alcohol during pregnancy have all been associated with PDA [18]. In contrast, maternal use of NSAID pain-relievers and antidepressants can cause fetal DA constriction [18, 19].

Furthermore, drugs commonly administered to neonates often have vasoactive properties and may inadvertently affect postnatal DA closure [18]. Several drugs have been shown to specifically dilate the DA or cause resistance to indomethacin therapy (Table 34.3). Of note, DA reopening has been reported after exposure to diazoxide, a K_{ATP} channel activator used to treat neonatal hyperinsulinism [20].

34.5 Clinical Implications and Future Directions

PDA remains a significant problem that is inefficiently managed with currently available therapies. Therefore, a greater emphasis must be placed on identifying other factors that can be targeted to regulate DA tone.

The identification of drug targets outside of the prostaglandin pathway is informed by the molecular findings, mouse models of PDA, and human genetic studies mentioned above. While these provide several pathways that could be targeted therapeutically, one with a high likelihood of success is K_{ATP} channels. The vascular form of K_{ATP} channels (i.e., Kir6.1/SUR2B) is enriched in smooth muscle cells of the DA [9, 21] making it a promising target for developing DA-preferring dilators and constrictors. Advances in molecular target-based high-throughput screening of large compound libraries have enabled the ability to discover small molecules that target specific K_{ATP} channel subtypes [22]. We recently performed a thallium flux-based high-throughput screen of compounds for modulators of Kir6.1/SUR2 and identified several novel-scaffold inhibitors of this channel (Denton,

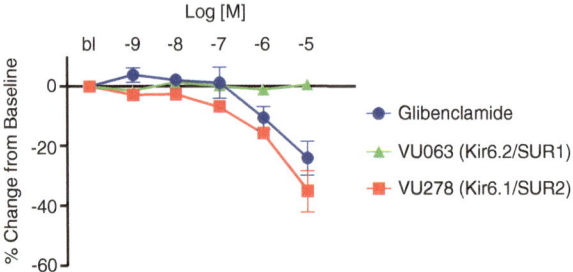

Fig. 34.1 Term-gestation mouse DAs were treated with increasing concentrations of gliben-clamide, VU063, or VU278. Changes in lumen diameter were measured and plotted as a percent change from the initial lumen diameter reading under baseline (bl) conditions. Glibenclamide and VU279 caused DA constriction while VU063 had no effect

unpublished data). The most potent inhibitor, termed VU278, exhibited preferential activity toward the vascular form of K_{ATP} channels (Kir6.1/SUR2) over the pancreatic beta/neuronal cell form (i.e. Kir6.2/SUR1). Using isolated vessel pressure myography assays, we evaluated the specificity and vasoactive potential of these drugs (Fig. 34.1). Fetal mouse DAs were exposed to increasing concentrations of glibenclamide (non-specific sulfonylurea receptor inhibitor), VU063 (pancreatic/neuronal Kir6.2/SUR1 activator) [22], or VU278 (vascular Kir6.1/SUR2 inhibitor). As expected, glibenclamide constricted the DA in a dose-dependent manner. Importantly, VU063 had no effect on the DA while VU278 induced constriction.

In conclusion, an emerging body of genetic, physiological, and pharmacological evidence paints a bright future for the treatment of PDA. Developing a comprehensive understanding of the molecular mechanisms and signaling pathways that regulate DA patency, coupled with focused efforts to develop specific pharmacological modulators of these new targets, is creating unprecedented opportunities for improving PDA outcomes. Among several potential drug targets emerging from these studies, vascular-specific Kir6.1/SUR2 channels hold significant promise due to their enriched expression in the DA and unique pharmacological properties. Ongoing efforts by our laboratories will explore the therapeutic potential of Kir6.1/SUR2B channels in regulating DA patency.

Acknowledgments This work was supported by R21HL132805 and AHA15SDG25280015 awarded to E.L.S. and by NIHR01DK082884 awarded to J.S.D.

References

1. Drayton MR, Skidmore R. Ductus arteriosus blood flow during first 48 hours of life. Arch Dis Child. 1987;62(10):1030–4.
2. Smith GC. The pharmacology of the ductus arteriosus. Pharmacol Rev. 1998;50(1):35–58.
3. Koch J, Hensley G, Roy L, Brown S, Ramaciotti C, Rosenfeld CR. Prevalence of spontaneous closure of the ductus arteriosus in neonates at a birth weight of 1000 grams or less. Pediatrics. 2006;117(4):1113–21.

4. Reese J, Shelton EL, Slaughter JC, McNamara PJ. Prophylactic indomethacin revisited. J Pediatr. 2017;186:11–14.e1.
5. Yun SW. Congenital heart disease in the newborn requiring early intervention. Korean J Pediatr. 2011;54(5):183–91.
6. Lewis TR, Shelton EL, Van Driest SL, Kannankeril PJ, Reese J. Genetics of the patent ductus arteriosus (PDA) and pharmacogenetics of PDA treatment. Semin Fetal Neonatal Med. 2018;23:232.
7. Bokenkamp R, DeRuiter MC, van Munsteren C, Gittenberger-de Groot AC. Insights into the pathogenesis and genetic background of patency of the ductus arteriosus. Neonatology. 2010;98(1):6–17.
8. Stoller JZ, Demauro SB, Dagle JM, Reese J. Current perspectives on pathobiology of the ductus arteriosus. J Clin Exp Cardiolog. 2012;8(1):S8-001.
9. Shelton EL, Ector G, Galindo CL, et al. Transcriptional profiling reveals ductus arteriosus-specific genes that regulate vascular tone. Physiol Genomics. 2014;46(13):457–66.
10. Nichols CG. KATP channels as molecular sensors of cellular metabolism. Nature. 2006;440(7083):470–6.
11. Toyoshima K, Momma K, Ishii T, Nakanishi T. Dilatation of the ductus arteriosus by diazoxide in fetal and neonatal rats. Pediatr Int. 2017;59(12):1246–51.
12. Waleh N, Reese J, Kajino H, et al. Oxygen-induced tension in the sheep ductus arteriosus: effects of gestation on potassium and calcium channel regulation. Pediatr Res. 2009;65(3):285–90.
13. Hajj H, Dagle JM. Genetics of patent ductus arteriosus susceptibility and treatment. Semin Perinatol. 2012;36(2):98–104.
14. Grange DK, Nichols CG, Singh GK. Cantu syndrome and related disorders. In: Adam MP, Ardinger HH, Pagon RA, et al., editors. GeneReviews®. Seattle, WA: University of Washington; 1993.
15. Kawase K, Sugiura T, Nagaya Y, et al. Single nucleotide polymorphisms in AGTR1, TFAP2B, and TRAF1 are not associated with the incidence of patent ductus arteriosus in Japanese preterm infants. Pediatr Int. 2016;58(6):461–6.
16. Christmann V, Liem KD, Semmekrot BA, van de Bor M. Changes in cerebral, renal and mesenteric blood flow velocity during continuous and bolus infusion of indomethacin. Acta Paediatr. 2002;91(4):440–6.
17. Lewis AB, Freed MD, Heymann MA, Roehl SL, Kensey RC. Side effects of therapy with prostaglandin E1 in infants with critical congenital heart disease. Circulation. 1981;64(5):893–8.
18. Reese J, Veldman A, Shah L, Vucovich M, Cotton RB. Inadvertent relaxation of the ductus arteriosus by pharmacologic agents that are commonly used in the neonatal period. Semin Perinatol. 2010;34(3):222–30.
19. Hooper CW, Delaney C, Streeter T, et al. Selective serotonin reuptake inhibitor exposure constricts the mouse ductus arteriosus in utero. Am J Physiol Heart Circ Physiol. 2016;311(3):H572–81.
20. Demirel F, Unal S, Cetin II, Esen I, Arasli A. Pulmonary hypertension and reopening of the ductus arteriosus in an infant treated with diazoxide. J Pediatr Endocrinol Metab. 2011;24(7–8):603–5.
21. Bokenkamp R, van Brempt R, van Munsteren JC, et al. Dlx1 and Rgs5 in the ductus arteriosus: vessel-specific genes identified by transcriptional profiling of laser-capture microdissected endothelial and smooth muscle cells. PLoS One. 2014;9(1):e86892.
22. Raphemot R, Swale DR, Dadi PK, et al. Direct activation of beta-cell KATP channels with a novel xanthine derivative. Mol Pharmacol. 2014;85(6):858–65.

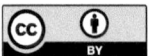

New Mediators in the Biology of the Ductus Arteriosus: Lessons from the Chicken Embryo

35

Saskia van der Sterren, Riazudin Mohammed, and Eduardo Villamor

Abstract

The chicken embryo is an ideal model for the study of new hypotheses on the developmental biology of ductus arteriosus (DA). A unique characteristic of chicken DA is that it is the result of the fusion of two vessels with different embryological origins, morphologies, and functionalities. The pulmonary side (PulmDA) consists almost exclusively of neural crest-derived cells, shows the structure of a muscular artery, and responds to O_2 with contraction whereas the aortic part is of mesodermal origin, shows the morphology of an elastic artery and relaxes in response to O_2. In addition the two parts of the DA show marked differences in responsiveness to other contractile and relaxant agents.

In mammals, the most accepted model of O_2-induced DA constriction involves a rise in O_2 modulating the function of the mitochondrial electron transport chain (the sensor), leading to an increased production of H_2O_2 (the mediator) that causes the inhibition of K_V channels (the effector) with Rho kinase acting as another downstream effector of the O_2-sensing system in the DA. In the chicken embryo, we verified the very same pathway, proving a conserved mechanism for O_2 sensing/signaling in mammalian and nonmammalian DA. Moreover, we demonstrated a developmentally regulated response to O_2, which is restricted to the mature PulmDA and involves parallel maturation of the three components: sensor, mediator, and effectors. Besides O_2, we used the chicken embryo model to investigate the possible ductal effects of vasoactive mediators such as ceramide, H_2S, isoprostanes, or platelet-derived vasoactive mediators.

Keywords

Ductus arteriosus · Oxygen sensing · H_2S · Isoprostanes · Ceramide

S. van der Sterren · R. Mohammed · E. Villamor (✉)
Department of Pediatrics, Maastricht University Medical Center (MUMC+),
School for Oncology and Developmental Biology (GROW), Maastricht, The Netherlands
e-mail: E.Villamor@mumc.nl

35.1   The Chicken Embryo as a Model for Ductus Arteriosus' Developmental Biology

Several mammalian models have helped to unravel the biology and pathobiology of the ductus arteriosus (DA) and to understand the factors responsible for its closure or patency after birth. However, these models are technically complex and experimental manipulations affect both the mother and the fetus [1, 2]. Therefore, there is a need for additional models, addressing these limitations. In the last years, the chicken embryo has emerged as a suitable model for the study of DA vascular biology [3–15].

A unique characteristic of chicken DA is that it is the result of the fusion of two vessels with different embryological origins, morphologies, and functionalities [1, 3, 6, 7]. The pulmonary side (PulmDA) consists almost exclusively of neural crest-derived cells, shows the structure of a muscular artery, and responds to O_2 with contraction whereas the aortic part (AoDA) is of mesodermal origin, shows the morphology of an elastic artery and relaxes in response to O_2 [1, 3, 6, 7]. The two parts of the DA show marked differences in responsiveness not only to O_2 but to other contractile and relaxant agents as well [4, 5]. These differences are summarized in Table 35.1. Another advantage of the chicken DA model is that we have an exhaustive developmental calendar. The developmental changes in PulmDA responsiveness to contractile and relaxant agents are summarized in Table 35.2.

Table 35.1 Effect of vasoactive mediators in the pulmonary (PulmDA) and the aortic (AoDA) side of chicken DA

Vasoactive agent	Nature or mechanism of action	Effect in PulmDA		Effect in AoDA	Ref.
Oxygen	Gaseous mediator	Contraction	$\neq$	Relaxation	[3]
KCl	Depolarizing agent	Contraction	$<$	Contraction	[3]
PGE$_2$	Prostaglandin	Contraction[a]	$>$	Contraction	[4]
Norepinephrine	Adrenoceptor agonist	Contraction	$>$	Contraction	[3]
U46619	TP receptor agonist	Contraction	$>$	Contraction	[3]
Isoproterenol	β-Adrenoceptor agonist	Relaxation	$>$	Relaxation	[4]
Forskolin	Adenylyl cyclase activator	Relaxation	$>$	Relaxation	[4]
Milrinone	Phosphodiesterase-3 inhibitor	Relaxation	$>$	Relaxation	[4]
Acetylcholine	Muscarinic agonist	Relaxation[b]	$<$	Relaxation	[5]
SNP	NO-donor	Relaxation	$<$	Relaxation	[5]
BAY 41-2272	sGC stimulator	Relaxation	$<$	Relaxation	[5]
CO$_2$	Gaseous mediator	Relaxation	$=$	Relaxation	[8]
15-E$_{2t}$-IsoP	Isoprostane	Contraction	$>$	Contraction	[14]
15-F$_{2t}$-IsoP	Isoprostane	Contraction	$>$	Contraction	[14]
H$_2$O$_2$	Reactive oxygen species	Contraction	$\neq$	Relaxation	[6]
Hydroxyfasudil	Rho-kinase inhibitor	Relaxation	$=$	Relaxation	[6]
Y27632	Rho-kinase inhibitor	Relaxation	$=$	Relaxation	[6]
CO	Gaseous mediator	Relaxation	$=$	Relaxation	[13]
H$_2$S	Gaseous mediator	Relaxation	$=$	Relaxation	[13]
17α-estradiol	Estrogen hormone	Relaxation	$=$	Relaxation	[15]
17β-estradiol	Estrogen hormone	Relaxation	$=$	Relaxation	[15]
Ceramide	Membrane sphingolipid	Contraction	$\neq$	Relaxation	[9]
Serotonin	Amine	Contraction	$>$	Contraction	[16]
Thrombin	Protease	Contraction	$>$	Contraction	[18]

[a]In the presence of TP receptor blockade, PGE$_2$ evokes relaxation
[b]Concentrations >3 µM of acetylcholine evoke contraction

Table 35.2 Developmental changes in the response of chicken DA (pulmonary side) to vasoactive mediators

Vasoactive agent	Nature/mechanism of action	15-day DA		19-day DA		21-day DA	Ref.
Oxygen	Gaseous mediator	No response	≠	Contraction	<	Contraction	[3]
KCl	Depolarizing agent	Contraction	<	Contraction	<	Contraction	[3]
4-AP	K_V-channel blocker	Contraction	<	Contraction	<	Contraction	[3]
Norepinephrine	Adrenoceptor agonist	No response	≠	Contraction	<	Contraction	[3]
Phenylephrine	α-Adrenoceptor agonist	No response	≠	Contraction	<	Contraction	[3]
U46619	TP receptor agonist	Contraction	<	Contraction	=	Contraction	[3]
Endothelin-1	Polypeptide	Contraction	<	Contraction	>	Contraction	[3]
ACh (≥3 μM)	Muscarinic agonist	Contraction	<	Contraction	>	Contraction	[10]
PGE_2	Prostaglandin	Relaxation	≠	Contraction	≠	No response	[4]
PGE_2 (+TP-blockade)	Prostaglandin	Relaxation	>	Relaxation	>	Relaxation	[4]
Acetylcholine (<3 μM)	Muscarinic agonist	Relaxation	>	Relaxation	>	Relaxation	[5]
SNP	NO-donor	Relaxation	=	Relaxation	>	Relaxation	[5]
Isoproterenol	β-Adrenoceptor agonist	Relaxation	=	Relaxation	>	Relaxation	[4]
BAY 41-2272	sGC stimulator	Relaxation	=	Relaxation	=	Relaxation	[5]
8-Br cGMP	cGMP analog	Relaxation	=	Relaxation	=	Relaxation	[5]
Forskolin	Adenylyl cyclase activator	Relaxation	=	Relaxation	=	Relaxation	[4]
Milrinone	Phosphodiesterase-3 inhibitor	Relaxation	<	Relaxation	=	Relaxation	[4]
H_2O_2	ROS	No response	≠	Contraction			[6]
BAY K8644	Calcium-channel activator	No response	≠	Contraction			[6]
Nifedipine	Calcium-channel blocker	Relaxation	<	Relaxation			[6]
Hydroxyfasudil	Rho-kinase inhibitor	Relaxation	<	Relaxation			[6]
Y27632	Rho-kinase inhibitor	Relaxation	<	Relaxation			[6]
H_2S	Gaseous mediator	Relaxation	=	Relaxation			[13]
CO	Gaseous mediator	Relaxation	=	Relaxation			[13]
15-E_{2t}-IsoP	Isoprostane	Contraction	<	Contraction			[14]
15-F_{2t}-IsoP	Isoprostane	Contraction	<	Contraction			[14]

35.2 Oxygen Sensing and Signaling in the Chicken DA

In mammals, the most accepted model of O_2-induced DA constriction involves a rise in O_2 modulating the function of the mitochondrial electron transport chain (the sensor), leading to an increased production of H_2O_2 (the mediator) that causes the inhibition of K_V channels (the effector) with Rho kinase acting as another downstream effector of the O_2-sensing system in the DA. In the chicken embryo the very same pathway has been verified, proving a conserved mechanism for O_2 sensing/signaling in mammalian and nonmammalian DA [1, 6, 7]. Moreover, we demonstrated a developmentally regulated response to O_2, which is restricted to the mature PulmDA and involves parallel maturation of the three components: sensor, mediator, and effectors [6].

35.3   New Mediators in the Biology of the DA

35.3.1 Role of Ceramide in DA Oxygen Sensing and Signaling

Ceramide is synthesized from membrane sphingomyelin by sphingomyelinases (SMases) which are activated by multiple membrane receptors and non-receptor stimuli. Using the chicken model, we observed that inhibition of the ceramide-generating enzyme neutral SMase reduced the hypoxic vasoconstriction in the pulmonary artery (PA) and the normoxic contraction of the DA [9]. Moreover, ceramide content and H_2O_2 production were increased by hypoxia in PAs and by normoxia in the DA. Accordingly, ceramide mimicked the contractile responses of hypoxia in PAs and those of normoxia in the DA. In addition, ceramide inhibited Kv currents in PA and DA smooth muscle cells. Finally, the role of nSMase in acute oxygen sensing was confirmed in human PA and DA [12]. However, the mechanisms matching the putative O_2 sensor(s) (i.e., mitochondria and/or NADPH oxidase) and ceramide remain unknown.

35.3.2 Vasoactivity of H₂S in the Chicken DA

Oxygen is not the only gaseous mediator with a relevant role in DA reactivity. CO_2 and non-respiratory gases, such as NO and CO, are also ductal vasoactive mediators [1, 16]. In the last years H_2S has been identified as an endogenous gaseous transmitter, playing multiple physiological roles in animal systems [13]. Furthermore, H_2S has been proposed as a vascular O_2 sensor. We have investigated the vasoactivity of H_2S and CO in the chicken DA. We observed that either H_2S or CO induces relaxation of chicken DA. However, this relaxation is not vessel-specific since PulmDA, AoDA, and chicken embryo pulmonary and femoral arteries were similarly relaxed by H_2S and CO [13]. Moreover, the presence of precursors/inhibitors of H_2S and CO synthesis did not significantly affect the response of the chicken DA to normoxia/hypoxia and did not affect endothelium-dependent or -independent relaxation [13]. Therefore, our results indicate that the gasotransmitters H_2S and CO are vasoactive in the chicken DA but they do not suggest an important role for endogenous H_2S or CO in the control of chicken ductal reactivity.

35.3.3 Response of Chicken DA to Isoprostanes

Isoprostanes (IsoPs) are a unique series of prostaglandin-like compounds formed in vivo from the free radical-catalyzed peroxidation of arachidonic acid independent of the cyclooxygenase enzymes [17]. Initially, IsoPs were recognized as valuable markers of oxidative stress and numerous pathological conditions have been shown to be associated with increases in urinary, plasma, and tissue levels of IsoPs. Later it became apparent that IsoPs exhibit significant bioactivity and could contribute to the functional consequences of oxidative stress and participate in oxygen signaling, particularly during the transition to extra-uterine life [17]. Surprisingly, until our study, the possible vascular effects of IsoPs in the DA had not been investigated. We observed that $15\text{-}E_{2t}\text{-}IsoP$ evoked a potent and efficacious, TP receptor-mediated, contraction in the chicken DA [18]. On the other hand, $15\text{-}F_{2t}\text{-}IsoP$ is probably acting as a partial agonist at TP receptors. The contractile response of the PulmDA to IsoPs increased with development and both $15\text{-}E_{2t}\text{-}IsoP$ and $15\text{-}F_{2t}\text{-}IsoP$ were particularly efficacious in contracting the PulmDA in comparison with the AoDA and the femoral or the pulmonary arteries [14]. Altogether, our data suggest that IsoPs, acting through TP receptors, may play a role in the control of chicken DA tone and could participate in its closure.

35.3.4 Role of Platelet-Derived Vasoactive Mediators in DA Biology

Several cohort studies have shown an association between low platelet counts in the first day(s) of life and patent DA (PDA) in preterm infants [19]. Activated platelets release different substances with vasoactive properties, like serotonin, thromboxane A_2 (TXA$_2$), platelet activating factor, or thrombin. The two former agonists are vasoactive in the chicken DA [10, 16]. In addition, we investigated the possible vasoactive effects of thrombin in the DA. Cellular effects of thrombin are mediated by protease-activated receptors (PARs), members of the G-protein-coupled receptors that carry their own ligand, which remains cryptic until unmasked by proteolytic cleavage. PAR-1 and PAR-2 have been shown to be involved in regulating vascular tone. Our preliminary results indicate that thrombin, acting through PAR-1, is a selective vasoconstrictor in the DA of the chicken, providing the first functional evidence for a role of PARs in DA biology [18]. Currently, we are analyzing the expression of PARs in the DA of several species (human, lamb, rat, mouse, and chicken).

35.4 Future Direction and Clinical Implications

The hope for future targeted therapies and for the prevention of patent DA (PDA) requires knowledge of the fundamental mechanisms controlling its development and pathogenesis [20]. In addition, new drugs or even those that are commonly used in the neonatal intensive care unit may have unexpected effects on the ability of the DA to spontaneously close, resulting in increased risks for PDA [20]. The chicken DA is a feasible model to test the possible ductal effects of drugs or therapeutic strategies to which the infants are exposed in utero or after birth.

References

1. Dzialowski EM, Sirsat T, van der Sterren S, et al. Prenatal cardiovascular shunts in amniotic vertebrates. Respir Physiol Neurobiol. 2011;178:66–74.
2. Itani N, Salinas CE, Villena M, et al. The highs and lows of programmed cardiovascular disease by developmental hypoxia: studies in the chicken embryo. J Physiol. 2018;596(15):2991–3006.

3. Agren P, Cogolludo AL, Kessels CG, et al. Ontogeny of chicken ductus arteriosus response to oxygen and vasoconstrictors. Am J Physiol Regul Integr Comp Physiol. 2007;292:R485–96.
4. Agren P, van der Sterren S, Cogolludo AL, et al. Developmental changes in the effects of prostaglandin E2 in the chicken ductus arteriosus. J Comp Physiol B. 2009;179:133–43.
5. Agren P, van der Sterren S, Cogolludo AL, et al. Developmental changes in endothelium-dependent relaxation of the chicken ductus arteriosus. J Physiol Pharmacol. 2008;59:55–76.
6. Cogolludo AL, Moral-Sanz J, van der Sterren S, et al. Maturation of O2 sensing and signaling in the chicken ductus arteriosus. Am J Physiol Lung Cell Mol Physiol. 2009;297:L619–30.
7. Greyner H, Dzialowski EM. Mechanisms mediating the oxygen-induced vasoreactivity of the ductus arteriosus in the chicken embryo. Am J Physiol Regul Integr Comp Physiol. 2008;295:R1647–59.
8. Moonen RM, Agren P, Cogolludo AL, et al. Response of chicken ductus arteriosus to hypercarbic and normocarbic acidosis. Neonatology. 2010;98:47–56.
9. Moreno L, Moral-Sanz J, Morales-Cano D, et al. Ceramide mediates acute oxygen sensing in vascular tissues. Antioxid Redox Signal. 2014;20:1–14.
10. Schuurman MJ, Villamor E. Endothelium-dependent contraction induced by acetylcholine in the chicken ductus arteriosus involves cyclooxygenase-1 activation and TP receptor stimulation. Comp Biochem Physiol A Mol Integr Physiol. 2010;157:28–34.
11. Van der Sterren S, Agren P, Zoer B. Morphological and functional alterations of the ductus arteriosus in a chicken model of hypoxia-induced fetal growth retardation. Pediatr Res. 2009;65:279–84.
12. Van der Sterren S, Kessels L, Perez-Vizcaino F, et al. Prenatal exposure to hyperoxia modifies the thromboxane prostanoid receptor-mediated response to H2O2 in the ductus arteriosus of the chicken embryo. J Physiol Pharmacol. 2014;65:283–93.
13. Van der Sterren S, Kleikers P, Zimmermann LJ, Villamor E. Vasoactivity of the gasotransmitters hydrogen sulfide and carbon monoxide in the chicken ductus arteriosus. Am J Physiol Regul Integr Comp Physiol. 2011;301:R1186–98.
14. van der Sterren S, Villamor E. Contractile effects of 15-E2t-isoprostane and 15-F2t-isoprostane on chicken embryo ductus arteriosus. Comp Biochem Physiol A Mol Integr Physiol. 2011;159:436–44.
15. Flinsenberg TW, van der Sterren S, van Cleef AN, et al. Effects of sex and estrogen on chicken ductus arteriosus reactivity. Am J Physiol Regul Integr Comp Physiol. 2010;298:R1217–24.
16. van Zogchel L, Villamor E. Serotonin is a selective vasoconstrictor of chicken embryo ductus arteriosus. Arch Dis Child. 2014;99:A620.
17. Belik J, González-Luis GE, Perez-Vizcaino F, et al. Isoprostanes in fetal and neonatal health and disease. Free Radic Biol Med. 2010;48:177–88.
18. Kartal K, Meekels J, Mohammed R, et al. Protease-activated receptor (PAR)-mediated contraction of the chicken ductus arteriosus. Arch Dis Child. 2012;97:A325.
19. Simon SR, Van Zogchel L, Bas-Suárez MP, et al. Platelet counts and patent ductus arteriosus in preterm infants: a systematic review and meta-analysis. Neonatology. 2015;108:143–51.
20. Stoller JZ, DeMauro SB, Dagle JM, et al. Current perspectives on pathobiology of the ductus arteriosus. J Clin Exp Cardiolog. 2012;8:S8-001.

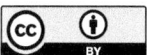

Constriction of the Ductus Arteriosus with K_{ATP} Channel Inhibitors

36

Kazuo Momma, Katsuaki Toyoshima, Emiko Hayama, and Toshio Nakanishi

Abstract

The cause of fetal death by sulfonylureas (SUs), used for diabetes in pregnancy in the early 1960s, remained unsolved for decades. In 1993, Nakanishi discovered constriction of ductus arteriosus (DA) strips in rabbit fetuses with glibenclamide, a SU and inhibitor of the K_{ATP} channel. Later, Momma showed dose-dependent fetal DA constriction by glibenclamide injected directly into the fetus in rats. Every first-generation SU constricted the fetal DA by oral administration to the pregnant rat. DA constriction with the clinical dose of these SUs was mild, whereas a 100 times larger dose was needed to close the DA completely. Coadministration of SUs and cylooxygenase inhibitors caused additive severe constriction and complete closure of the fetal DA. These data suggested that the aforementioned high fetal death rate (63% in 1962) with chlorpropamide was due to the coadministration of this SU and aspirin-like drugs.

Keywords

Ductus arteriosus · K_{ATP} channel inhibitor · Glibenclamide · Sulfonylurea · Premature closure of ductus arteriosus

K. Momma (✉) · E. Hayama · T. Nakanishi
Department of Pediatric Cardiology, Tokyo Women's Medical University, Tokyo, Japan
e-mail: kmomma@iris.ocn.ne.jp; nakanishi.toshio@twmu.ac.jp

K. Toyoshima
Division of Pediatric Cardiology, Tokyo Women's Medical University, Tokyo, Japan

Division of Neonatology, Kanagawa Children's Medical Center, Yokohama, Japan

© The Editor(s) (if applicable) and The Author(s) 2020
T. Nakanishi et al. (eds.), *Molecular Mechanism of Congenital Heart Disease and Pulmonary Hypertension*, https://doi.org/10.1007/978-981-15-1185-1_36

36.1 Transplacental Fetal Death by Sulfonylureas

Sulfonylureas (SUs) were used for diabetes treatment in the early 1950s. In 1962, it was reported from South Africa that chlorpropamide, a first-generation SU (an inhibitor of the K_{ATP} channel) administered to diabetic pregnant women caused 63% fetal death rate during the latter half of gestation [1]. Fetal autopsies revealed no malformations and the mechanism of death remained uncertain. In 1964, a survey of diabetic pregnant patients in the United Kingdom confirmed the association of chlorpropamide and tolbutamide with fetal death. Although the mechanism of fetal death was unknown, the use of these SUs became contraindicated during pregnancy from then onward.

36.2 Closure of Fetal Ductus Arteriosus with Non-Steroidal Anti-Inflammatory Drugs

Aspirin was discovered in 1901. Cardiac catheterization and angiography was the major cardiovascular diagnostic methods in the 1960s. In 1969, the first case of trans-placental premature fetal DA closure was reported by Arcilla [2]. In this case, a full-term mother had severe arthritis and she took massive doses of salicylates for 11 days. The neonate was severely cyanotic, and cardiac catheterization and angiography at 4 h postpartum revealed pulmonary hypertension, atrial right-to-left shunting, and a closed DA at the aortic end. Since 1978, we studied fetal rat DA with a rapid whole-body freezing method, and we showed transplacental constriction of the fetal DA with all 50 non-steroidal anti-inflammatory drugs (NSAIDs) [3–5] (Fig. 36.1). Experimentally, constriction was absent in mid-gestation, but it increased in late gestation [6].

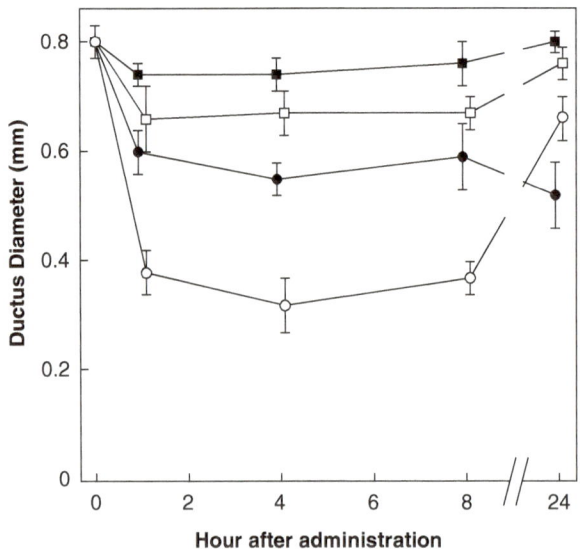

Fig. 36.1 Fetal DA diameters following orogastric administration of non-steroidal anti-inflammatory drugs to the near-term rat. Time course of fetal DA constriction by 14 mg/kg Acetoaminophen (black squares) and 14 mg/kg Aspirin (white squares), 0.7 mg/kg Indomethacin (black circles), and 6 mg/kg Ibuprofen (white circles) to d21 pregnant rats (mean ± SEM)

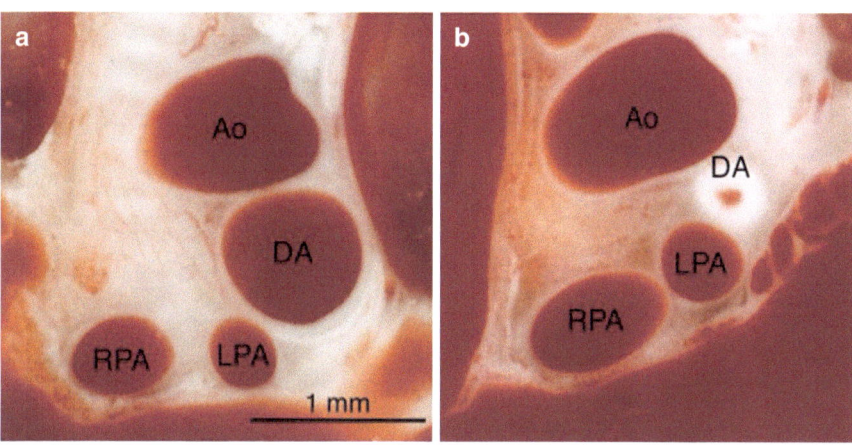

Fig. 36.2 Frontal sections of the frozen rat fetus through aortic arch (Ao), ductus arteriosus (DA), and right and left pulmonary artery (RPA, LPA). The inner diameter of the Ao, DA, and main pulmonary artery (PA) were 0.8 mm, respectively. The DA/PA ratio was 1.0 in the control (**a**). A large dose (100 mg/kg, injected into the fetal abdomen) of glibenclamide constricted the DA severely in 30 min, the DA inner diameter diminished to 0.1 mm, and the DA/PA ratio was 0.1 (**b**)

36.3   Constriction of Ductus Arteriosus with Glibenclamide

In 1993, Nakanishi discovered constriction of DA strips in rabbit fetuses with glibenclamide, a second-generation SU and inhibitor of the K_{ATP} channel. Glibenclamide passed into the placenta slowly [7]. Since 2012, we studied direct intraperitoneal injection of glibenclamide into the rat fetus and demonstrated dose-dependent DA constriction in the preterm and term fetus [8]. The DA constriction with the clinical doses was mild, and the DA inner diameter decreased to 70% in 30 min. The DA closed completely with a 100 times larger dose compared to the clinical dose (Figs. 36.2 and 36.3).

36.4   Constriction of Fetal DA with Other Sulfonylureas

Since 2010, we demonstrated transplacental constriction of the fetal DA with first-generation sulfonylureas in the rat model (Table 36.1). Every SU constricted the fetal DA mildly in 4 h after orogastric administration of the drug to the near-term rats. The fetal DA constriction was severe, or the DA closed completely with 100 times larger doses (Table 36.1). Rat fetuses survived with clinical doses of SUs with associated mild DA constriction, whereas fetal death increased with closure of the DA. Severe DA constriction with 100 times larger doses of SUs persisted up to 24 h later.

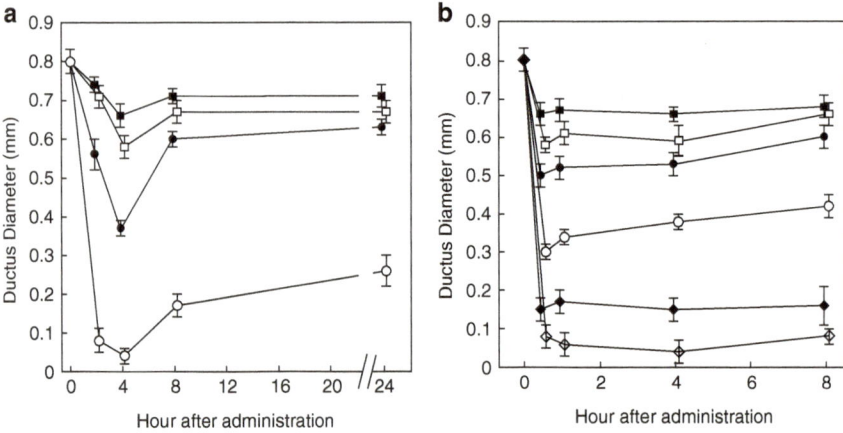

Fig. 36.3 Time courses of fetal DA constriction with maternal orogastric administration of chlor-propamide (**a**), and those with fetal intraperitoneal injection of glibenclamide (**b**) in rats. Time course of fetal DA constriction in rats exposed to chlorpromide, 1 mg/kg (black squares), 10 mg/kg (white squares), 100 mg/kg (black circles), and 1000 mg (white circles) (mean ± SEM)

Table 36.1 Constriction of fetal ductus arteriosus with sulfonylureas (SU) in rats

Sulfonylurea	Clinical dose mg/kg	Test dose mg/kg	Route	Fetal rat DA constriction
Tolbutamide	10–40	A:10 B:1000	OG	Experimentally with orogastric administration to the mother rat, clinical doses (A) induced mild
Chlorpropamide	2–10	A:10 B:1000	OG	DA constriction and DA/PA decreased from 1.0 to 0.9–0.7 in 3 h. Large doses (B) induced severe DA
Glyclopyramide	2–5	A:10 B:1000	OG	constriction and DA/PA decreased to 0.2–0.0 (complete closure)
Acetohexamide	10–20	A:10 B:1000	OG	
Glibenclamide	0.02–0.1–1	A:1 B:100	IP	IP of clinical doses (A) induced mild DA constriction. IP of large doses (B) induced severe
Glimepiride	0.01–0.1	A:1 B:100	IP	DA constriction

First-generation SUs were administered orogastrically (OG) to the near-term pregnant rats. Second-generation SUs were injected intraperitoneally (IP) to the fetal rats

36.5 Fetal DA Closure with Combined Administration of Cyclooxygenase Inhibitors and SUs

We studied the combined effects of indomethacin and glibenclamide in the fetal DA model (Fig. 36.4). Indomethacin (0.1, 1, and 10 mg/kg) was administered orogastrically to 19th day and 21st day rats. Glibenclamide (1 mg/kg) was

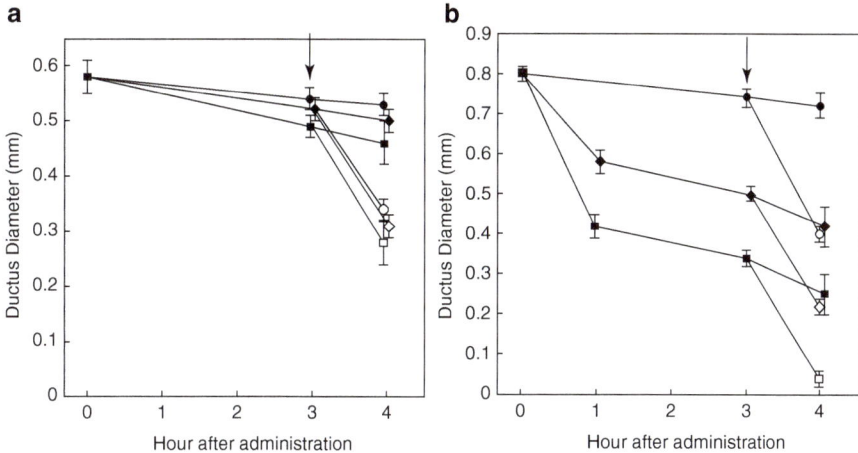

Fig. 36.4 Fetal rat DA constriction in 4 h with three doses, 0.1 mg/kg (white circles), 1 mg/kg (white diamonds), and 10 mg/kg (white squares), of indomethacin with orogastric administration to preterm rats on the 19th day (**a**) and to near-term rats on 21st day (**b**). Glibenclamide (1 mg/kg) was injected to the fetus intraperitoneally at 3 h after administration of indomethacin

administered to the fetus at 3 h, and the fetal DA was studied at 4 h. As shown in Fig. 36.4, indomethacin and glibenclamide constricted the DA additively. These data suggest that the aforementioned high fetal death rate with chlorpropamide was due to the additional intake of cyclooxygenase inhibitors (COX-I), used as analgesics and antipyretics, combined with the SU effects of K_{ATP} channel inhibition.

36.6   Early Fetal Exposure to COX-I

Fetal DA contractility in the presence of oxygen is the basic mechanism of neonatal DA closure. In 1986, we discovered in rat experiments the following paradoxical phenomenon: early exposure to COX-Is impaired fetal DA contractility to late administration of COX-Is or oxygen, respectively [9]. The same phenomenon was reported in clinical patent DA in premature infants [10]. The molecular mechanism of this paradox was only clarified recently [11, 12]. We created a rat model with this paradox [13]: the fetal rats with exposure to large doses of indomethacin during the latter 30% of the total fetal gestational period showed much reduced DA contractility. Moreover, they showed eight times slower DA closure in the postpartum period. In this fetus model, DA constriction with glibenclamide was weak, and the DA constricted only moderately with a large dose (1000 mg/kg) of glibenclamide.

36.7   Effects of Massive Doses of Glibenclamide in Newborn Rat

As is shown in Fig. 36.3, glibenclamide constricted the fetal DA only mildly with clinical doses, and closed the DA completely with massive doses. The effects of massive doses of glibenclamide were studied with orogastric administration in one-day-old newborn rats under maternal nursing. Large doses of glibenclamide (100 mg and 1000 mg/kg) were well tolerated, and more than 90% of these rats survived with normal weight gain up to 3 weeks. Severe hypoglycemia, as low as 30 mg/dL of plasma glucose, developed and persisted for up to 3 days. The hypoglycemia was treated with large doses of orogastric glucose. Laboratory tests at 1 day after gliben-clamide administration revealed hypoglycemia, but other parameters were normal.

36.8   Future Direction and Clinical Implications

Recent studies of cord bloods at birth in neonates of diabetic mothers with gliben-clamide treatment revealed the presence of the drug in concentrations at about 50% of the maternal levels [14]. This suggests mild DA constriction and increased risk of premature DA closure in the fetus of mothers treated with glibenclamide. The clinical application of glibenclamide to close patent DA in premature infants is difficult because of the associated prolonged hypoglycemia when used in large doses, and a decreased constrictive effect in DA with early exposure to COX-Is.

References

1. Jackson WPU, Campbell GD, Noteloviz M. Tolbutamide and chlorpropamide during pregnancy in human diabetes. Diabetes. 1962;11(Suppl):98–101.
2. Archilla RA, Thilenius OG, Ranniger K. Congestive heart failure from suspected ductus closure in utero. J Pediatr. 1969;75:74–8.
3. Momma K, Takeuchi H. Constriction of fetal ductus arteriosus by non-steroidal anti-inflammatory drugs. Prostaglandins. 1983;26:631–43.
4. Momma K, Hagiwara H, Konishi T. Constriction of fetal ductus arteriosus by non-steroidal anti-inflammatory drugs. Study of additional 34 drugs. Prostaglandins. 1984;28:527–36.
5. Momma K, Takao. Transplacental cardiovascular effects of four popular analgesics in rats. Am J Obstet Gynecol. 1990;162:1304–10.
6. Momma K, Takao A. In vivo constriction of the ductus arteriosus by non-steroidal anti-inflammatory drugs in near-term and preterm fetal rats. Pediatr Res. 1987;22:567–72.
7. Nakanishi T, Gu H, Hagiwara N, et al. Mechanisms of oxygen-induced contraction of ductus arteriosus isolated from the fetal rabbit. Circ Res. 1993;72:1218–28.
8. Momma K, Monma M, Toyoshima K, et al. Fetal and neonatal ductus arteriosus is regulated with ATP-sensitive potassium channel. In: Nakanishi T, et al., editors. Etiology and morphogenesis of congenital heart disease. Tokyo: Springer Japan; 2016. p. 263–5.
9. Konishi T, Momma K, Takao A. Inhibited maturation of fetal ductus arteriosus by indomethacin in rats. Jpn J Neonatol. 1986;22:430–5.. (in Japanese).
10. Norton ME, Merrill J, Cooper BAB, et al. Neonatal complication after the administration of indomethacin for preterm labor. N Engl J Med. 1993;329:1602–7.

11. Yokoyama U, Minamisawa S, Quan H, et al. Chronic activation of the prostaglandin receptor EP4 promotes hyaluronan-mediated neointimal formation in the ductus arteriosus. J Clin Invest. 2006;116:3026–34.
12. Reese J, Waleh SD, Poole SD, et al. Chronic in utero cyclooxygenase inhibition alters PGE_2-regulated ductus arteriosus contractile pathways and prevents postnatal closure. Pediatr Res. 2009;66:155–61.
13. Momma K, Toyoshima K, Ito K, et al. Delayed neonatal closure of the ductus arteriosus following early in utero exposure to indomethacin in the rat. Neonatology. 2007;96:69–79.
14. Schwartz RA, Rosenn B, Katarina A, et al. Glyburide transport across the human placenta. Obstet Gynecol. 2015;125:583–8.

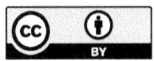

New Insights on How to Treat Patent Ductus Arteriosus

37

Utako Yokoyama, Rika Aoki, Shujiro Fujita, Shiho Iwasaki, Kazuo Seki, Asou Toshihide, Munetaka Masuda, Susumu Minamisawa, and Yoshihiro Ishikawa

Abstract

The ductus arteriosus (DA) must be closed after birth for the establishment of adult circulation. Extremely preterm infants, however, frequently have patent ductus arteriosus (PDA), which associates with significant morbidity and mortality. At birth, the separation of the fetus from its maternal environment constitutes a dramatic change for the infant. Initiation of respiration changes serum composition and oxygen tension resulting in the closure of the DA. We found that serum osmolality was significantly decreased early after birth in rats, and that the hypo-osmolality sensor transient receptor potential melastatin (TRPM) 3 had increased expression in the rat DA compared to the aorta. Our data suggest that a decrease

U. Yokoyama (✉) · Y. Ishikawa
Cardiovascular Research Institute, Yokohama City University, Yokohama, Japan
e-mail: utako@yokohama-cu.ac.jp

R. Aoki
Cardiovascular Research Institute, Yokohama City University, Yokohama, Japan

Department of Pediatrics, Yokohama City University, Yokohama, Japan

S. Fujita · S. Iwasaki
Department of Pediatrics, Yokohama City University, Yokohama, Japan

K. Seki
Perinatal Center, Yokohama City University Medical Center, Yokohama, Japan

A. Toshihide
Department of Surgery, Kanagawa Children's Medical Center, Yokohama, Japan

M. Masuda
Department of Cardiovascular Surgery, Yokohama City University, Yokohama, Japan

S. Minamisawa
Department of Cell Physiology, The Jikei University School of Medicine, Tokyo, Japan

in serum osmolality promotes DA closure via TRPM3 and that an increase in osmolality dilates the DA. For extremely preterm infants, recent recommendations include immediate amino acid supplementation. We examined plasma amino acid composition and found an association between low glutamate concentration and PDA. Our data suggest that glutamate induces DA contraction through the AMPA receptor GluR-mediated noradrenaline production. Based on these data, maintaining proper levels of serum osmolality and amino acid composition may improve the therapeutic outcome of PDA in extremely preterm infants.

Keywords
Ductus arteriosus · Smooth muscle · TRP channel · AMPA receptor

37.1   Introduction

In the fetus, the ductus arteriosus (DA) diverts ventricular output away from the high-resistance pulmonary vascular bed into the systemic circulation. Although its patency is essential for fetal circulation, once pulmonary circulation is established, the DA must be closed.

Despite considerable progress in medical management for preterm infants, 25% of PDA in extremely preterm infants is still resistant to pharmacological therapies, i.e., cyclooxygenase inhibitors, which have been the only pharmacological therapeutic strategy since the mid-1970s [1–3]. Therefore, novel strategies for PDA in extremely preterm infants are required.

At birth, dynamic changes occur in serum components. A previous study demonstrated that serum osmolality decreased transiently after birth, but recovered over the next few days in full-term human neonates [4]. However, the significance of this transient decrease in osmolality has never been addressed. Amino acid composition is also changed after birth. Amino acid administration beginning immediately after birth has recently been suggested [5]. However, the role of amino acids on DA regulation has not been reported. Therefore, we investigated the roles of serum osmolality and amino acid composition in DA closure.

37.2   Novel Mechanisms Regulating DA Closure

37.2.1 Decreased Serum Osmolality Promotes DA Contraction

Under physiological conditions, body-fluid osmolality is tightly regulated to near 300 mOsm/kg through the intake or excretion of water and salt [6]. Hypotonicity is sensed, partly, by the transient receptor potential (TRP) channels, such as TRP vanilloid 4 (TRPV4) [7] or TRP melastatin 3 (TRPM3) [8, 9], which acts as a Ca^{2+} channel. Because changes in intracellular Ca^{2+} are associated with DA contraction [10–12], we focused on TRP channels.

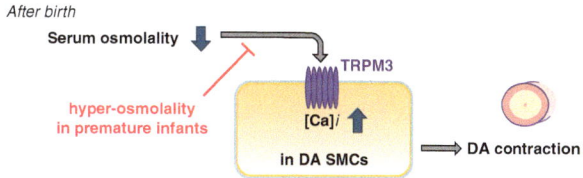

Fig. 37.1 Proposed diagram for the role of serum osmolality after birth. Transient decrease in serum osmolality induces DA contraction via TRPM3. $[Ca]_i$: intracellular Ca^{2+}

We found that rats exhibited a similar transient hypo-osmolality after birth as in humans. Hypotonic stimulation induced constriction of DA rings and increased Ca^{2+} transient in DA smooth muscle cells. TRPM3 was highly expressed in the rat DA, and TRPM3-targeted siRNA abolished the Ca^{2+} response to hypo-osmolality. The TRPM3 stimulator, pregnenolone sulfate, induced rat DA constriction ex vivo and in vivo. Contrary to these findings, intra-peritoneal hypertonic fluid administration impaired rat DA closure.

In humans, neonatal serum hypo-osmolality was observed in relatively mature preterm infants (≥28 weeks). In extremely preterm infants (<28 weeks), however, this hypo-osmolality was not observed. Instead, a rapid increase in osmolality occurred after birth in extremely preterm infants. The degree of osmolar increase was greater in patients with PDA.

These data suggest that a transient decrease in serum osmolality may promote DA closure during the first few days of life (Fig. 37.1) [13].

37.2.2 Glutamic Acid Contributes to DA Closure

First, we analyzed amino acid composition in human neonates. Aminogram results in human neonates at day 2 revealed that the plasma glutamate concentration was significantly lower in extremely preterm infants (<28 weeks gestation) with PDA than in those without PDA and relatively mature preterm infants (28–29 weeks gestation).

It has been shown that glutamate stimulates noradrenaline release [14, 15]. Many adrenergic nerve terminals were shown in the muscular walls of the human DA, and fluorometric results revealed the presence of noradrenaline in the human DA [16]. A previous report demonstrated that noradrenaline induced significant constriction of the DA even in the 20-week human fetus [16]. Moreover, a recent study demonstrated that glutamate induces noradrenaline release through glutamate inotropic receptor alpha-amino-3-hydroxy-5-methyl-4-isoxazolepropionate (AMPA) type subunit 1 (GluR1) [17]. As a result, we investigated the role of glutamate in DA closure.

In the rat, GluR1 mRNA was highly expressed in the DA compared to the aorta on gestational day 19 (preterm) and gestational day 21 (term). GluR1 proteins were co-localized with tyrosine hydroxylase-positive autonomic nerve terminals in the rat and human DA. Intraperitoneal administration of glutamate promoted

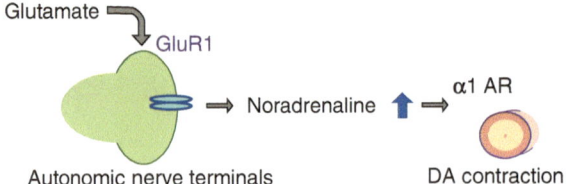

Fig. 37.2 Proposed diagram for the role of glutamate in the DA. Glutamate stimulates autonomic nerve terminals of the DA, resulting in noradrenaline release. This noradrenaline promotes DA contraction via α1 adrenergic receptor (α1 AR)

noradrenaline production in the rat DA. Glutamate administration induced DA contraction in both preterm (gestational day 20) and term rat fetuses in vivo. Glutamate-induced DA contraction was attenuated by the Ca^{2+}-sensitive GluR receptor antagonist NASPM or the adrenergic receptor α1 blocker, prazosin.

These data suggest that glutamate induces DA contraction through GluR-mediated noradrenaline production (Fig. 37.2) [18].

37.3   Future Direction and Clinical Implications

PDA often causes serious problems in very premature infants, depending on the degree of left-to-right shunting. It has been reported that more than 50% of infants with birth weights <1000 g receive pharmacological therapy consisting of cyclo-oxygenase (COX) inhibitors or surgical ligation of the DA. Because the current pharmacological and surgical therapies for treating PDA are not always ideal, it is highly desirable to find a relatively simple and noninvasive strategy that would prevent PDA from occurring.

Our study demonstrated that serum osmolality is transiently decreased after birth, and this decrease may be a physiological mechanism to facilitate DA contraction. The significance of this transient decrease in serum osmolality has been largely overlooked. It may be time to reconsider the importance of serum osmolality. Keeping their serum osmolality at the proper, but not elevated, level may be important among preterm infants at risk for PDA.

Our data also suggest that glutamate promoted DA contraction in preterm infants. The composition of amino acid mixtures varies between commercially available solutions. Of note, glutamate concentration is markedly different compared to the other components among commercially available amino acid solutions (0.8–10.0 g/L). Supplementation of glutamate might help to prevent PDA in extremely preterm infants, and the importance of amino acid composition, i.e., glutamate, may need to be considered in postnatal circulatory adaptation.

Acknowledgments The authors are grateful to Yuka Sawada for technical assistance. This study was funded by MEXT/JSPS KAKENHI (U.Y., JP17K19403, JP16H05358, JP15H05761; S.I., JP17K16276; J.S., JP16H07107; Y.I., JPH1605300), and the Yokohama Foundation for the Advancement of Medical Science (J.S.), the Japan Agency for Medical Research and Development (AMED) (Y.I., 66890007, 56689113), and the Kitsuen Research Foundation (Y.I., 71890005).

References

1. Friedman WF, Hirschklau MJ, Printz MP, Pitlick PT, Kirkpatrick SE. Pharmacologic closure of patent ductus arteriosus in the premature infant. N Engl J Med. 1976;295:526–9.
2. Kiefer AS, Wickremasinghe AC, Johnson JN, Hartman TK, Hintz SR, Carey WA, Colby CE. Medical management of extremely low-birth-weight infants in the first week of life: a survey of practices in the United States. Am J Perinatol. 2009;26:407–18.
3. Yokoyama U. Prostaglandin E-mediated molecular mechanisms driving remodeling of the ductus arteriosus. Pediatr Int. 2015;57:820–7.
4. Feldman W, Drummond KN. Serum and urine osmolality in normal full-term infants. Can Med Assoc J. 1969;101:73–4.
5. Koletzko B, Goulet O, Hunt J, Krohn K, Shamir R, Parenteral Nutrition G, Guidelines Working N. European Society for Clinical, Metabolism, H. European Society of Paediatric Gastroenterology, Nutrition, R. European Society of Paediatric, 1. Guidelines on Paediatric Parenteral Nutrition of the European Society of Paediatric Gastroenterology, Hepatology and Nutrition (ESPGHAN) and the European Society for Clinical Nutrition and Metabolism (ESPEN), supported by the European Society of Paediatric Research (ESPR). J Pediatr Gastroenterol Nutr. 2005;41(Suppl 2):S1–87.
6. Bourque CW, Oliet SH. Osmoreceptors in the central nervous system. Annu Rev Physiol. 1997;59:601–19.
7. Liedtke W, Friedman JM. Abnormal osmotic regulation in trpv4−/− mice. Proc Natl Acad Sci U S A. 2003;100:13698–703.
8. Grimm C, Kraft R, Sauerbruch S, Schultz G, Harteneck C. Molecular and functional characterization of the melastatin-related cation channel TRPM3. J Biol Chem. 2003;278:21493–501.
9. Oberwinkler J, Phillipp SE. TRPM3. Handb Exp Pharmacol. 2007;179:253–67.
10. Nakanishi T, Gu H, Hagiwara N, Momma K. Mechanisms of oxygen-induced contraction of ductus arteriosus isolated from the fetal rabbit. Circ Res. 1993;72:1218–28.
11. Akaike T, Jin MH, Yokoyama U, Izumi-Nakaseko H, Jiao Q, Iwasaki S, Iwamoto M, Nishimaki S, Sato M, Yokota S, Kamiya Y, Adachi-Akahane S, Ishikawa Y, Minamisawa S. T-type Ca²⁺ channels promote oxygenation-induced closure of the rat ductus arteriosus not only by vasoconstriction but also by neointima formation. J Biol Chem. 2009;284:24025–34.
12. Yokoyama U, Minamisawa S, Adachi-Akahane S, Akaike T, Naguro I, Funakoshi K, Iwamoto M, Nakagome M, Uemura N, Hori H, Yokota S, Ishikawa Y. Multiple transcripts of Ca²⁺ channel alpha1-subunits and a novel spliced variant of the alpha1C-subunit in rat ductus arteriosus. Am J Physiol Heart Circ Physiol. 2006;290:H1660–70.
13. Aoki R, Yokoyama U, Ichikawa Y, Taguri M, Kumagaya S, Ishiwata R, Yanai C, Fujita S, Umemura M, Fujita T, Okumura S, Sato M, Minamisawa S, Asou T, Masuda M, Iwasaki S, Nishimaki S, Seki K, Yokota S, Ishikawa Y. Decreased serum osmolality promotes ductus arteriosus constriction. Cardiovasc Res. 2014;104:326–36.
14. Pittaluga A, Raiteri M. N-methyl-D-aspartic acid (NMDA) and non-NMDA receptors regulating hippocampal norepinephrine release. I. Location on axon terminals and pharmacological characterization. J Pharmacol Exp Ther. 1992;260:232–7.
15. Wang JK, Andrews H, Thukral V. Presynaptic glutamate receptors regulate noradrenaline release from isolated nerve terminals. J Neurochem. 1992;58:204–11.
16. Aronson S, Gennser G, Owman C, Sjoberg NO. Innervation and contractile response of the human ductus arteriosus. Eur J Pharmacol. 1970;11:178–86.
17. Chourbaji S, Vogt MA, Fumagalli F, Sohr R, Frasca A, Brandwein C, Hortnagl H, Riva MA, Sprengel R, Gass P. AMPA receptor subunit 1 (GluR-A) knockout mice model the glutamate hypothesis of depression. FASEB J. 2008;22:3129–34.
18. Fujita S, Yokoyama U, Ishiwata R, Aoki R, Nagao K, Masukawa D, Umemura M, Fujita T, Iwasaki S, Nishimaki S, Seki K, Ito S, Goshima Y, Asou T, Masuda M, Ishikawa Y. Glutamate promotes contraction of the rat ductus arteriosus. Circ J. 2016;80:2388–96.

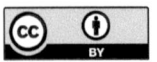

Antenatal Administration of Betamethasone Contributes to Intimal Thickening of the Ductus Arteriosus

38

Takahiro Kemmotsu, Utako Yokoyama, Junichi Saito,
Satoko Ito, Azusa Uozumi, Shiho Iwasaki,
Shigeru Nishimaki, Shuichi Ito, Munetaka Masuda,
Toshihide Asou, and Yoshihiro Ishikawa

Keywords

Ductus arteriosus · Glucocorticoid · Intimal thickening

Antenatal betamethasone (BTM) is a standard therapy to reduce respiratory distress syndrome [1], and some reports indicate that BTM decreases prevalence of patent ductus arteriosus in preterm infants [2]. Closure of the ductus arteriosus (DA) requires morphological remodeling, i.e., intimal thickening (IT) formation [3]. However, the role of BTM in IT formation of the preterm DA has not been reported.

T. Kemmotsu
Department of Pediatrics, Yokohama City University, Yokohama, Japan

Cardiovascular Research Institute, Yokohama City University, Yokohama, Japan

U. Yokoyama (✉) · J. Saito · S. Ito · Y. Ishikawa
Cardiovascular Research Institute, Yokohama City University, Yokohama, Japan
e-mail: utako@yokohama-cu.ac.jp; yishikaw@med.yokohama-cu.ac.jp

A. Uozumi · S. Nishimaki · S. Ito
Department of Pediatrics, Yokohama City University, Yokohama, Japan

S. Iwasaki
Perinatal Center, Yokohama City University Medical Center, Yokohama, Japan

M. Masuda
Department of Surgery, Yokohama City University, Yokohama, Japan

T. Asou
Department of Cardiovascular Surgery, Kanagawa Children's Medical Center, Yokohama, Japan

First, we analyzed the expression of glucocorticoid receptor (GR) in preterm and term DA tissues. Quantitative RT-PCR of rat DA tissues (day 19 and day 21 of gestation) and immunohistochemistry of the human DA tissue (day 7, coarctation of the aorta) showed that GR was highly expressed in the human and rat DAs. We then performed DNA microarray analysis using smooth muscle cells of preterm rat DA (DASMCs) on day 20 of gestation stimulated with or without BTM. Among all of the genes detected in preterm DASMCs, the gene X was markedly increased by BTM stimulation, which was confirmed by quantitative RT-PCR in rat preterm DASMCs, but not in preterm rat aortic smooth muscle cells. A scratch assay demonstrated that BTM promoted preterm DASMC migration, which was attenuated by the gene X-targeted siRNA.

Furthermore, we examined whether BTM increased IT formation in vivo. Maternal rats were administered intravenously with BTM or normal saline (control) on day 18 and 19 of gestation, and fetal rat DA tissues were obtained on day 20 of gestation. The ratio of IT to tunica media was significantly higher in BTM treatment group ($n = 5$, $p < 0.05$).

In conclusion, these data suggest that antenatal BTM administration promotes IT of the DA through the gene X-mediated DASMC migration.

Acknowledgment This study was funded by MEXT/JSPS KAKENHI (S.I., 43008732; U.Y., 16H05358, 15H05761; J.S., 16H07107; Y.I., H1605300, 16K15205), Yokohama Foundation for Advancement of Medical Science (J.S.), and AMED (Y.I., 66890011, 66890023, 17ek0109240h0001, A261TS).

References

1. Roberts D, et al. Antenatal corticosteroids for accelerating fetal lung maturation for women at risk of preterm birth. Cochrane Datebase Syst Rev. 2006;19(3):CD004454.
2. Been JV, et al. Antenatal steroids and neonatal outcome after chorioamnionitis: a meta-analysis. BJOG. 2011;118(2):113–22.
3. Yokoyama U, et al. Regulation of vascular tone and remodeling of the ductus arteriosus. J Smooth Muscle Res. 2010;46(2):77–87.

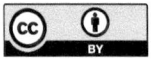

Prostaglandin E-EP4-Mediated Fibulin-1 Up-regulation Plays a Role in Intimal Thickening of the Ductus Arteriosus

39

Satoko Ito, Utako Yokoyama, Junichi Saito,
Munetaka Masuda, Toshihide Asou,
and Yoshihiro Ishikawa

Keywords
Ductus arteriosus · Cell migration · Intimal thickening

The normal closure of the ductus arteriosus (DA) consists of two steps: vasoconstriction and intimal thickening (IT). We have revealed that prostaglandin E2 (PGE_2)-EP4 signaling plays a critical role in IT formation via smooth muscle cell (SMC) migration through hyaluronic acid [1]. In this study, we found that fibulin-1 was the most significantly up-regulated gene by EP4 stimulation in DA smooth muscle cells (SMCs).

It has been reported that fibulin-1 has binding domains for ADAMTS-1 (a disintegrin and metalloprotease with thrombospondin motif type 1) and versican [2, 3], which participates in cell migration, and this fibulin-1-binding protease ADAMTS-1 promotes versican fragmentation [4, 5]. Furthermore, coupling of fragmented versican and hyaluronic acid promotes cell migration [6]. We speculated that fibulin-1 promotes DASMC migration and induces IT of the DA with ADAMTS-1 and versican. We aimed to examine the role of PGE_2-EP4-signaling-mediated fibulin-1 in IT of the DA.

S. Ito · U. Yokoyama (✉) · J. Saito · Y. Ishikawa
Cardiovascular Research Institute, Yokohama City University, Yokohama, Japan
e-mail: utako@yokohama-cu.ac.jp

M. Masuda
Department of Surgery, Yokohama City University, Yokohama, Japan

T. Asou
Department of Cardiovascular Surgery, Kanagawa Children's Medical Center, Yokohama, Japan

Based on the microarray analysis showing that fibulin-1 was the most increased gene by EP4 stimulation in DASMCs, we performed RT-PCR and confirmed similar findings. EP4 stimulation did not increase fibulin-1 in aortic SMCs. Protein expression of fibulin-1 was markedly increased by EP4 stimulation in DASMCs. Immunohistochemistry of rat DA tissues showed that fibulin-1, ADAMTS-1, and fragmented versican were co-localized in the area of IT. VersicanV1 mRNA expression was significantly higher in endothelial cells than in DASMCs, and ADAMTS-1 was expressed in both endothelial cells and DASMCs. EP4 stimulation significantly increased binding of hyaluronic acid to fragmented versicanV1 protein in DASMCs. A Scratch assay showed that EP4 promoted DASMC migration, which was attenuated by fibulin-1-targeted siRNA and ADAMTS-1-targeted siRNA.

In conclusion, PGE_2-EP4-mediated fibulin-1 integrates extracellular matrices such as ADAMTS-1, versican V1, and hyaluronic acid to promote SMC migration of the DA.

Acknowledgment This study was funded by MEXT/JSPS KAKENHI (SI, 43008732; U.Y., 16H05358, 15H05761; J.S., 16H07107; Y.I., H1605300, 16K15205), Yokohama Foundation for Advancement of Medical Science (J.S.), and the Japan Agency for Medical Research and Development (AMED) (Y.I., 66890011, 66890023, 17ek0109240h0001, A261TS).

References

1. Yokoyama U, et al. Chronic activation of the prostaglandin receptor EP4 promotes hyaluronan-mediated neointimal formation in the ductus arteriosus. J Clin Invest. 2006;116:3026–34.
2. Argraves WC. Fibulin, a novel protein that interacts with the fibronectin receptor beta subunit cytoplasmic domain. Cell. 1989;58(4):623–9.
3. Lee NV. Fibulin-1 acts as a cofactor for the matrix metalloprotease ADAMTS-1. J Biol Chem. 2015;280(41):34796–804.
4. Jonsson-Rylander AC, et al. Role of ADAMTS-1 in atherosclerosis; remodeling of carotid artery, immunohistochemistry, and proteolysis of versican. Thromb Vasc Biol. 2005;25(10):2075–80.
5. Nandadasa S, et al. The multiple, complex roles of versican and its proteolytic turnover by ADAMTS proteases during embryogenesis. Matrix Biol. 2014;35:34–41.
6. Wight TN. Provisional matrix: arole for versican and hyaluronan. Matrix Biol. 2017;60-61:38–56.

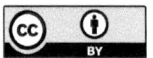

Transcriptional Profiles in the Chicken Ductus Arteriosus During Hatching

40

Satoko Shinjo, Toru Akaike, Eriko Ohmori, Ichige Kajimura, Nobuhito Goda, and Susumu Minamisawa

Keywords

Ductus arteriosus · Microarray analysis · Chicken

The ductus arteriosus (DA) of oviparous animals differs from mammals' in the embryonic gas exchange system and its anatomy. We performed transcriptional analysis of chicken DA, attempting to elucidate the similarity and diversity in the mechanism of DA closure among species.

Chicken DA proximal to the pulmonary arteries (proximal DA) closes after hatching while the DA proximal to the aorta (distal DA) remains open even after hatching [1]. Histological analysis revealed that the ductal wall of the proximal DA became thicker with fragmented elastic fibers from embryonic day (ED) 19. Therefore, we performed microarray analysis with proximal DA, distal DA, and aorta from chicken embryo at ED19. Clustering analysis found that the expression pattern of distal DA was similar to that of proximal DA than that of aorta although

S. Shinjo · T. Akaike · I. Kajimura
Department of Cell Physiology, The Jikei University School of Medicine, Minato, Tokyo, Japan

E. Ohmori · S. Minamisawa (✉)
Department of Cell Physiology, The Jikei University School of Medicine, Minato, Tokyo, Japan

Department of Life Science and Medical Bioscience, School of Advanced Science and Engineering, Waseda University, Shinjuku, Tokyo, Japan
e-mail: sminamis@jikei.ac.jp

N. Goda
Department of Life Science and Medical Bioscience, School of Advanced Science and Engineering, Waseda University, Shinjuku, Tokyo, Japan

distal DA has a similar structure to aorta. Subsequent pathway analysis with DAVID [2] revealed that proximal DA had enhanced expression of the melanogenetic genes compared with distal DA and aorta (Table 40.1). This result appears reasonable because proximal DA shares its developmental origin, neural crest, with melano-cytes. Although several known genes such as transcription factor AP-2 beta (tfap2b) [3] were highly expressed in proximal and distal DA, we newly found proximal-DA-dominant genes. Further investigation would be required to understand the role of these genes in DA closure not only for the chick but also for mammals.

Table 40.1 KEGG pathway analysis by DAVID from chicken DA microarray

Gene symbol	Gene name	Proximal DA/aorta	Distal DA/aorta	Note
Proximal DA dominant pathways				
Melanogenesis/tyrosine metabolism				
DCT	Dopachrome tautomerase (dopachrome delta-isomerase, tyrosine-related protein 2)	1.44*	1.06	
EDNRB2	Endothelin receptor B subtype 2	1.31*	1.07	(1)
TYR	Tyrosinase (oculocutaneous albinism IA)	1.54*	0.94	(1)
TYRP1	Tyrosinase-related protein 1	1.48*	1.03	
WNT11	Wingless-type MMTV integration site family, member 11	1.33*	1.14	
Arachidonic acid metabolism				
CYP2C45	Cytochrome P-450 2C45	1.44*	1.02	
HPGDS	Hematopoietic prostaglandin D synthase	1.56*	1.02	
PTGS2	Prostaglandin-endoperoxide synthase 2 (prostaglandin G/H synthase and cyclooxygenase)	1.31*	1.21	
DA dominant pathways				
Focal adhesion/ECM-receptor interaction				
FIGF	c-fos-Induced growth factor (vascular endothelial growth factor D)	1.50*	1.29*	(2)
KDR	Kinase insert domain receptor (a type III receptor tyrosine kinase)	1.34*	1.32*	(2)
LAMA4	Laminin subunit alpha 4	1.33*	1.24	
LAMB1	Laminin, beta 1	1.36*	1.27*	
TNC	Tenascin C	2.15*	1.82*	
VWF	von Willebrand factor	1.39*	1.31*	
CHAD	Chondroadherin	1.24	1.22*	
ITGA1	Integrin, alpha 1	1.28	1.21*	
VEGF signaling pathway				
HSPB1	Heat shock 27kDa protein 1	1.34*	1.21*	
KDR	Kinase insert domain receptor (a type III receptor tyrosine kinase)	1.34*	1.32*	
PTGS2	Prostaglandin-endoperoxide synthase 2 (prostaglandin G/H synthase and cyclooxygenase)	1.31*	1.21*	
PLCG2	Phospholipase C, gamma 2 (phosphatidylinositol-specific)	1.17	1.20*	

The asterisk indicates that the component genes appeared in the result of DAVID analysis
(1) Only appeared in "melanogenesis,"
(2) Only appeared in "focal adhesion"

Acknowledgment This work was supported by grants from the Ministry of Education, Culture, Sports, Science and Technology of Japan (T.A., S.M.), MEXT-Supported Program for the Strategic Research Foundation at Private Universities (S.M.), the Vehicle Racing Commemorative Foundation (S.M.), The Jikei University Graduate Research Fund (S.M.), and the Miyata Cardiology Research Promotion Foundation (S.M.).

References

1. Belanger C, Copeland J, et al. Morphological changes in the chicken ductus arteriosi during closure at hatching. Anat Rec (Hoboken). 2008;291:1007–15. https://doi.org/10.1002/ar.20720.
2. Huang da W, Sherman BT, et al. Systematic and integrative analysis of large gene lists using DAVID bioinformatics resources. Nat Protoc. 2009;4:44–57. https://doi.org/10.1038/nprot.2008.211.
3. Zhao F, Bosserhoff AK, et al. A heart-hand syndrome gene: Tfap2b plays a critical role in the development and remodeling of mouse ductus arteriosus and limb patterning. PLoS One. 2011;6:e22908. https://doi.org/10.1371/journal.pone.0022908.

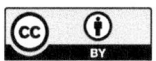

Inhibition of Cyclooxygenase Contracts Chicken Ductus Arteriosus

41

Toru Akaike and Susumu Minamisawa

Keywords

Ductus arteriosus · Prostaglandin · Chicken

Ductus arteriosus (DA) is an essential fetal artery that connects the main pulmonary artery and the descending aorta. Mammalian DA closes right after birth through vasoconstriction via a decrease in circulating prostaglandin E_2 (PGE_2) [1]. Avian DA also closes after birth although avians have no placenta that is a source of PGE_2 in mammals. Previous studies have demonstrated that the PGE_2 signal pathway is not involved in the constriction of isolated chicken DA [2]. However, the in vivo effect of PGE_2 in avian DA has been little investigated.

We first measured blood concentration of PGE_2 in chicken at embryonic day 19 (just before hatching) by enzyme immunoassay to confirm whether PGE_2 circulated in the chicken blood during a perinatal period. Plasma PGE_2 was significantly high in chicken compared to rat. PGE_2 was strongly produced in chicken DA compared to chicken aorta and rat DA. Next, we determined the expression of prostaglandin E receptors (EP1, EP2, EP3 and EP4) in chicken DA. EP2 and EP3 receptors in fetal chicken DA were significantly higher than that of fetal chicken aorta. Especially, the EP2 receptor was significantly up-regulated before hatching and down-regulated after hatching. Finally, we performed a rapid whole-body freezing method to evaluate DA closure in vivo. We measured the internal diameter of DA two hours after in ovo injection of indomethacin, which is a non-selective cyclooxygenase inhibitor. Indomethacin constricted chicken DA at embryonic day 19 but did not constrict chicken aorta. These data suggest that, similar to mammals, PGE_2 acts as a vasodilative factor on DA closure in avians.

T. Akaike · S. Minamisawa (✉)

Department of Cell Physiology, The Jikei University School of Medicine, Minato, Tokyo, Japan

e-mail: sminamis@jikei.ac.jp

We demonstrated that factors of the PGE_2 signal were detected in chicken DA and inhibition of cyclooxygenase contracted chicken DA. We concluded that the PGE_2 signal may play an important role in acute vasodilatation of chicken DA closure.

Acknowledgment This work was supported by grants from the Ministry of Education, Culture, Sports, Science and Technology of Japan (T.A., S.M.), MEXT-Supported Program for the Strategic Research Foundation at Private Universities (S.M.), the Vehicle Racing Commemorative Foundation (S.M.), The Jikei University Graduate Research Fund (S.M.), and the Miyata Cardiology Research Promotion Foundation (S.M.).

References

1. Yokoyama U, Minamisawa S, Ishikawa Y. Regulation of vascular tone and remodeling of the ductus arteriosus. J Smooth Muscle Res. 2010;46:77–87.
2. Agren P, van der Sterren S, Cogolludo AL, et al. Developmental changes in the effects of prostaglandin E2 in the chicken ductus arteriosus. J Comp Physiol B. 2009;179(2):133–43.

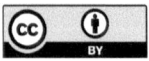

Prostaglandin E$_2$ Receptor EP4 Inhibition Constricts the Rat Ductus Arteriosus

42

Toshiki Sakuma, Toru Akaike, and Susumu Minamisawa

Keywords
Ductus arteriosus · Prostaglandin · EP4 antagonist

Patent ductus arteriosus (PDA) often occurs in premature infants [1]. At present, the cyclooxygenase inhibitor indomethacin is used to treat patients with PDA by inhibiting prostaglandin E$_2$ synthesis. However, its efficiency is frequently limited [2] and adverse effects are problematic [3]. We have demonstrated that the prostaglandin E$_2$ receptor EP4 specifically expresses in the rat ductus arteriosus (DA) [4]. Therefore, we hypothesized that EP4 inhibition promoted closure of the DA with fewer side effects.

We first examined the effect of the EP4 antagonist RQ-15986 (CJ-042794) on isometric tension of the ex vivo DA at embryonic day 19 (e19) and 21 (e21). RQ-15986 at a dose of $10-^4$ M significantly increased the isometric tension of the DA up to $57 \pm 14\%$ and $78 \pm 11\%$ of 120mM KCl contraction at e19 and e21, respectively. The constrictive effect of RQ-15986 was greater on the DA than on the aorta. Second, we tested the effect of RQ-15986 on in vivo DA. RQ-15986 was intraperitoneally injected into fetuses at e19 and e21. We measured the inner diameter of the vessels by a rapid whole-body freezing method. RQ-15986 constricted the DA but not the aorta in a dose-dependent manner. The contraction percentage was greater at e21 than at e19. Finally, RQ-15986 did not constrict the marginal artery of the colon.

T. Sakuma
The Jikei University School of Medicine, Minato, Tokyo, Japan

T. Akaike · S. Minamisawa (✉)
Department of Cell Physiology, The Jikei University School of Medicine, Minato, Tokyo, Japan
e-mail: sminamis@jikei.ac.jp

We demonstrated that RQ-15986 constricted the DA with fewer side effects. We concluded that EP4 inhibition would be a promising alternative strategy to treat a patient with PDA.

Acknowledgment This work was supported by grants from the Ministry of Education, Culture, Sports, Science and Technology of Japan (T.A., S.M.), MEXT-Supported Program for the Strategic Research Foundation at Private Universities (S.M.), the Vehicle Racing Commemorative Foundation (S.M.), The Jikei University Graduate Research Fund (S.M.), and the Miyata Cardiology Research Promotion Foundation (S.M.).

References

1. Lee SK, McMillan DD, Ohlsson A, et al. Variations in practice and outcomes in the Canadian NICU network: 1996-1997. Pediatrics. 2000;106(5):1070–9.
2. Heymann MA, Rudolph AM, Silverman NH. Closure of the ductus arteriosus in premature infants by inhibition of prostaglandin synthesis. N Engl J Med. 1976;295(10):530–3.
3. Van Overmeire B, Smets K, Lecoutere D, et al. A comparison of ibuprofen and indomethacin for closure of patent ductus arteriosus. N Engl J Med. 2000;343(10):674–81.
4. Yokoyama U, Minamisawa S, Shioda A, et al. Prostaglandin E2 inhibits elastogenesis in the ductus arteriosus via EP4 signaling. Circulation. 2014;129(4):487–96.

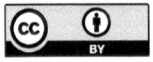

Dilatation of the Ductus Arteriosus by Diazoxide in Fetal and Neonatal Rats

43

Katsuaki Toyoshima, Kazuo Momma, Tetsuko Ishii, and Toshio Nakanishi

Keywords

Diazoxide · Ductus arteriosus · Rat

43.1 Background

We previously reported that ATP-sensitive potassium (K_{ATP}) channels regulate ductal constriction in response to oxygen [1]. Diazoxide is a K_{ATP} channel opener while the usefulness of diazoxide for hyperinsulinemic hypoglycemia is well established. Yoshida et al. reported DA reopening in very low-birth-weight infants [2]. The objectives of this study were to elucidate the effect of K_{ATP} channel openers on the DA in neonatal rats as well as the different effects in preterm and full-term fetal rats [3].

43.2 Methods

Near-term rat pups delivered via a cesarean section were housed at 33 °C. After rapid whole-body freezing, the ductus arteriosus (DA) diameter was measured using a microscope and a micrometer. Full-term pregnant rats (gestational day 21) were

K. Toyoshima (✉)
Division of Pediatric Cardiology, Tokyo Women's Medical University, Shinjuku, Tokyo, Japan

Division of Neonatology, Kanagawa Children's Medical Center, Yokohama, Kanagawa, Japan
e-mail: ktoyoshima@kcmc.jp

K. Momma · T. Ishii · T. Nakanishi
Department of Pediatric Cardiology, Tokyo Women's Medical University, Tokyo, Japan
e-mail: nakanishi.toshio@twmu.ac.jp

© The Editor(s) (if applicable) and The Author(s) 2020
T. Nakanishi et al. (eds.), *Molecular Mechanism of Congenital Heart Disease and Pulmonary Hypertension*, https://doi.org/10.1007/978-981-15-1185-1_43

intraperitoneally injected with diazoxide (10 and 100 mg/kg) 4 h before delivery, and the neonatal DA diameter was measured at 0, 30, or 60 min after birth. The newborn rats were also intraperitoneally injected with diazoxide (10 and 100 mg/kg) at birth or 60 min after birth. DA was measured at 0, 30, or 60 min after injection. In the fetal study, *constricted by COX and NOS inhibition* the *dilating* effects of diazoxide was studied by simultaneous administration of indomethacin (10 mg/kg) and L-nitroarginine methyl ester (100 mg/kg) in gestational day 21 and 19.

43.3   Results

DA closure was delayed in rats exposed to prenatal diazoxide. Both doses of transplacentally administered diazoxide induced significant and dose-dependent inhibitory effect in postnatal DA constriction. Intraperitoneal injection of diazoxide at 60 min after birth induced DA reopening in a dose-dependent manner.

Diazoxide (10 mg/kg) dilatated the fetal DA in both near-term and preterm fetal rats. The effect of diazoxide in dilating the DA at preterm was the same as at full-term fetal rats.

43.4   Conclusion

K_{ATP} channel openers attenuate postnatal DA constriction and dilatate a closing DA in neonatal rats. If the DA is affected in a similar manner in human neonates, then PDA could be warranted for use with K_{ATP} channel openers to treat infants with hyperinsulinemic hypoglycemia, especially preterm infants.

References

1. Nakanishi T, et al. Mechanisms of oxygen-induced contraction of ductus arteriosus isolated from the fetal rabbit. Circ Res. 1993;72(6):1218–28.
2. Yoshida K, et al. High prevalence of severe circulatory complications with diazoxide in premature infants. Neonatology. 2014;105(3):166–71.
3. Toyoshima K, et al. Dilatation of the ductus arteriosus by diazoxide in fetal and neonatal rats. Pediatr Int. 2017;59(12):1246–51.

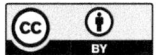

The Effect of Long-term Administration of Prostaglandin E1 on Morphological Changes in Ductus Arteriosus

44

Ryuma Iwaki, Hironori Matsuhisa, Susumu Minamisawa, Toru Akaike, Masato Hoshino, Naoto Yagi, Kiyozo Morita, Gen Shinohara, Yukihiro Kaneko, Syuichi Yoshitake, Masashi Takahashi, Takuro Tsukube, and Yoshihiro Oshima

Abstract

The morphological and histopathological effects of PGE_1 infusion for ductus arteriosus were clarified through novel modality XPCT and immunohistochemical analyses, EP4, and LOX expression. Recognition of microstructural changes of ductal tissue induced by extended administration of PGE_1 is profound to establish the safety usage of PGE_1 for HLHS patients with staged Norwood repair.

Keywords

Ductus arteriosus · Prostaglandin E_1 · Hypoplastic left heart syndrome · X-ray phase contrast tomography

R. Iwaki (✉) · H. Matsuhisa · Y. Oshima
Department of Cardiovascular Surgery, Kobe Children's Hospital, Kobe, Japan

S. Minamisawa · T. Akaike
Department of Cell Physiology, The Jikei University School of Medicine, Tokyo, Japan

M. Hoshino · N. Yagi
Japan Synchrotron Radiation Research Institute (SPring-8), Sayo, Japan

K. Morita · G. Shinohara
Department of Cardiovascular Surgery, The Jikei University School of Medicine, Tokyo, Japan

Y. Kaneko · S. Yoshitake
Division of Cardiovascular Surgery, National Center for Child Health and Development, Tokyo, Japan

M. Takahashi
Division of Thoracic and Cardiovascular Surgery, Niigata University Graduate School of Medical and Dental Sciences, Niigata, Japan

T. Tsukube
Division of Cardiovascular Surgery, Japanese Red Cross Kobe Hospital, Kobe, Japan

44.1 Introduction

Prostaglandin E_1 (PGE_1) is essential to maintain the ductus arteriosus (DA) in ductal-dependent congenital heart diseases. Recently, relatively long-term administration of PGE_1 has become common, especially in patients with hypoplastic left heart syndrome (HLHS). Staged Norwood approach which consists of PGE_1 infusion, bilateral pulmonary artery banding and Norwood procedure provided excellent survival benefit. However, microstructural changes in DA after long-term PGE_1 administration remain unknown. Therefore, we sought to investigate the features of DA after long-term PGE_1 infusion using synchrotron-based X-ray phase contrast tomography (XPCT), a novel modality to inspect biological soft tissue and pathological scrutiny including DA-specific immunostaining.

44.2 Methods

Seventeen DA tissues from HLHS patients were obtained during the Norwood procedure. The median duration of PGE_1 was 48 days (range 3–123). Radiographic microstructural analysis of DA was performed using XPCT at SPring-8 (Hyogo, Japan). Histological changes focused on elastic fiber and smooth muscle formation were evaluated by Elastica van Gieson staining. Expressions of prostaglandin E_2 receptor (EP4) and LOX, a cross-linking enzyme that forms insoluble mature elastic fibers, were evaluated by immunohistochemical analyses.

44.3 Results

The XPCT study showed sclerotic changes in ductal media. There was a significant correlation between the duration of PGE_1 infusion and the mass density of ductal media (R: 0.723, $p = 0.001$). The histological study showed that the duration of PGE_1 infusion was positively correlated with the elastic fiber formation (R: 0.795, $P = 0.002$) and negatively correlated with smooth muscle formation in a disorganized manner (R: –0.83, $P < 0.001$). EP4 was disappeared in DAs that were administered PGE_1 over 20 days. LOX expression was observed in all DAs, especially LOX strongly emerged in specimens where elastic fiber formation was immature.

44.4 Conclusion

Long-term administration of PGE_1 induced disorganized elastogenesis and density growth of the ductal media. In addition, downregulation of EP4 and LOX expression might emphasize this hypothesis. These results suggested that the dosage of PGE_1 could be decreased after a definite period of administration.

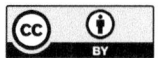

Significance of SGK1 as a Protein Kinase Transcriptionally Regulated by ALK1 Signaling in Vascular Endothelial Cells

45

Osamu Nakagawa, Yusuke Watanabe, Yukihiro Harada, Toru Tanaka, and Teruhisa Kawamura

Keywords

Serum/glucocorticoid-regulated kinase 1 · AGC family kinases · ALK1 signaling · Endothelial transcription · Vascular development

Bone morphogenetic protein 9 (BMP9)/BMP10-ALK1 receptor signaling is essential for endothelial differentiation and vascular morphogenesis and is implicated in hereditary hemorrhagic telangiectasia and pulmonary arterial hypertension [1]. The ALK1 signal induces SMAD1/5/9-dependent transcription of its own signaling components, transcription factors and membrane ligands/receptors. In addition, we recently identified Serum/glucocorticoid-regulated kinase 1 (SGK1) to be transcriptionally regulated by ALK1 signaling in vascular endothelial cells [2] (Fig. 45.1a). The ALK1 signal is known to evoke post-translational activation of protein kinases such as TAK1 and ERK as a non-canonical pathway, but SGK1 is the first example of protein kinases whose expression is controlled by the SMAD-dependent pathway (Fig. 45.1b).

O. Nakagawa (✉) · Y. Watanabe · T. Tanaka
Department of Molecular Physiology, National Cerebral and Cardiovascular Center Research Institute, Osaka, Japan
e-mail: osamu.nakagawa@ncvc.go.jp

Y. Harada
Department of Molecular Physiology, National Cerebral and Cardiovascular Center Research Institute, Osaka, Japan

Laboratory of Stem Cell and Regenerative Medicine, Department of Biomedical Sciences, College of Life Sciences, Ritsumeikan University, Shiga, Japan

T. Kawamura
Laboratory of Stem Cell and Regenerative Medicine, Department of Biomedical Sciences, College of Life Sciences, Ritsumeikan University, Shiga, Japan

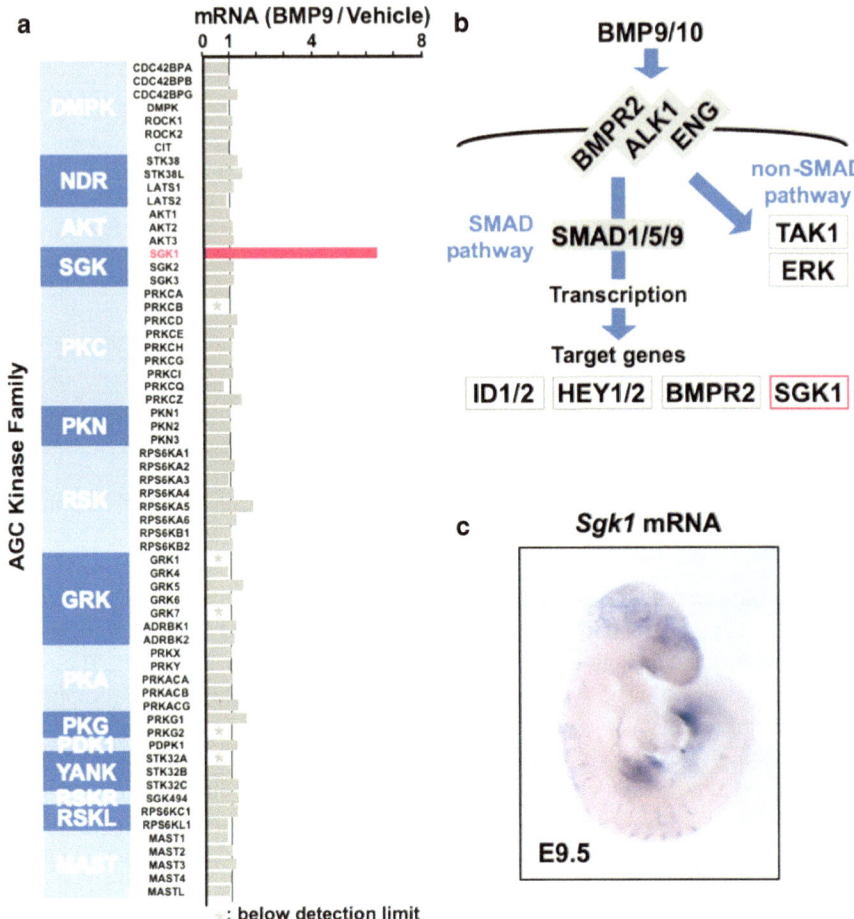

Fig. 45.1 (**a**) Specific induction of SGK1 mRNA expression by ALK1 signaling. Microarray results of the AGC family kinases using human umbilical artery endothelial cells at 2 hours after BMP9 stimulation (10 ng/mL) are shown. (**b**) A schematic of the SMAD-dependent and -independent pathways of ALK1 signaling and representative downstream targets. (**c**) Endothelial expression of *Sgk1* mRNA during embryonic development. The in situ hybridization result of a mouse embryo (embryonic day 9.0) is shown

SGK1 belongs to the AGC (named after PKA, PKG and PKC) superfamily of protein kinases often involved in cardiovascular development and disease [3]. The microarray screen using BMP9-stimulated endothelial cells demonstrates that only SGK1 shows significant increase in mRNA expression among the AGC kinases (Fig. 45.1a). SGK1 plays pivotal roles in renal sodium reabsorption and T cell differentiation as well as cardiovascular diseases such as hypertension and cardiac arrhythmia [3]. Furthermore, *Sgk1* null mice with a particular genetic background exhibit severe abnormalities of vascular development and embryonic lethality [4], suggesting its role in the mechanisms of angiogenesis defects due to ALK1 signaling deficiency. While *Sgk1* mRNA is clearly enriched in vascular endothelial cells of mouse embryos (Fig. 45.1c), nothing was known as to how its specific expression was achieved in vivo. It is important to identify an *Sgk1* endothelial enhancer and examine whether SMAD cooperates with endothelial transcription factors to control the *Sgk1* expression. Moreover, the expression and kinase activity of SGK1 are regulated not only by its transcription but also by mRNA turnover, protein degradation and phosphorylation. It will be of significance to clarify how SGK1 function is optimized in developing vasculature.

Acknowledgment This work was supported in part by the grants from the Ministry of Education, Culture, Sports, Science and Technology, the Smoking Research Foundation and the Novartis foundation (Japan).

References

1. Garcia de Vinuesa A, Abdelilah-Seyfried S, Knaus P, et al. BMP signaling in vascular biology and dysfunction. Cytokine Growth Factor Rev. 2016;27:65–79.
2. Araki M, Hisamitsu T, Kinugasa-Katayama Y, et al. Serum/glucocorticoid-regulated kinase 1 as a novel transcriptional target of bone morphogenetic protein-ALK1 receptor signaling in vascular endothelial cells. Angiogenesis. 2018;21:415–23.
3. Di Cristofano A. SGK1: the dark side of PI3K Signaling. Curr Top Dev Biol. 2017;123:49–71.
4. Catela C, Kratsios P, Hede M, et al. Serum and glucocorticoid-inducible kinase 1 (SGK1) is necessary for vascular remodeling during angiogenesis. Dev Dyn. 2010;239:2149–60.

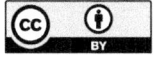

Fabrication of Implantable Human Arterial Graft by Periodic Hydrostatic Pressure

46

Junichi Saito, Utako Yokoyama, Toshio Takayama,
Hiroaki Ito, Tomomi Tadokoro, Yoshinobu Sugo,
Kentaro Kurasawa, Miyuki Ogawa, Etsuko Miyagi,
Hideki Taniguchi, Makoto Kaneko, and Yoshihiro Ishikawa

Keywords

Tissue engineering · Periodic hydrostatic pressure · Human vascular graft · Implantation · Mechanoresponse

Structural heart disease is the most common congenital anomaly, affecting almost 1% of live births [1]. Approximately 25% of newborns with congenital heart disease (CHD) require surgical or trans-catheter intervention in the first year of life [2]. Artificial materials such as polytetrafluoroethylene are used for the surgical repair of CHD, but these materials lack growth potential and lead to stenosis according to patient's growth. Therefore, biological tissue-engineered blood vessels are desired for pediatric patients. Recently, we fabricated implantable "scaffold-free" grafts consisting of rat vascular smooth muscle cells by periodic hydrostatic pressure (PHP) [3]. Here we aimed to fabricate implantable human grafts and examine the molecular response to PHP.

J. Saito · U. Yokoyama (✉) · Y. Ishikawa (✉)
Cardiovascular Research Institute, Yokohama City University, Yokohama, Japan
e-mail: utako@yokohama-cu.ac.jp; yishikaw@med.yokohama-cu.ac.jp

T. Takayama · H. Ito · M. Kaneko
Department of Mechanical Engineering, Osaka University, Suita, Japan

T. Tadokoro · H. Taniguchi
Department of Regenerative Medicine, Yokohama City University, Yokohama, Japan

Y. Sugo · K. Kurasawa · M. Ogawa · E. Miyagi
Department of Obstetrics and Gynecology, Yokohama City University, Yokohama, Japan

© The Editor(s) (if applicable) and The Author(s) 2020
T. Nakanishi et al. (eds.), *Molecular Mechanism of Congenital Heart Disease and Pulmonary Hypertension*, https://doi.org/10.1007/978-981-15-1185-1_46

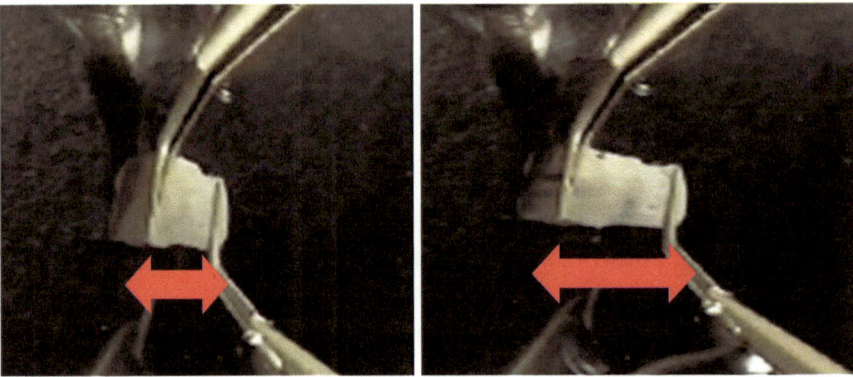

Fig. 46.1 Layered hUASMC showed elasticity

We seeded human umbilical arterial smooth muscle cells (hUASMCs) on a culture disk to make the first cell layer. Twenty-four hours after seeding, cells were exposed to PHP for 24 h, and then cells for the next layer were seeded on the top of the first layer, followed by repeating the same procedure to construct ten layered cell sheets. The multi-layered construct exhibited high elasticity (Fig. 46.1) and was successfully implanted at the aorta of nude rat. Echocardiography confirmed patency, and histological analysis demonstrated complete endothelialization.

We previously demonstrated that PHP promoted actin polymerization and fibronectin fibrillogenesis [3]. We further investigated the molecular response to PHP. hUASMCs were exposed to PHP and subjected to a microarray analysis. A microarray analysis revealed PHP-response genes, which are related to angiogenesis and stabilization of fibronectin. These genes were increased in a pressure-dependent manner, and co-localized with focal adhesion. These mechanoresponse molecules may contribute to construct the multi-layered cell sheets.

Acknowledgment This work was supported by JSPS KAKENHI (U.Y., JP17K19403, JP16H05358; M.K., JP15H05761) and AMED (Y.I., 66890007).

References

1. Van Der Linde D, Konings EE, Slager MA, et al. Birth prevalence of congenital heart disease worldwide: a systematic review and meta-analysis. J Am Coll Cardiol. 2011;58:2241–7.
2. Simeone RM, Oster ME, Cassell CH, et al. Pediatric inpatient hospital resource use for congenital heart defects. Birth Defects Res A Clin Mol Teratol. 2014;100:934–9433.
3. Yokoyama U, Tonooka Y, Koretake R, et al. Arterial graft with elastic layer structure grown from cells. Sci Rep. 2017;7:140.

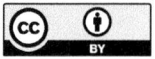

Optimum Preparation of *Candida albicans* Cell Wall Extra (CAWE) for the Mouse Model of Kawasaki Disease

47

Yukako Yoshikane, Tamaki Cho, Mitsuhisa Koga, Seiji Haraoka, and Atsushi Ogawa

Keywords

Kawasaki disease · Animal model · *Candida albicans*

Kawasaki disease is the most common acute systemic vasculitis of unknown etiology in children [1] and can cause inflammation of the coronary arteries leading to aneurysms. *Candida albicans* extract is one of the materials commonly used to induce coronary arteritis in a mouse model of Kawasaki disease [2, 3]. Here we report an optimized method for preparing *C. albicans* cell wall extra (CAWE).

1. 80% of the mice administered CAWE that had been alkalinized at 87 °C showed massive inflammation around the origin of the coronary arteries. By contrast, the mice administered CAWE that had been alkalinized at 97 °C showed no inflammation.
2. 60% of the mice administered CAWE adjusted to 640 μg protein/mouse died within 2 days whereas 100% of the mice administered CAWE adjusted to 320 μg protein/mouse exhibited inflammation but survived.

Y. Yoshikane (✉) · A. Ogawa
Department of Pediatrics, Fukuoka University, Chikushi Hospital, Fukuoka, Fukuoka, Japan
e-mail: yyoshika@fukuoka-u.ac.jp

T. Cho
Department of Oral Microbiology, Fukuoka Dental College, Fukuoka, Fukuoka, Japan

M. Koga
Faculty of Pharmaceutical Sciences, Fukuoka University, Fukuoka, Fukuoka, Japan

S. Haraoka
Department of Pathology, Fukuoka University, Chikushi Hospital, Fukuoka, Fukuoka, Japan

In conclusion, high heat processing causes poor pathogenicity and high protein content causes excessive pathogenicity. Therefore, CAWE that has been heat processed at 87 °C and adjusted to 320 μg protein/mouse is optimal for the mouse model of Kawasaki disease.

Acknowledgment We thank Kate Fox, DPhil, from Edanz Group (www.edanzediting.com/ac) for editing a draft of this manuscript.

References

1. Kawasaki T, Kosaki F, Okawa S, Shigematsu I, Yanagawa H. A new infantile acute febrile mucocutaneous lymph node syndrome (MLNS) prevailing in Japan. Pediatrics. 1974;54:271–6.
2. Murata H. Experimental candida-induced arteritis in mice. Relation to arteritis in the mucocutaneous lymph node syndrome. Microbiol Immunol. 1979;23:825–31.
3. Takahashi K, Oharaseki T, Wakayama M, Yokouchi Y, Naoe S, Murata H. Histopathological features of murine systemic vasculitis caused by Candida albicans extract—an animal model of Kawasaki disease. Inflamm Res. 2004;53:72–7.

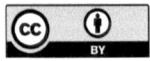

Part IV

Development and Regeneration of the Cardiovascular System

Perspective for Part IV

48

H. Scott Baldwin

The advances that have been made in understanding the developmental processes and molecular pathways that control cardiac development have been enormous in the last several decades. It was the original goal of the first Takao Symposia in 1978 to promote the scientific understanding of cardiac morphogenesis to form a foundation for investigating the mechanisms of congenital heart disease. However, even the ambitious investigators who attended that first meeting would not have anticipated the rapid progress that has occurred in this field. Furthermore, few would have predicted that there would be serious discussion about exploiting developmental paradigms to promote cardiac stem cell differentiation as an approach to attain cardiac regeneration. In this section we get a glimpse of some exciting new developments in these areas that have been the direct result of insights presented at and encouraged by the Takao Symposia.

One of the major advances in understanding the early stages of cardiac development has been the discovery that the entire heart does not arise from a single developmental field but rather the right ventricle, outflow track, and portions of the atria were derived from a second population of cells, now known as the second heart field (SHF), and the left ventricle appears to be primarily derived from anterior or the first heart field (FHF) derivatives. In this volume, Narematsu and Nakajima (Chap. 59) show that these distinct heart fields demonstrate differential response to the mutagen retinoic acid as early exposure of the FHF result in Transposition of the Great Vessels (TGA) and the double outlet right ventricle while exposure of the SHF at the same age results in persistence of the truncus arteriosus (PTA). Robert Kelley, one of the

H. S. Baldwin (✉)
Department of Pediatrics (Cardiology) and Cell and Development Biology,
Vanderbilt University Medical Center, Nashville, TN, USA
e-mail: scott.baldwin@vanderbilt.edu

T. Nakanishi et al. (eds.), *Molecular Mechanism of Congenital Heart Disease and Pulmonary Hypertension*, https://doi.org/10.1007/978-981-15-1185-1_48

initial investigators to identify and delineate the SHF, and colleagues (Chap. 49) utilized an intricate combination of immunohistochemistry, Cre lineage tracing, transcriptome analysis, and novel in vivo morphological analysis to identify the heterogenous nature of the SHF cell populations. They specifically detailed the epithelial like characterization of cell populations important in defining the transitional cell populations at both the arterial and venous poles of the SHF that are critical for normal morphogenesis. Kodo et al. (Chap. 58) added to the characterization of this heterogenous SHF population by demonstrating that expression of the neurovascular molecule, semaphorin 3c, within the arterial pole of the SHF is essential for correct navigation of the cardiac neural crest cell (cNCC) populations essential for OFT development. Watanabe and Nakagawa (Chap. 60) expand the studies on novel factors regulating SHF and NCC interaction by showing that, Hey1, a downstream target of Notch 1 and Alk1 signaling is critical in aortic arch formation as null animals display an increased incidence or right sided aortic arch, interrupted aortic arch, aberrant origin of the right sub-clavian artery. Further adding to the complexity of understanding the heterogeneity of SHF progenitor cell components, Kokubo et al. (Chap. 50) used a new lineage tracing model based on expression of secreted frizzled-related protein 5 (*Sfrp5*) to identify a novel progenitor cell population that contributes to the OFT, sinus venosus, left atria, and also to the left ventricle, which was previously thought to be primary, if not exclusively, derived from FHF progenitors. These studies raise the intriguing possibility of a single progenitor cell population that contributes to both the SHF and FHF. Regional heterogeneity of cardiac gene expression in distinct regions of the heart may not only be important for developmental regulation but may also play an important role in pathology of the mature organism. In a fascinating study, Steimle et al. (Chap. 51) used transcriptional profiling to examine genetic differences that may actually regulate early post-natal cardiac function as well as cardiac function in the adult. They were able to identify discrete differences in gene expression between the left atrial appendage and the peri-pulmonary vein region of the left atria which is believed to be the nidus for many forms of atrial fibrillation.

With the development of induced pluripotent stem (iPS) cell technology, scientific interest in factors that regulate cardiac stem cell differentiation into functional components of the mature heart has expanded well beyond the focus on early events of cardiac ontogeny as these cells could provide a foundation for future cell based regenerative therapies. New methods to identify differentiated progenitor cells *in vitro* will be required for clinical utilization of iPS cells. Kawaguchi et al. (Chap. 61) showed that c-kit, a stem cell factor receptor often used for identifying cardiac progenitor cell populations, demonstrated robust expression in iPS cells grown on feeder cells but was subsequently downregulated following mesodermal and myocardial differentiation. They suggested that this factor might affect the early stages of cardiomyocyte differentiation. In an elegant study, Morita and Takeuchi (Chap. 57) developed transgenic iPSCs that could be induced to differentiation in functional cardiomyocytes, without the addition of extrinsic growth factors, by induction of two critical factors that they identified in a single cell screening of early cardiac progenitors. While iPS cells can be differentiated into cells that express myocardial markers, a major limitation has been achieving myocyte maturation that would achieve clinical utility. As such Brockmeier and co-workers (Chap. 55) present a novel *in vitro* model to quantify myocardial contractility of both embryonic stem cell (ESC) and iPS derived cardiomyocytes by assessing the ability of these cells to integrate, *in situ*, with both normal and damaged myocardial tissue slices instrumented for measurement of isometric force transduction. This system allows for precise pharmacologic manipulation and they found that ESCs and IPS cells showed quantifiable increases in force/contractility as measured in the system and few differences were noted between the two cell types. However, neither generates contractile forces comparable to native heart tissue and their work points to development of the sarcoplasmic reticulum as a limiting feature of ESC and iPSC differentiation strategies. In a "tour de force", Keller and colleagues (Chap. 54) go beyond an isolated single cell iPSC strategy in favor of the use of multiple cell lineages in 3D matrix formulations to form implantable engineered cardiac tissues (ECTs) from several sources including human iPS cells. They showed that these ECT tissues had improved maturation, could be optically paced, and were capable of improving the myocardial function after infarction. They describe several recent modifications that enhance the potential use in human tissue engineering strategies. To further expand the utility of iPSCs, Hayama et al. (Chap. 62) were able to determine that iPSCs could be derived from immortalized B cell lines and successfully differentiated into cardiomyocytes. This dramatically expands the potential of the iPS methodology to evaluate human diseases as these cell lines have been utilized to identify genetic mutations associated with an array of CHDs and thus now provide a new source for *in vitro* disease modeling. The utility of iPSCs in modeling human diseases is further illustrated by the work of Furutani et al. (Chap. 63) who developed an *in vitro* model to study Long QT Syndrome 3 by generating iPSCs from patient derived immortalized B-cell lines.

While significant attention has been paid to the early stages of cardiac morphogenesis including organization of the first and second heart fields as discussed above, heart tube looping, septation, and valve formation during latter stages of cardiac morphogenesis have been inaccessible to laboratory investigation because of the early embryonic demise of many genetic mutants. However, newer Cre mediated deletion strategies allowing temporal and tissue specific deletion of genes have been increasingly utilized to interrogate gene regulation in later gestational events. Qu and Baldwin (Chap. 52) offer novel insights into the important dynamic process of ventricular trabeculation. Using Cre mediated endocardial specific deletion of the receptor tyrosine kinase Tie2, they showed that signaling via this RTK is required for endocardial proliferation and development of the endocardial "sprouts" that define the trabeculae. Perhaps equally important, they showed that endothelial Tie2 mediated paracrine signaling suppresses myocardial proliferation, thus regulating the proper number of myocytes in the developing ventricle. Ishida et al. (Chap. 56) showed that following trabeculation, Glial cell line-derived neurotrophic factor receptor alpha (*Gfra*) is required in subsequent stages of ventricular compaction as *Gfra1&2* compound mutants developed a no-compaction cardiomyopathy. Furthermore, this phenotype was the result of perturbation in non-canonical Notch signaling. Nogimori et al. (Chap. 64) turned to human genetic studies to document the clinical variability in the process of left ventricular non-compaction by comparing one case of Gata4 mutation which was only mildly symptomatic with a patient harboring a TBX20 mutation who showed severe pulmonary hypertension and diastolic dysfunction. In a fascinating study, Steimle et al. (Chap. 51) used transcriptional profiling to examine genetic differences that may actually regulate post-natal cardiac function after birth and in the adult. They were able to identify discrete differences in gene expression between the left atrial appendage and the peripulmonary vein region of the left atria which is believed to be the nidus for many forms of atrial fibrillation.

The advances that have occurred since the first Takao Symposia have truly been impressive. Yet as Nakagama and Inuzuka remind us (Chap. 65) there are still significant challenges that remain in elucidating the pathogenesis of CHD and particularly challenging is developing vertebrate models that recapitulate human CHD to distinguish truly causal genetic variants from benign mutants. In addition, Dr. Bittel (Chap. 53) elegantly describes a potential role of non-coding RNAs in the etiology of Tetralogy of Falot further complicating the possible genetic mechanisms leading to CHD. It is clear that the mechanisms of normal and abnormal cardiac development are much more complicated than ever imagined. But based on the progress seen since the first Takao Symposia, we can be optimistic that the mechanisms and treatments for CHD will ultimately be unraveled.

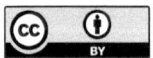

Advances in the Second Heart Field

49

Robert G. Kelly

Abstract

The deployment of progenitor cells from the second heart field (SHF) to the poles of the cardiac tube drives heart tube elongation during looping morphogenesis. Defects in this process underlie a spectrum of common forms of congenital heart defects (CHDs) affecting the cardiac poles, including conotruncal and atrioventricular septal defects. In this chapter recent findings will be reviewed concerning sequential steps in SHF development: the early emergence of the SHF lineage, the epithelial properties of SHF cells during heart tube elongation, and the importance of the transition zone as progenitor cells differentiate at the cardiac poles. Together these studies define critical regulatory nodes at successive stages of SHF deployment, providing new insights into mechanisms of heart development and the origins of CHD.

Keywords

Second heart field · Cardiac progenitor cells · Heart development · Congenital heart defects · Tbx1

49.1 Introduction

The second heart field (SHF) contributes cardiac progenitor cells to the poles of the vertebrate heart as it elongates during looping morphogenesis [1]. This process occurs between E8 and E10.5 of mouse gestation or between weeks 3–5 of

R. G. Kelly (✉)

Aix-Marseille Université, CNRS UMR 7288, IBDM, Marseille, France

e-mail: Robert.Kelly@univ-amu.fr

© The Editor(s) (if applicable) and The Author(s) 2020

T. Nakanishi et al. (eds.), *Molecular Mechanism of Congenital Heart Disease and Pulmonary Hypertension*, https://doi.org/10.1007/978-981-15-1185-1_49

human development. The embryonic heart thus grows by a process of progenitor cell recruitment, separating proliferation of multipotent cardiac progenitor cells in the SHF from differentiated cells of the first heart field (FHF) in the early heart tube. Correct SHF deployment is essential to maximally elongate the heart tube and for subsequent alignment and septation of the future cardiac chambers [2]. Failure of SHF addition at the arterial pole results in conotruncal CHD, including ventricular septal defects, overriding aorta and tetralogy of Fallot, while defects of SHF addition at the venous pole result in primum type atrial and atrioventricular septal defects. Dissecting the mechanisms regulating SHF deployment is therefore a critical step towards understanding the origins of common forms of CHD.

In this chapter we will briefly summarize recent advances in SHF biology, focusing on three successive steps of progenitor cell deployment: (1) emergence of SHF lineages in the early mouse embryo, (2) evidence that the epithelial properties of SHF cells play an important role in controlling the progenitor cell niche during heart tube elongation, and (3) new insights into events at the cardiac poles as SHF cells transit through a transition zone to acquire a differentiated phenotype.

49.2   Emergence of SHF Lineages in the Early Embryo

Clonal analyses have shown that FHF and SHF cells segregate extremely early in the developing embryo, at or before the time of gastrulation, and prior to the activation of *Mesp1*, one of the earliest transcription factors expressed in the cardiac lineage [3, 4]. Single cell RNA sequencing data of nascent precardiac mesoderm in the *Mesp1* lineage has recently revealed early segregation of anterior and posterior SHF populations, ultimately contributing to the arterial and venous poles of the heart, respectively. This study demonstrated that different cardiac progenitor cells emerge from a population of multipotent heterogeneous precardiac mesoderm, through which pseudotime trajectories to distinct emergent fates can be mapped (Fig. 49.1a) [5]. Moreover these data provide evidence of transcriptional priming of anterior and posterior SHF sub-populations, consistent with clonal analysis and vital dye labeling experiments indicating that these cells emerge from common progenitor cells in the early embryo. Progressive segregation of arterial and venous pole progenitor cells has been shown to depend on the transcription factor Tbx1, encoded by the major gene for 22q11.2 deletion syndrome (22q11.2DS, also known as Takao or DiGeorge Syndrome) [6]. CHDs affecting both conotruncal development and atrioventricular septation are observed in *Tbx1* null embryos and 22q11.2DS patients, consistent with a requirement for Tbx1 in both anterior and posterior SHF sub-populations. Moreover, the SHF itself lies within a larger population of evolutionarily conserved cardiopharyngeal mesoderm giving rise to skeletal muscles of the head and neck as well as myocardium; segregation of the heart and head muscle fate within cardiopharyngeal mesoderm occurs after the segregation of FHF and SHF lineages [7].

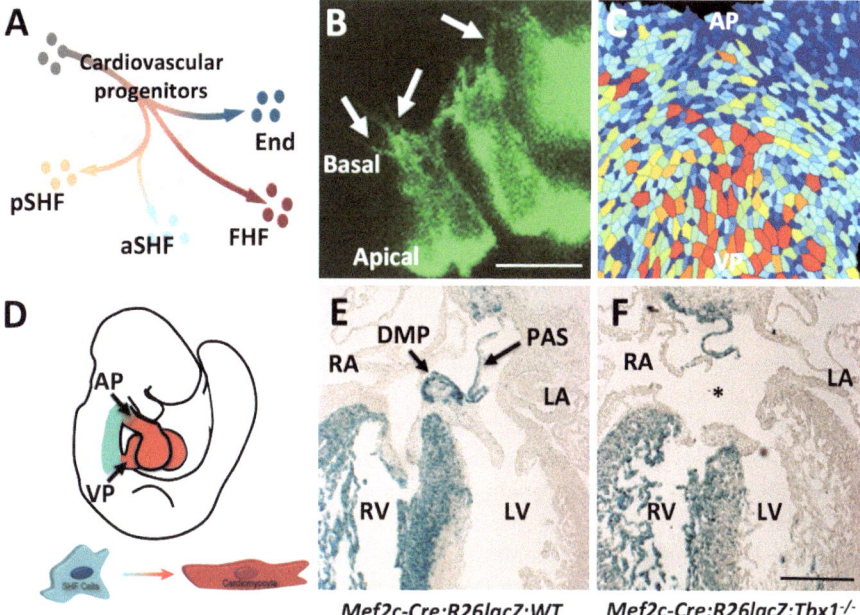

Fig. 49.1 Advances in the second heart field. (**a**) Early segregation of SHF cells in nascent cardiac mesoderm visualized by single cell gene expression analysis (adapted from [5]). (**b**) Actin enriched basal filopodia (arrows) in epithelial SHF cells visualized using Utrophin-GFP (adapted from [10]). (**c**) Segmentation of the apical surface of cells in the dorsal pericardial wall showing an increased cell size (red) and elongation in the posterior region (adapted from [15]). (**d**) Cartoon showing the transition zones (arrows) between proliferating progenitor cells (green) and differentiated cardiomyocytes (red) at the arterial and venous poles. (**e**, **f**) Failure of dorsal mesenchymal protrusion (DMP) development results in atrioventricular septal defects (asterisk) in *Tbx1* null hearts (adapted from [6]). *aSHF* anterior second heart field, *pSHF* posterior second heart field, *FHF* first heart field, *End* endocardium, *AP* arterial pole, *VP* venous pole, *PAS* primary atrial septum, *RA* right atrium, *LA* left atrium, *RV* right ventricle, *LA* left ventricle. Scale bars: **b**, 10 μm; **e**, **f**: 200 μm

49.3   Epithelial Properties of the SHF Cell Regulate the Progenitor Cell Niche

Inducible *Cre* recombinase alleles allowing genetic tracing of early differentiating cardiomyocytes (*Smooth muscle actin*) or progenitor cells (*Six2*) reveal the progressive contribution of SHF cells to the early heart tube [8, 9]. Whereas FHF cells differentiate in epithelial splanchnic mesoderm in the anterior lateral region of the embryo, SHF cells are situated in medial splanchnic mesoderm forming the dorsal pericardial wall (DPW). SHF cells also have an epithelial phenotype with a smooth apical surface with adherence and tight junctions facing the pericardial cavity [10]. In contrast to typical epithelia, the basolateral side of DPW cells is characterized by a mesenchymal-like convoluted cell membrane with actin-enriched filopodial structures (Fig. 49.1b). Confocal time-lapse

imaging of living SHF cells in thick slice culture has revealed that these filopodia are highly dynamic and contact the underlying endodermal and mesenchymal cells [10]. Phospho-Tyrosine accumulates in the basal filopodia of SHF
cells, consistent with activation of intercellular signaling receptors and a potential signaling role in maintaining the progenitor cell niche. Filopodia formation
is impaired in mouse embryos lacking *Tbx1*, associated with elevated levels of
the apical determinant atypical PKCz and abnormal SHF deployment. Exposure
of embryos to a physiological activator of aPKCz phenocopies the filopodial
phenotype of *Tbx1* null embryos, reducing proliferation and enhancing differentiation in the SHF [10].

N-cadherin is also required in the SHF to maintain the progenitor cell niche.
Conditional loss of N-cadherin results in elevated differentiation and reduced
proliferation associated with decreased Wnt β-catenin signaling [11]. Non-
canonical Wnt signaling also plays important roles in SHF development. In particular, loss of *Wnt5a*, expressed in splanchnic mesoderm in the posterior SHF,
results in arterial pole defects similar to those observed in *Tbx1* null embryos
[12]. Furthermore, *Wnt5a* has been shown to be a direct target gene of Tbx1 in
the SHF [13]. The regional expression of *Wnt5a* has been proposed to drive mesenchymal cell intercalation in the DPW, creating a pushing force promoting SHF
deployment to the arterial pole [14]. Increased cell adhesion in the anterior SHF
may reinforce this process by creating a pulling force, supported by missexpres-
sion experiments in transgenic mice [14] and evidence that E-cadherin accumulates in the apical membrane of cells in the anterior but not posterior SHF [10].

Ventral views of the dorsal pericardial wall epithelium have shown that cells in
the posterior region are under greater epithelial tension than cells close to the arterial pole. This is observed as an increase in the cell size, cell elongation oriented
towards the arterial pole and accumulation of active actomyosin complexes along
the long membrane of elongated cells (Fig. 49.1c) [15]. Moreover this is associated with elevated proliferation in the posterior SHF, oriented distribution of
daughter cells after cell division, and clonal growth patterns directed towards the
arterial pole of the heart, likely promoting heart tube elongation. A biomechanical
feedback loop between SHF deployment and tension in the DPW, driven by the
process of heart tube elongation itself, may accelerate terminal stages of SHF
deployment [15]. Cells in the DPW are initially attached to the heart tube along
its entire length by the dorsal mesocardium. Rupture of this transient mesentery
isolates the SHF from the looping heart tube with the exception of the cardiac
poles. Elevated epithelial tension in the posterior SHF is observed only after addition of SHF cells is restricted to the cardiac poles and tension is dependent on
heart tube elongation [15]. Interestingly, elevated nuclear accumulation of the
transcriptional co-factor YAP in the posterior region of the SHF may provide a
link between epithelial tension and proliferation [15]. Ongoing work aims to
refine this working model by characterizing the sources of tension and the pathways by which this impacts on proliferation in the SHF.

49.4   SHF Cells at the Cardiac Poles Pass Through a Transition Zone

As SHF cells contribute to the cardiac poles they pass through a transition zone (TZ), or zone of commitment (Fig. 49.1d). The TZ is characterized by a cardiomyoblast phenotype, altered cell shape and actin cytoskeleton remodeling associated with sarcomere assembly and the onset of differentiation [16–18]. Cells in the TZ are distinguished by reduced *FlnA* and *Hopx* expression, the latter associated with modulating intercellular signals controlling the switch from proliferation to differentiation [17, 18]. Downregulation of the SHF transcriptional program is mediated by the cardiac transcription factor Nkx2-5 that competes with the SHF activator Isl1 to repress transcription at the *Fgf10* locus [19]. Similarly, binding of Nkx2-5 to sites in the *Popdc2* gene initially bound by Meis1 is associated with spatiotemporal progression of cells through the TZ [20]. Defects in TZ development result in failure to fully extend the outflow tract and subsequent ventriculoarterial alignment defects. For example, the planar cell polarity gene *Vangl2* controls the epithelial properties of cells in the TZ, and outflow tract alignment defects including double outlet right ventricle are observed in conditional mutant embryos [16]. At the venous pole, SHF cells give rise to the dorsal mesenchymal protrusion (DMP) contributing to the muscular base of the primary atrial septum [21]. Multiple transcription factors, including Tbx5, Osr1, Gata, and Fox factors, as well as several intercellular signaling pathways, have been implicated in DMP development [21, 22]. Defects in the development of the DMP underlie atrial primum type CHD, a class of atrioventricular septal defect. Such defects, in addition to failure of subpulmonary myocardium development at the arterial pole, are observed in *Tbx1* null hearts and constitute part of the CHD spectrum in *TBX1* haploinsufficent 22q11.2DS patients (Fig. 49.1e, f) [6, 23].

49.5   Future Directions and Clinical Implications

The studies discussed above identify critical regulatory nodes at successive stages of SHF deployment, providing new insights into the mechanisms of heart morphogenesis. Further analysis using dynamic approaches, single cell transcriptomic and epigenetic studies and lineage analysis will refine our understanding of these steps and generate a more complete blueprint of SHF deployment with which to dissect the origins of CHD and develop future preventive and, potentially, therapeutic approaches.

Acknowledgements Research in the author's laboratory is supported by the Fondation pour la Recherche Médicale (DEQ20150331717), the Association Française contre les Myopathies, a grant from the Fondation Leducq (Transatlantic Network of Excellence 15CVD01) and the Agence National pour la Recherche (Heartbox project).

References

1. Kelly RG. The second heart field. Curr Top Dev Biol. 2012;100:33–65. https://doi.org/10.1016/B978-0-12-387786-4.00002-6.
2. Epstein JA. Franklin H. Epstein Lecture. Cardiac development and implications for heart disease. N Engl J Med. 2010;363(17):1638–47. https://doi.org/10.1056/NEJMra1003941.
3. Devine WP, Wythe JD, George M, Koshiba-Takeuchi K, Bruneau BG. Early patterning and specification of cardiac progenitors in gastrulating mesoderm. Elife. 2014;3 https://doi.org/10.7554/eLife.03848.
4. Lescroart F, Chabab S, Lin X, Rulands S, Paulissen C, Rodolosse A, Auer H, Achouri Y, Dubois C, Bondue A, Simons BD, Blanpain C. Early lineage restriction in temporally distinct populations of Mesp1 progenitors during mammalian heart development. Nat Cell Biol. 2014;16(9):829–40. https://doi.org/10.1038/ncb3024.
5. Lescroart F, Wang X, Lin X, Swedlund B, Gargouri S, Sanchez-Danes A, Moignard V, Dubois C, Paulissen C, Kinston S, Gottgens B, Blanpain C. Defining the earliest step of cardiovascular lineage segregation by single-cell RNA-seq. Science. 2018;359(6380):1177–81. https://doi.org/10.1126/science.aao4174.
6. Rana MS, Theveniau-Ruissy M, De Bono C, Mesbah K, Francou A, Rammah M, Dominguez JN, Roux M, Laforest B, Anderson RH, Mohun T, Zaffran S, Christoffels VM, Kelly RG. Tbx1 coordinates addition of posterior second heart field progenitor cells to the arterial and venous poles of the heart. Circ Res. 2014;115(9):790–9. https://doi.org/10.1161/CIRCRESAHA.115.305020.
7. Diogo R, Kelly RG, Christiaen L, Levine M, Ziermann JM, Molnar JL, Noden DM, Tzahor E. A new heart for a new head in vertebrate cardiopharyngeal evolution. Nature. 2015;520(7548):466–73. https://doi.org/10.1038/nature14435.
8. Choquet C, Marcadet L, Beyer S, Kelly RG, Miquerol L. Segregation of central ventricular conduction system lineages in early SMA+ cardiomyocytes occurs prior to heart tube formation. J Cardiovasc Dev Dis. 2016;3(1) https://doi.org/10.3390/jcdd3010002.
9. Zhou L, Liu J, Xiang M, Olson P, Guzzetta A, Zhang K, Moskowitz IP, Xie L. Gata4 potentiates second heart field proliferation and Hedgehog signaling for cardiac septation. Proc Natl Acad Sci U S A. 2017;114(8):E1422–31. https://doi.org/10.1073/pnas.1605137114.
10. Francou A, Saint-Michel E, Mesbah K, Kelly RG. TBX1 regulates epithelial polarity and dynamic basal filopodia in the second heart field. Development. 2014;141(22):4320–31. https://doi.org/10.1242/dev.115022.
11. Soh BS, Buac K, Xu H, Li E, Ng SY, Wu H, Chmielowiec J, Jiang X, Bu L, Li RA, Cowan C, Chien KR. N-cadherin prevents the premature differentiation of anterior heart field progenitors in the pharyngeal mesodermal microenvironment. Cell Res. 2014;24(12):1420–32. https://doi.org/10.1038/cr.2014.142.
12. Sinha T, Li D, Theveniau-Ruissy M, Hutson MR, Kelly RG, Wang J. Loss of Wnt5a disrupts second heart field cell deployment and may contribute to OFT malformations in DiGeorge syndrome. Hum Mol Genet. 2015;24(6):1704–16. https://doi.org/10.1093/hmg/ddu584.
13. Chen L, Fulcoli FG, Ferrentino R, Martucciello S, Illingworth EA, Baldini A. Transcriptional control in cardiac progenitors: Tbx1 interacts with the BAF chromatin remodeling complex and regulates Wnt5a. PLoS Genet. 2012;8(3):e1002571. https://doi.org/10.1371/journal.pgen.1002571.
14. Li D, Sinha T, Ajima R, Seo HS, Yamaguchi TP, Wang J. Spatial regulation of cell cohesion by Wnt5a during second heart field progenitor deployment. Dev Biol. 2016;412(1):18–31. https://doi.org/10.1016/j.ydbio.2016.02.017.
15. Francou A, De Bono C, Kelly RG. Epithelial tension in the second heart field promotes mouse heart tube elongation. Nat Commun. 2017;8:14770. https://doi.org/10.1038/ncomms14770.
16. Ramsbottom SA, Sharma V, Rhee HJ, Eley L, Phillips HM, Rigby HF, Dean C, Chaudhry B, Henderson DJ. Vangl2-regulated polarisation of second heart field-derived cells is required for

outflow tract lengthening during cardiac development. PLoS Genet. 2014;10(12):e1004871. https://doi.org/10.1371/journal.pgen.1004871.

17. Jain R, Li D, Gupta M, Manderfield LJ, Ifkovits JL, Wang Q, Liu F, Liu Y, Poleshko A, Padmanabhan A, Raum JC, Li L, Morrisey EE, Lu MM, Won KJ, Epstein JA. HEART DEVELOPMENT. Integration of Bmp and Wnt signaling by Hopx specifies commitment of cardiomyoblasts. Science. 2015;348(6242):aaa6071. https://doi.org/10.1126/science.aaa6071.

18. Metais A, Lamsoul I, Melet A, Uttenweiler-Joseph S, Poincloux R, Stefanovic S, Valiere A, Gonzalez de Peredo A, Stella A, Burlet-Schiltz O, Zaffran S, Lutz PG, Moog-Lutz C. Asb2alpha-filamin A axis is essential for actin cytoskeleton remodeling during heart development. Circ Res. 2018;122:e34. https://doi.org/10.1161/CIRCRESAHA.117.312015.

19. Watanabe Y, Zaffran S, Kuroiwa A, Higuchi H, Ogura T, Harvey RP, Kelly RG, Buckingham M. Fibroblast growth factor 10 gene regulation in the second heart field by Tbx1, Nkx2-5, and Islet1 reveals a genetic switch for down-regulation in the myocardium. Proc Natl Acad Sci U S A. 2012;109(45):18273–80. https://doi.org/10.1073/pnas.1215360109.

20. Dupays L, Shang C, Wilson R, Kotecha S, Wood S, Towers N, Mohun T. Sequential binding of MEIS1 and NKX2-5 on the Popdc2 gene: a mechanism for spatiotemporal regulation of enhancers during cardiogenesis. Cell Rep. 2015;13(1):183–95. https://doi.org/10.1016/j.celrep.2015.08.065.

21. Briggs LE, Kakarla J, Wessels A. The pathogenesis of atrial and atrioventricular septal defects with special emphasis on the role of the dorsal mesenchymal protrusion. Differentiation. 2012;84(1):117–30. https://doi.org/10.1016/j.diff.2012.05.006.

22. Xie L, Hoffmann AD, Burnicka-Turek O, Friedland-Little JM, Zhang K, Moskowitz IP. Tbx5-hedgehog molecular networks are essential in the second heart field for atrial septation. Dev Cell. 2012;23(2):280–91. https://doi.org/10.1016/j.devcel.2012.06.006.

23. Momma K. Cardiovascular anomalies associated with chromosome 22q11.2 deletion syndrome. Am J Cardiol. 2010;105(11):1617–24. https://doi.org/10.1016/j.amjcard.2010.01.333.

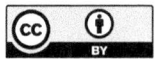

Novel Cardiac Progenitors for All Components of the Heart Except for the Right Ventricle

Hiroki Kokubo, Masayuki Fujii, Akane Sakaguchi, Masao Yoshizumi, and Yumiko Saga

Abstract

Mammalian heart is first recognized as the cardiac crescent at the egg cylinder stage, which had been thought to form all components of the heart. Recently, several lineage-tracing experiments using dye-labeling and mouse genetic technique have demonstrated that another cardiac progenitor population, called the second heart field, contributes to the outflow tract, the right ventricle, and a part of the atria. This finding has provided a great impetus for the understanding of cardiac morphogenesis, but it has also raised additional questions such as the potential existence of unique cardiac progenitors that give rise to the left ventricle and the conduction system. Here, we show that a novel cardiac progenitor population is identified by expression and lineage tracing analysis of the *Sfrp5* gene. We found that *Sfrp5* gene expression was constantly seen in the venous pole of the forming heart, which is later differentiated into the myocardium of the sinus venosus, a precursor of the sinoatrial node. Descendants of *Sfrp5*-expressing cells were found to contribute not only to the sinus venosus, but also to the left ventricle, atria, and the outflow tract by lineage-tracing analysis using *Sfrp5-Cre* and *-Ert2Cre* mice. These results indicate that *Sfrp5*-expressing cells could include progenitors for the sinus venosus, atria, the left ventricle, and the outflow tract, but not in the right ventricle, implying that the origin of the right ventricle essential for pulmonary circulation could be unique from progenitors for other components in mammalian cardiac development. In this session, we would like to discuss a new understanding of cardiac progenitor distribution.

H. Kokubo (✉) · M. Fujii · M. Yoshizumi
Department of Cardiovascular Physics Medicine, Hiroshima University, Hiroshima, Japan
e-mail: hkokubo@hiroshima-u.ac.jp

A. Sakaguchi · Y. Saga
Determent of Mammalian Development, National Institute of Genetics, Mishima, Japan

Keywords
Sfrp5 · Heart development

Mammalian cardiac development starts with the cardiac crescent, which forms the primary heart tube and then the four-chambered heart along with the progressive differentiation of progenitors into cardiomyocytes [1–3]. In this process, two independent pulmonary and systemic circulatory systems are established. For the establishment of these systems, remodeling of the ancestral heart into these two separate systems might occur with the production and rearrangement of progenitor cells. Recent findings pertaining to another cardiac lineage called the secondary heart field (SHF) modified the classical view of cardiac development that the myocardium was derived from a single source. The SHF emerges in the splanchnic mesoderm to supply cells at both the arterial and venous poles of the heart tube, including the right ventricle (RV), most of the atria and outflow tract (OFT). However, the progenitor population that forms the first heart field (FHF), which gives rise to the left ventricle (LV) and the rest of the atria and the sinus venosus (SV) are still ambiguous. Since Wnt signalling is one of the most important regulatory pathways in vertebrate cardiogenesis [4–8], we focused on the Secreted frizzled-related protein (Sfrp) sub-family, known to encode secreted decoy receptors for Wnt signalling, and analyze its expression and lineage during cardiac development [9].

We first observed expression of *Sfrp5*. At E7.5, *Sfrp5* was detected in the lateral and caudal region of the *Mlc2a* and *Nkx2-5* expressing region in the cardiac crescent. This region was distinct from the *Isl1* and *Hcn4*-expressing region, but mostly overlapped with the region marked by *Tbx5*. These observations suggest that *Sfrp5* expression seems to be restricted in undifferentiated FHF progenitors existing in the lateral sides of the cardiac crescent. During the heart tube looping stage (E8.0–E8.5), *Sfrp5* was continuously expressed in the venous pole of the heart. This *Sfrp5*-expressing area was distinct from the expression area of *Mlc2a* and *Nkx2-5*, indicating that *Sfrp5* is exclusively expressed in the undifferentiated cardiomyocytes. At E9.5, *Sfrp5* expression was restricted to the Tbx18 and WT1 expressing the ventral venous pole, suggesting that *Sfrp5* is expressed in progenitors of such SV and epicardium.

Since *Sfrp5* expression was found in progenitors of the FHF at E7.5, and also detected continuously in the progenitors of the SV and the epicardium, we hypothesize that *Sfrp5*-expressing cells include progenitors for the LV, the atrium, the SV and the epicardium. To test this possibility, we performed lineage analysis of *Sfrp5*-expressing cells by crossing the *Sfrp5*-Cre line with Rosa26R or CAG-floxed-CAT-eGFP reporter mice [10]. We found that β-galactosidase (LacZ) labeled cells were detected in the OFT, LV, atria, and venous pole, but not in the RV at E9.5. Labeled cells overlapped with TnT in the OFT, LV, and atria, suggesting that descendants of *Sfrp5*-expressing cells differentiated into the chamber myocardium in addition to the SV. At E13.5, LacZ-stained cells were mostly found in the LV and also in the WT1-expressing pericardium and the CD31-expressing endocardium. Labelled cells were found in part of the interventricular septum but rarely in the RV. These observations suggest that *Sfrp5* is expressed in progenitors of the SV, pericardium, epicardium, endocardium, and the OFT, as well as in all chamber myocardium except for the RV.

Since *Sfrp5* expression is restricted in the venous pole of the heart at E8.5, which does not include the chamber myocardium, we speculated that cells expressing *Sfrp5* prior to E8.5 might include progenitors of the FHF. To evaluate the fate of *Sfrp5*-expressing cells at specific developmental stages, we crossed a tamoxifen inducible *Sfrp5*- ERT2 Cre mouse line with reporter mice and found that LacZ staining revealed that cells labelled at E7.5 were found in the OFT, LV, atria, SV, and venous pole but not in the RV. Moreover, labelled cells at E8.5 and E9.5 were still found in the atria, indicating that *Sfrp5*-expressing cells at the venous pole may supply cardiomyocytes for the inflow tract. These data suggest that *Sfrp5*-expressing cells at E7.5 include common progenitors for the SV, OFT, and all chamber myocardium except for the RV.

Although the expression pattern of *Sfrp5* was distinct from that of *Isl1*, an SHF marker at E7.5, descendants of *Sfrp5*-expressing cells were found in the OFT, which was thought to be derived from the SHF. This observation gave rise to a hypothesis that the expression of *Sfrp5* precedes that of *Isl1* in the splanchnic mesoderm. To test this possibility, we performed lineage-tracing analysis using *Isl1*-Cre and CAG-floxed-CAT-mRFP reporter/*Sfrp5*-venusYFP mice and found that the YFP signal in the ventral venous pole rarely overlapped with derivatives of *Isl1*-expressing cells. Instead, in *Sfrp5*-Cre/CAG-floxed-CAT-eGFP-reporter mice, GFP-labelled cells expressed *Isl1* in the dorsal splanchnic mesoderm and part of the OFT. These findings indicate that part of the SHF lineage is derived from *Sfrp5*-expressing cells to contribute to the OFT and atria.

Based on our findings, we propose a model for the contribution of *Sfrp5*-expressing cardiac precursors to heart development (Fig. 50.1). We found that *Sfrp5*-expressing cells at E7.5 contributed to the OFT, the LV, the atria, and the SV, but not to the RV, by fate mapping experiments using *Sfrp5*-Cre and -ERT2Cre mice. This observation indicates the possibility that the FHF lineage and the SV might share a common origin. Given that *Isl1* lineages contribute to all myocardium except for the LV [11, 12], the fate of *Isl1* lineages to the RV or *Sfrp5* lineages to the LV may be exclusively determined during the earliest stages of cardiogenesis.

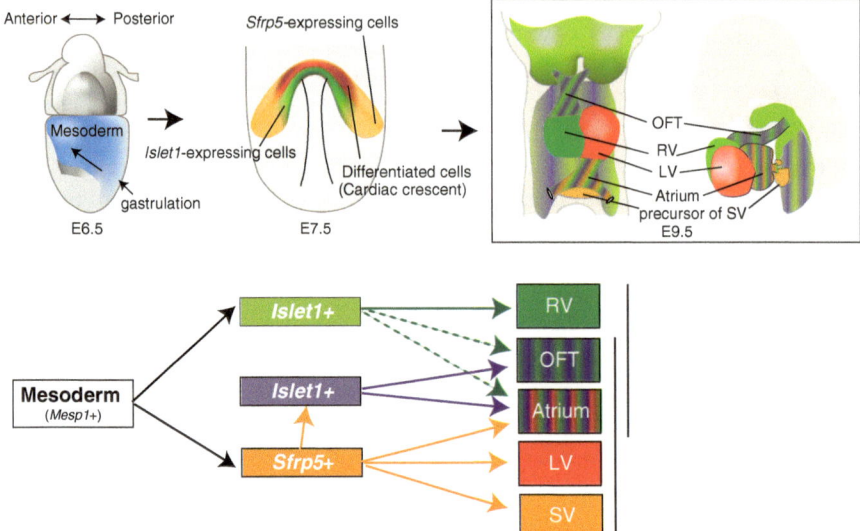

Fig. 50.1 A new model for heart development: Crescent shaped heart primordium is divided into two layers along the mediolateral axis. The medial side of heart crescent, expressing *Islet1*, forms splanchnic mesoderm and its decedents contribute to all cardiac components except the LV. On the other hand, the lateral side of heart crescent, expressing *Sfrp5*, localizes in the mesenchymal cells in the inflow tract to form the SV, and its decedents contribute to all cardiac components except the RV

References

1. Moorman AF, Christoffels VM, Anderson RH, van den Hoff MJ. The heart-forming fields: one or multiple? Philos Trans R Soc Lond B Biol Sci. 2007;362:1257–65, G5L17245615197K8 [pii]. https://doi.org/10.1098/rstb.2007.2113.
2. Buckingham M, Meilhac S, Zaffran S. Building the mammalian heart from two sources of myocardial cells. Nat Rev Genet. 2005;6:826–35. https://doi.org/10.1038/nrg1710.
3. Abu-Issa R, Kirby ML. Heart field: from mesoderm to heart tube. Annu Rev Cell Dev Biol. 2007;23:45–68. https://doi.org/10.1146/annurev.cellbio.23.090506.123331.
4. Brade T, Manner J, Kuhl M. The role of Wnt signalling in cardiac development and tissue remodelling in the mature heart. Cardiovasc Res. 2006;72:198–209. https://doi.org/10.1016/j.cardiores.2006.06.025.
5. Cohen ED, Tian Y, Morrisey EE. Wnt signaling: an essential regulator of cardiovascular differentiation, morphogenesis and progenitor self-renewal. Development. 2008;135:789–98. https://doi.org/10.1242/dev.016865.
6. Gessert S, Kuhl M. The multiple phases and faces of wnt signaling during cardiac differentiation and development. Circ Res. 2010;107:186–99. https://doi.org/10.1161/CIRCRESAHA.110.221531.
7. Qyang Y, et al. The renewal and differentiation of Isl1+ cardiovascular progenitors are controlled by a Wnt/beta-catenin pathway. Cell Stem Cell. 2007;1:165–79., 10.1016/j.stem.2007.05.018.
8. Ueno S, et al. Biphasic role for Wnt/beta-catenin signaling in cardiac specification in zebrafish and embryonic stem cells. Proc Natl Acad Sci U S A. 2007;104:9685–90. https://doi.org/10.1073/pnas.0702859104.

9. Fujii M, et al. Sfrp5 identifies murine cardiac progenitors for all myocardial structures except for the right ventricle. Nat Commun. 2017;8:14664. https://doi.org/10.1038/ncomms14664.
10. Soriano P. Generalized lacZ expression with the ROSA26 Cre reporter strain. Nat Genet. 1999;21:70–1. https://doi.org/10.1038/5007.
11. Moretti A, et al. Multipotent embryonic isl1+ progenitor cells lead to cardiac, smooth muscle, and endothelial cell diversification. Cell. 2006;127:1151–65. https://doi.org/10.1016/j.cell.2006.10.029.
12. Laugwitz KL, Moretti A, Caron L, Nakano A, Chien KR. Islet1 cardiovascular progenitors: a single source for heart lineages? Development. 2008;135:193–205. https://doi.org/10.1242/dev.001883.

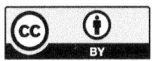

Regional and *TBX5*-Dependent Gene Expression in the Atria: Implications for Pulmonary Vein Development and Atrial Fibrillation

51

Jeffrey D. Steimle, Brigitte Laforest,
Rangarajan D. Nadadur, Michael T. Broman,
and Ivan P. Moskowitz

Abstract

Atrial fibrillation, characterized by irregular atrial depolarization leading to an uncoordinated contraction of the atrial muscle, is the most common cardiac arrhythmia. The T-box transcription factor *TBX5* regulates atrial rhythm and has been genetically associated with human atrial fibrillation by both familial and genome-wide association studies. Over the last 30 years, the pulmonary veins and peri-pulmonary region of the left atrium have been implicated as a physical locus that frequently initiates atrial fibrillation. Regional gene expression differences within the atria have been reported that may reflect distinct ontogeny of these regions and impact arrhythmia mechanisms. In this study, we investigated transcriptional differences between regions of the adult left atrium in the mouse. We performed and compared transcriptional profiling of the left atrial appendage and peri-pulmonary vein atrium of the adult mouse. We identified novel markers and transcriptional differences between the two regions, including of multiple known AF genes. Furthermore, we compared *Tbx5*-dependent genes between each region and identified *Hcn4* as a novel dysregulated gene in the peri-pulmonary vein atrium. Regional and *Tbx5*-dependent gene expression

J. D. Steimle · R. D. Nadadur · I. P. Moskowitz (✉)
Departments of Pediatrics, Pathology, and Human Genetics, University of Chicago, Chicago, IL, USA
e-mail: imoskowitz@uchicago.edu

B. Laforest · M. T. Broman
Department of Medicine, University of Chicago, Chicago, IL, USA

T. Nakanishi et al. (eds.), *Molecular Mechanism of Congenital Heart Disease and Pulmonary Hypertension*, https://doi.org/10.1007/978-981-15-1185-1_51

differences between the left atrial appendage and peri-pulmonary vein atrium are considered in the context of the genetic basis of atrial fibrillation.

Keywords
Atrial fibrillation · Arrhythmia · TBX5 · Cardiac conduction · Pulmonary vein · Atrium · Gene regulatory network · PITX2 · HCN4 · SHOX2

51.1 Introduction

51.1.1 Atrial Fibrillation and the Pulmonary Vein

Atrial fibrillation (AF) is the most common sustained cardiac arrhythmia, affecting more than 7 million Americans and 33 million people worldwide [1]. AF is characterized by an irregular pattern of atrial depolarization, resulting in rapid and disorganized atrial conduction and lack of effective atrial chamber contraction. The rhythm abnormality in AF manifests with circulatory deficits and systemic thromboembolism that greatly increase morbidity and mortality. Patients with AF have an increased risk of developing major complications including heart failure and stroke. In addition, the prevalence of AF is expected to rise significantly as the population ages. AF has become a major clinical and economic burden, owing to the limitations and side effects associated with current AF therapies. Although AF most often manifests in the context of pre-existing cardiac pathologies, idiopathic or lone AF forms indicated a heritable component [2]. Over the last decade, genome-wide association studies (GWAS) have identified over one hundred AF-associated loci [3, 4]. These advances in understanding the genetic basis of AF portend an understanding of the complex molecular pathways provoking AF.

The current paradigm of AF requires two arrhythmogenic components: (1) ectopic (triggered) atrial myocardial activity such as early or delayed afterdepolarizations and (2) a fibrillogenic substrate that propagates these triggers throughout the atrial chambers [5]. The most common source of triggered activity is the pulmonary veins, which connect the lungs to the left atria [6, 7]. It has been shown that the pulmonary vein (PV) and peri-pulmonary vein (PPV) myocardium can demonstrate automaticity which can trigger atrial depolarization [8]. A pacemaker current has been observed in the PV-left atrial junction in atrial fibrillation, and gene expression contributing to myocardial automaticity, such as the HCN4 channel protein, is observed in the pulmonary veins [9]. A common treatment for AF is to isolate the PV myocytes from the atrial myocardium by catheter ablation, severing the electrical connectivity between these two populations and preventing inappropriate PV depolarizations from initiating global atrial depolarization and atrial arrhythmias [6, 7].

An important advance in the understanding of the pathophysiology of AF has been the demonstration that the pulmonary vein plays an important role in the initiation of AF [6, 10]. Other initiating foci include the superior vena cava and the left atrium; however, the pulmonary vein remains the most common source of focal activity. This observation has stimulated consideration of the distinctions between the myocardium of the pulmonary/peri-pulmonary vein region and other regions of the atrium. However, the gene expression profile promoting focal activity around the PVs in humans has been difficult to elucidate, owing to the limitations of tissue samples from patients. The molecular identity of the PV myocardium, including specific ion channels and transcription factors expressed in this tissue, has only recently been described. Analysis of a whole-lung transcriptome data set uncovered a set of 24 transcripts, including sarcomeric structural proteins, genes regulating sarcomere assembly, ion transport proteins and hormone signaling in the pulmonary cardiomyocyte gene network [11]. Some of these genes have been linked to AF in humans, suggesting that perturbation of this transcriptional network might lead to altered calcium handling, altered myocardium contractile force and electrophysiological properties which may contribute to the initiation of atrial arrhythmias.

51.1.2 *TBX5* and Pulmonary Vein Development

Holt-Oram syndrome is an autosomal dominant disorder caused by mutations in the T-box family transcription factor *TBX5* [12–14], occurring in approximately 1 in 100,000 live births [15, 16]. The clinical diagnosis of Holt-Oram syndrome includes completely penetrant upper-limb malformations and variable congenital heart defects, most commonly septal and cardiac conduction defects [17]. Specifically, the conduction defects can manifest as long PR interval, AV and bundle branch block, bradycardia, sick sinus syndrome and atrial fibrillation with or without overt structural defects [18, 19]. The observation that conduction abnormalities can occur in the absence of structural heart defects was an early indication that TBX5 may play a direct role in controlling gene expression essential for normal cardiac conduction. Recently, GWAS have implicated *TBX5* in altered cardiac conduction speed (PR and QRS intervals) and AF in structurally normal hearts. Although strict clinical diagnosis of Holt-Oram Syndrome does not involve defects of the pulmonary veins [14, 17], pulmonary vein abnormalities are often associated with Holt-Oram syndrome and *TBX5* mutations [20–22]. Furthermore, homozygous mutation of *Tbx5* in the mouse germline [23] results in complete morphological failure of the cardiopulmonary progenitors, which would normally generate portions of the atria, the atrial septum, pulmonary vein myocardium and smooth muscle cells and airways smooth muscle cells [24, 25]. These observations suggested that *TBX5* may drive gene expression important for the development of the pulmonary vasculature in the embryo and for the suppression of atrial arrhythmias in the pulmonary veins or peri-pulmonary vein atrial myocardium in the adult.

Here, we describe regional differences between the transcriptome of the left atrial appendage and the peri-pulmonary vein of the left atrium from adult mice. RNA sequencing revealed previously known and novel regional differences, including several genes implicated in atrial fibrillation. We further compared *Tbx5*-depedent transcripts between the left atrial appendage and the peri-pulmonary vein of the left atrium from adult mice. Important distinctions were observed between the two regions including *Hcn4*, which demonstrated differential *Tbx5*-dependence. Our data suggests that underlying regional differences in the transcriptome of the atrial myocardium may enlighten susceptibility to atrial fibrillation.

51.2   Results

51.2.1 Comparison of Peri-Pulmonary Vein and Atrial Appendage Transcriptomes

We investigated transcriptional differences between regions of the left atrium in 7-week-old mice. The left atrium was microdissected into two parts: the left atrial appendage (LAA) and the peri-pulmonary vein (PPV) (Fig. 51.1a). Transcriptional profiling was performed by RNA sequencing (RNA-seq; $n = 4$ in each group) as previously described [26]. Principal component analysis (PCA) demonstrated that atrial region was responsible for the first principal component, accounting for 32% of the variation between samples (Fig. 51.1b). Differential expression testing between the PPV and LAA samples identified 747 significantly different genes (|log2FC| > 1; FDR < 0.01) with 582 expressed more strongly in the PPV samples and 165 expressed more strongly in the LAA samples (Fig. 51.1c, full table available at GEO accession GSE128870). Gene ontology (GO) terms and Kyoto Encyclopedia of Genes and Genomes (KEGG) pathways were examined using metascape (http://metascape.org) for both the LAA and PPV genes [27]. GO terms associated with the PPV indicated a preponderance of genes associated with immune cells. We observed GO terms that were unambiguously related to the immune system and only containing genes associated with the PPV, including phagocytosis (GO:0006909), inflammatory response (GO:0006954), humoral immune response (GO:0006959), lymphocyte differentiation (GO:0030098) and cytokine-cytokine receptor interaction (mmu04060). Although these 141 genes are of potential interest, they were separated from the remaining 441 PPV genes to focus on those genes previously verified as myocardially expressed or those with unknown roles or expression domains (Fig. 51.1c).

Because of the relationship between the left atria, pulmonary vein and AF, we examined region-specific gene expression against a list of 235 AF associated genes [3, 28–30]. Of the 606 genes that demonstrated regionalized expression in our RNA-seq, 19 have been associated with AF (Fig. 51.1d). Specifically, *Adrb1*, *Nkx2-5*, *Tmem182*, *Nppa*, *Nppb*, *Gja5* and *Kcnh7* are more strongly expressed in the LAA while *Ntrk2*, *Tubb4a*, *Cacna1d*, *Tbx3*, *Scn3b*, *Shox2*, *Kcne4*, *Hcn4*, *Adra1a*, *Adrb3*, *Tubb3* and *Cacna2d2* have higher expression in the PPV.

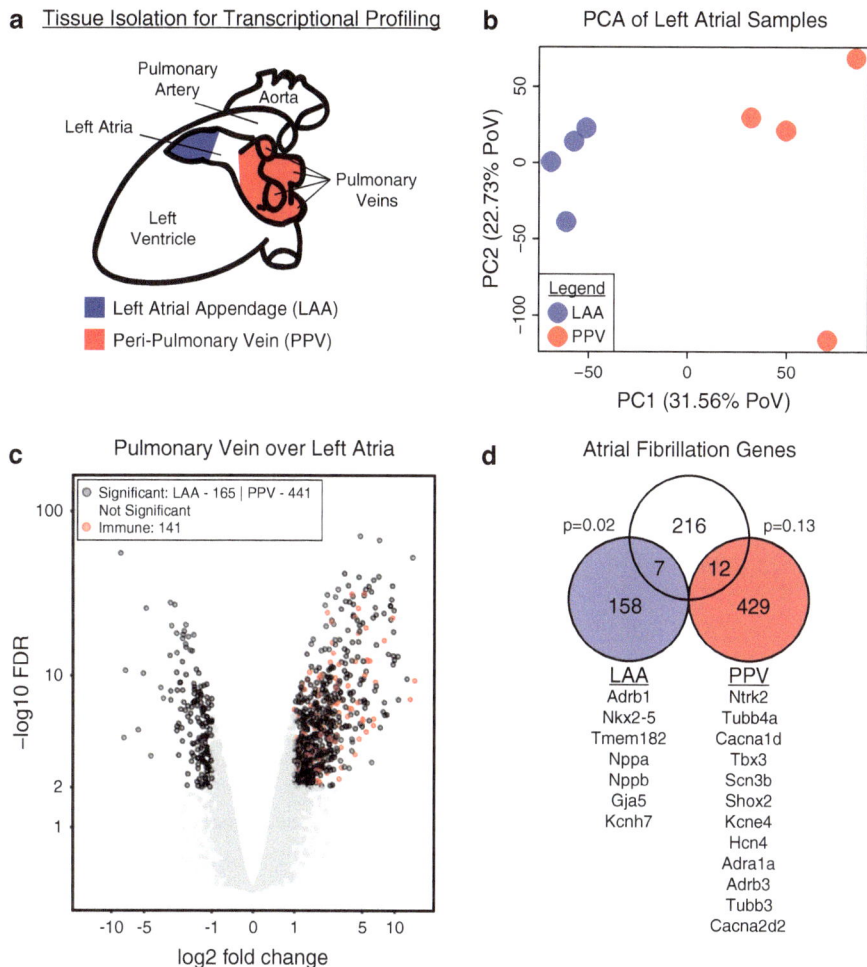

Fig. 51.1 Transcriptional comparison of the left atrial appendage and peri-pulmonary vein atrium. (**a**) The left atrial appendage (LAA, blue) and the peri-pulmonary vein region of the left atrium (PPV, red) were microdissected from 7-week-old adult mice. (**b**) Principal component analysis comparing the LAA (blue) and PPV (red) transcriptomes. (**c**) Volcano plot showing log2(fold-change PPV/LAA). One hundred and sixty five were associated with LAA and 582 were associated with the PPV (|log2FC|>1 and FDR < 0.01). Of the PPV genes, 141 genes were associated with GO terms related to the immune system (red) and removed from downstream analysis. (**d**) Overlap of genes associated with atrial fibrillation and either the LAA (7 genes) or PPV (12 genes). *P*-values derived from Fisher's exact test

51.2.2 *Tbx5*-Dependent Transcriptome of Peri-Pulmonary Vein Atrium Identifies Genes Involved with Cardiac Conduction

We hypothesized that *Tbx5*-dependent gene expression may vary between different regions in the left atria. Previous work has demonstrated that *Tbx5* regulates a gene regulatory network for atrial identity and its removal from the adult mouse results in atrial fibrillation [26]. *Tbx5* is robustly expressed in both the LAA and PPV tissues with an average TPM of 79.7 ± 9.9 SEM and 97.1 ± 18.4 SEM, respectively putting *Tbx5* within the top 8% of all genes expressed in either area of the left atrium (TPM > 1). To investigate differential *Tbx5*-dependent regional gene expression in the left atrium of the adult mouse, we performed *Tbx5*-dependent transcriptional profiling of the PPV tissue and compared it to previously described *Tbx5*-dependent transcriptional profiling of the left atrial appendage [26]. We performed RNA-seq on the PPV of an adult-specific conditional knockout of *Tbx5* [26]. Control ($R26^{creERT2/creERT2}$; $Tbx5^{+/+}$) and conditional mutant ($R26^{creERT2/creERT2}$; $Tbx5^{flox/flox}$) animals were treated with tamoxifen at 6-weeks old and tissue was harvested one week later prior to the onset or atrial arrhythmias (Fig. 51.1a) [26]. PCA analysis demonstrated clustering along PC1 and PC2 of samples (cumulative variation > 50%). PC1 demonstrated clustering associated with genotype (control versus conditional *Tbx5* mutant), and PC2 demonstrated clustering associated with LA region (LAA versus PPV), indicating that genotype differences drove the majority of variance followed by regional atrial differences (Fig. 51.2a).

We identified 338 significantly dysregulated genes (|log2FC| > 1; FDR < 0.01) comparing the PPV between *Tbx5* conditional mutant and controls (Fig. 51.2b, GEO accession GSE128870). Of these, 149 were up-regulated and 189 were down-regulated in the *Tbx5* mutants (Fig. 51.2b). Utilizing metascape [27], we identified seven representative GO terms associated with the up-regulated genes and two representative GO terms associated with the down-regulated genes (Fig. 51.2c).

***

Fig. 51.2 *Tbx5* conditional knockout from the peri-pulmonary vein reveals *Tbx5*-dependence of multiple unique features. (**a**) Principal component analysis comparing the left atrial appendage (LAA, blue) and peri-pulmonary vein (PPV, red) transcriptomes from control ($R26^{creERT2/creERT2}$; $Tbx5^{+/+}$, "Tbx5Ctrl", circles) and *Tbx5* conditional knockout ($R26^{creERT2/creERT2}$; $Tbx5^{flox/flox}$, "Tbx5CKO", squares) adult mice. (**b**) Volcano plot comparing the PPV *Tbx5* CKO and control samples. One hundred and forty nine genes were significantly up-regulated and 189 were significantly down-regulated (|log2FC|>1 and FDR< 0.01). (**c**) Summary GO terms representing all GO terms associated with up- and down-regulated genes (red and blue, respectively) with greater than five associated genes and −log10(*P*-value) greater than 5. (**d**) Full GO term list represented by "multicellular organismal signaling" with percent of genes identified (bar) and corresponding −log10(*P*-value) (dot). (**e**) Correlation of fold changes between the LAA and PPV samples. Colors and shapes represent whether the genes residuals were in the outermost one-thousandth quantiles (purple square, red circle, blue triangle, dark grey circle) or not (light grey circle). Furthermore, colors and shapes represent whether those outliers were significantly different in both datasets (purple square), the PPV only (red circle), the LAA only (blue triangle) or neither (dark grey circle)

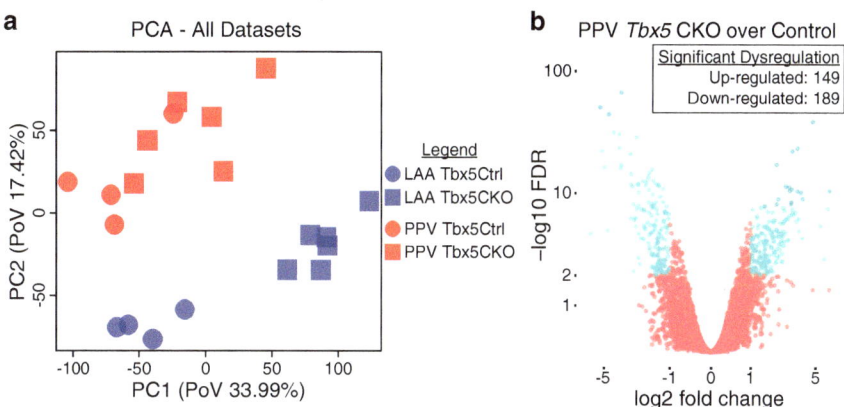

a PCA - All Datasets

b PPV *Tbx5* CKO over Control

Significant Dysregulation
Up-regulated: 149
Down-regulated: 189

Legend
LAA Tbx5Ctrl
LAA Tbx5CKO
PPV Tbx5Ctrl
PPV Tbx5CKO

c Representative GO Terms Associated with Up- and Down-Regulated Genes
5+ gene associations and -log10(P-value) > 5

	Category	Term	Description	-log10(P-value)
Up	GO BP	GO:0051301	cell division	27.64
	KEGG Pathway	mmu05322	Systemic lupus erythematosus	19.45
	Reactome Gene Sets	R-MMU-983231	Factors involved in megakaryocyte development and platelet production	13.25
	GO BP	GO:0030261	chromosome condensation	10.96
	GO BP	GO:0061640	cytoskeleton-dependent cytokinesis	10.36
	GO BP	GO:0008608	attachment of spindle microtubules to kinetochore	9.75
	GO BP	GO:0140013	meiotic nuclear division	9.03
Down	GO BP	GO:0035637	multicellular organismal signaling	8.00
	KEGG Pathway	mmu04921	Oxytocin signaling pathway	5.47

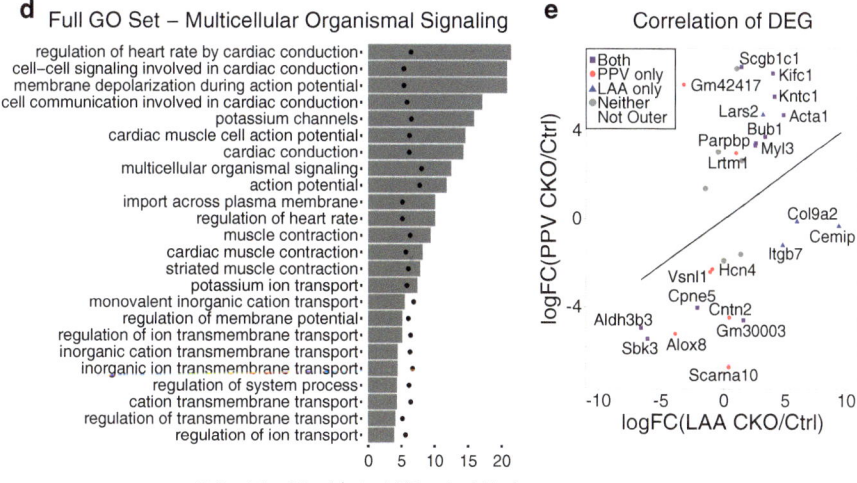

d Full GO Set – Multicellular Organismal Signaling

regulation of heart rate by cardiac conduction
cell–cell signaling involved in cardiac conduction
membrane depolarization during action potential
cell communication involved in cardiac conduction
potassium channels
cardiac muscle cell action potential
cardiac conduction
multicellular organismal signaling
action potential
import across plasma membrane
regulation of heart rate
muscle contraction
cardiac muscle contraction
striated muscle contraction
potassium ion transport
monovalent inorganic cation transport
regulation of membrane potential
regulation of ion transmembrane transport
inorganic cation transmembrane transport
inorganic ion transmembrane transport
regulation of system process
cation transmembrane transport
regulation of transmembrane transport
regulation of ion transport

% Contained (bar) | –log10(P–value) (dot)

e Correlation of DEG

Both
PPV only
LAA only
Neither
Not Outer

Scgb1c1
Kifc1
Gm42417
Kntc1
Lars2
Acta1
Bub1
Parpbp
Myl3
Lrtm1

Col9a2
Cemip
Itgb7
Vsnl1
Hcn4
Cpne5
Cntn2
Aldh3b3
Gm30003
Sbk3
Alox8
Scarna10

logFC(PPV CKO/Ctrl)

logFC(LAA CKO/Ctrl)

The down-regulated GO terms are reminiscent of the LAA previously reported [26]. In particular, examining the full set of GO terms under "multicellular organismal signaling," we identified multiple GO terms associated with the regulation of cardiac conduction, including ion channels, action potential and transmembrane signaling (Fig. 51.2d).

We identified 1492 significantly dysregulated genes in the LAA conditional mutant and control, with 770 up-regulated and 722 down-regulated, similar to our prior analysis of this dataset [26]. Although the numbers of significantly dysregulated genes were different between the PPV and LAA, the dysregulation between the LAA and PPV experiments were significantly correlated (p-value < 2.2E-16, Fig. 51.2e), suggesting that the removal of *Tbx5* had broadly similar effects in the LAA and PPV regions. In order to identify genes demonstrating distinct *Tbx5*-dependent effects between the atrial sub-regions, we correlated the *Tbx5*-dependent changes between the LAA and PPV samples. We identified the 28 genes with residuals in the outermost one-thousandth quantiles (Table 51.1). Amongst those genes, we identified 11 genes that were significantly different in both experiments with 10/11 demonstrating changes in the same direction, 4 genes that were significantly increased in only the LAA samples (*Cemip, Col9a2, Itgb7, Lars2*), 7 genes that were significantly different in only the PPV samples (increased: *Gm42417, Lrtm1*; decreased: *Alox8, Cntn2, Hcn4, Scarna10, Vsnl1*) and 6 genes that were not significantly different in either sample. Interestingly, among the genes that were in the outermost one-thousandth quantiles, we identified *Hcn4*, which encodes the potassium channel essential for the depolarizing "funny current" of the sinoatrial node. *Hcn4* was significantly down-regulated only in the PPV and was also significantly more expressed in the PPV samples than the LAA (Fig. 51.1d).

51.3 Discussion

51.3.1 The Genetics of Atrial Fibrillation Implicates Developmental Transcription Factors

Most genetic loci implicated in AF encode ion channels that affect arrhythmia trigger or substrate. Initial transcriptional studies of AF have focused on a restricted set of candidates, associating remodeling with changes in ion channels and components of cellular signaling cascades [31, 32]. Early transcriptomic or proteomic investigation of AF has been limited to animal models and/or chronic AF [33–36]. For example, animal models based on disruption of specific ion channels do not exhibit spontaneous AF in the absence of concomitant cardiac pathophysiology [37]. However, a recent transcriptomic study using the left atrial appendage of patients with AF revealed that AF susceptibility was associated with decreased expression of transcription factors involved in inflammation, oxidation and the cellular stress response [38]. This study further suggested that remodeling of ion channel expression occurs later in the onset of the disease. Accumulating evidence suggests that transcription factors are important contributors to the pathogenesis of AF [39].

Table 51.1 Genes displaying distinct *Tbx5*-dependent expression patterns

Gene symbol	LAA—Tbx5CKO/Ctrl	PPV—Tbx5CKO/Ctrl	Short description
Acta1	Increased	Increased	Skeletal muscle alpha-actin associated with myopathies [65]
Bub1	Increased	Increased	Spindle assembly checkpoint and centromeric cohesion [66]
Kifc1	Increased	Increased	Mitotic kinesin protein involved in centromsome duplication [67]
Kntc1	Increased	Increased	Kinetochore-binding mitotic checkpoint gene [68]
Myl3	Increased	Increased	Ventricular and slow skeletal muscle myosin light chain [69]
Parpbp	Increased	Increased	Inhibits inappropriate homologous recombination in mitosis [70]
Scgb1c1	Increased	Increased	Secretoglobin protein associated with anti-inflammatory function [71]
Aldh3b3	Decreased	Decreased	Removes lipid-derived aldehydes generated by oxidative stress [72]
Cpne5	Decreased	Decreased	Calcium-dependent, phospholipid-binding proteins [73]
Sbk3	Decreased	Decreased	Uncharacterized cardiac expressed, SH3 domain binding kinase [74]
Gm30003	Increased	Decreased	Lung-expressed predicted gene [75]
Cemip	Increased	NS	Depolymerizes hyaluronic acid [76]
Col9a2	Increased	NS	Type IX collagen found with type II fibrillar collagen [77]
Itgb7	Increased	NS	Leukocyte associated integrin beta subunit [78]
Lars2	Increased	NS	Mitochondrial leucyl-tRNA synthetase [79]
Gm42417	NS	Increased	Predicted gene [80]
Lrtm1	NS	Increased	Transmembrane protein with homology to *Slit3* [81]
Alox8	NS	Decreased	Peroxidizes polyunsaturated fatty acids [82]
Cntn2	NS	Decreased	Membrane junction protein associated with axons [83]
Hcn4	NS	Decreased	Hyperpolarization-activated current/"funny" current [84]
Scarna10	NS	Decreased	Small Cajal body-specific RNA 10 ([85])
Vsnl1	NS	Decreased	Neuronal calcium sensor [86]
Gm13938	NS	NS	Antisense lncRNA [80]
Gm33051	NS	NS	Kidney-expressed antisense lncRNA [75]
Igf2	NS	NS	Fetal growth hormone signaling and tissue differentiation [87]
Rab3c	NS	NS	Calcium-triggered vesicle transport [88]
Slc27a2	NS	NS	Fatty acid transport [89]
Snhg3	NS	NS	Competing endogenous RNA to miR-182-5p [90]

The 28 genes identified as outliers in the outermost one-thousandth quartiles when comparing the *Tbx5*-dependent gene changes in the LAA and the PPV. The genes are listed with whether they were significantly increased (red), decreased (blue) or not significant (NS) in each of the two comparisons. Furthermore, a short description of each gene is provided

GWAS of AF have identified numerous transcription factor loci that play funda-mental roles during cardiac development, including *TBX5, NKX2-5, GATA4* and *PITX2*. The implication of transcription factor genes essential for cardiac develop-ment in in AF raises the fundamental question of whether AF is a function or a result of a developmental defect, for example, of the pulmonary veins, or a later manifes-tation of altered transcriptional control of cardiac rhythm genes in the adult. The first GWAS of AF identified a susceptibility locus on chromosome 4q25 adjacent to *PITX2* [40]. There is evidence that *Pitx2c* affects adult gene expression in the atrium. *PITX2* is expressed both in the left atrium and the pulmonary myocardial sleeve and that its levels are decreased in patients with AF [41, 42]. Atrial-specific deletion of *Pitx2c* leads to hallmarks of AF, which is also observed in *Pitx2c* hetero-zygous mice or adult-specific deletion of this gene [41, 43, 44]. Furthermore, micro-array analysis of *Pitx2c* heterozygous mice revealed impaired gap and tight junction gene expression, consistent with the hypothesis that structural genes are remodeled later in the onset of AF [44].

We previously demonstrated that adult-specific deletion of *Tbx5* causes sponta-neous and sustained AF with atrial gene regulatory network dysfunction [26]. TBX5 drives the atrial expression of *Pitx2*, and TBX5 and PITX2 co-modulate the expres-sion of cardiac rhythm effector genes, including *Ryr2* and *Atp2a2*. These findings indicated that interactions between TBX5 and PITX2 provide tight control of an atrial rhythm gene regulatory network and that perturbation of this network trig-gered AF susceptibility. This example suggested that cardiac TFs implicated in AF by genetic association may co-regulate a gene regulatory network for atrial rhythm homeostasis in the adult atrium.

51.3.2 Transcription Factors and AF: A Pulmonary Vein Developmental Relationship?

The requirement of developmental TFs in the adult for normal cardiac rhythm con-trol does not rule out the possibility that developmental defects caused by their deficiency in the embryo also contributes to AF susceptibility. During embryonic development, the cardiopulmonary progenitors give rise to parts of the atria, pulmo-nary vein and lungs [25]. Distinct functional characteristics between the PPV and LAA regions may reflect distinct developmental ontogeny. The myocardium of the pulmonary veins has a distinct developmental origin from that of the atrial free walls [45]. Subsequently, the myocardium surrounding the pulmonary veins is dis-tinct from that of other regions in the atrium [46]. These developmental distinctions may set the stage for regional gene expression differences within the mature atrium of the adult that normally maintains atrial rhythm but which make the PPV region susceptible to trigger formation when faced with environmental or genetic insult.

Mutations in *NKX2-5, PITX2C and TBX5* increase susceptibility to AF, and all of these transcription factors (TF) play critical roles during cardiovascular develop-ment [26, 47–50]. Each of these TFs are expressed in the pulmonary veins, suggest-ing that perturbations of the transcription program in the PV myocardium may underlie the pathogenesis of AF. The caudal myocardium, including the developing pulmonary vein myocardium, expresses *Tbx5*, *Pitx2c*, *Nkx2-5* and *Gja5* (Cx40) at high levels [51, 52] consistent with a fast-conducting atrial myocardial phenotype. In a *Nkx2-5* haploinsufficient mouse model, *Gja5* levels are decreased whereas *Hcn4* levels are increased in the pulmonary vein myocardium. *Nkx2-5* and *Pitx2c* are both required for the development and maintain identity of the pulmonary myocardium [45, 53]. The changes in gene expression observed in *Nkx2-5* haploinsufficient mice could be reflective of a loss of fast conduction and acquisition of pacemaking conduction phenotype. This type of transition provided a conceivable model for how genetic changes could result in automaticity in the PPV region that resulted in arrhythmia initiation.

Absence of the lungs and pulmonary vasculature in *Tbx5* knockout mice suggests that it may play an essential developmental role specifically within the pulmonary veins as well [24]. We observed that a decrement in *Tbx5* in the PPV region decreased *Hcn4* expression, which is not overtly consistent with this transformation model. On the other hand, we observed that many genes with important roles in myocardial automaticity, including *Tbx3*, *Shox2*, *Cacna1d*, *Cacna2d2* and *Hcn4* were more highly expressed in the PPV than the LAA region, and remained more highly expressed in the context of adult-specific *Tbx5* conditional deletion. Furthermore, other *Tbx5*-dependent genes in the PPV region are classical fast conduction genes, including *Scn5a*, *Gja5* and *Kcnk3*. Reduction in the expression of these fast conduction genes in the context of retained high expression of automaticity genes such as *Hcn4* could diminish fast conduction physiology and allow the emergence of myocardial automaticity, providing a nidus for the initiation of atrial arrhythmias including AF.

51.4   Methods

51.4.1 Animal Experiments and Ethics Statement

All murine experiments were performed under University of Chicago Institutional Animal Care and Use Committee (IACUC) protocol number 71737. Mice harboring the ROSA26 tamoxifen-inducible cre recombinase transgene, *Gt(ROSA)26Sor^{tm1(cre/ERT2)Tyj}* (*R26^{creERT2}*), were bred with mice harboring the *Tbx5^{tm1Jse}* allele (*Tbx5^{flox}*) to generate *Tbx5* conditional mutants, *R26^{creERT2/creERT2}*; *Tbx5^{flox/flox}*, and controls, *R26^{creERT2/creERT2}*; *Tbx5^{+/+}* [23, 54]. Tamoxifen was administered by intraperitoneal injection for three consecutive days at 6 weeks of age and tissue samples were harvested 1 week after treatment as previously reported [26].

51.4.2 Transcriptional Profiling and Analysis

Transcriptional profiling was performed on the peri-pulmonary vein region of the left atrium (Fig. 51.1a). Total RNA was extracted from four controls and six conditional mutants. Following rRNA removal (Ribo-Zero rRNA Removal Kit, Illumina), libraries were prepared using the TruSeq RNA Sample prep kit v2 (Illumina). Samples were pooled in equimolar ratios and sequenced on the Illumina HiSeq4000 platform. Library preparation and sequencing were performed by the Genomics Core Facility at the University of Chicago.

The peri-pulmonary vein samples were compared with the previously published corresponding left atrial appendage samples [26]. Both the peri-pulmonary vein and left atrial appendage samples were analyzed in parallel as described below.

Between 20 and 22 million reads were generated for each replicate (14–19 million reads for left atrial appendage) and aligned to the GRCm38/mm10 build of the *Mus musculus* genome (retrieved from UCSC May 23, 2012) using TopHat v2.1.1 [55, 56]. Reads were filtered to remove poorly aligned (MAPQ<10), duplicated and unmapped reads using BamTools v2.4.1 [57]. Post-alignment, post-filtered reads were assigned to transcripts using StringTie v1.3.3 [58, 59].

Downstream analysis was performed using R v3.4.0 [60]. Differential expression testing was performed using edgeR v3.18.1 [61] and limma v3.32.10 [62]. Low level genes were removed within each condition using median log-transformed counts per gene per million mapped reads (cpm) cutoff of 1. A generalized linear model (GLM) framework was used to test for differential expressed genes between $Tbx5^{fl/fl};R26^{cre-ERT2}$ conditional mutants and $Tbx5^{+/+};R26^{cre-ERT2}$ controls for each tissue and between controls of the left atrial appendage and peri-pulmonary vein tissues. Data was plotted using the ggplot2 v2.3.0 [63] and scales v0.5.0 [64] packages. GO term analysis was performed using metascape (http://metascape.org) [27]. The raw and processed data as well as the full outputs were deposited in GEO at accession number GSE128870.

References

1. Nishida K, Datino T, Macle L, Nattel S. Atrial fibrillation ablation: translating basic mechanistic insights to the patient. J Am Coll Cardiol. 2014;64(8):823–31.
2. Tucker NR, Ellinor PT. Emerging directions in the genetics of atrial fibrillation. Circ Res. 2014;114(9):1469–82.
3. Fatkin D, Santiago CF, Huttner IG, Lubitz SA, Ellinor PT. Genetics of Atrial Fibrillation: State of the Art in 2017. Heart Lung Circ. 2017;26(9):894–901.
4. Nielsen JB, et al. Genome-wide Study of Atrial Fibrillation Identifies Seven Risk Loci and Highlights Biological Pathways and Regulatory Elements Involved in Cardiac Development. Am J Hum Genet. 2018;102(1):103–15.
5. Andrade J, Khairy P, Dobrev D, Nattel S. The clinical profile and pathophysiology of atrial fibrillation: relationships among clinical features, epidemiology, and mechanisms. Circ Res. 2014;114(9):1453–68.
6. Haissaguerre M, et al. Spontaneous initiation of atrial fibrillation by ectopic beats originating in the pulmonary veins. N Engl J Med. 1998;339(10):659–66.
7. Jais P, et al. A focal source of atrial fibrillation treated by discrete radiofrequency ablation. Circulation. 1997;95(3):572–6.
8. Chen YJ, Chen SA, Chang MS, Lin CI. Arrhythmogenic activity of cardiac muscle in pulmonary veins of the dog: implication for the genesis of atrial fibrillation. Cardiovasc Res. 2000;48(2):265–73.

9. Nguyen BL, Fishbein MC, Chen LS, Chen PS, Masroor S. Histopathological substrate for chronic atrial fibrillation in humans. Heart Rhythm. 2009;6(4):454–60.
10. Chen SA, et al. Initiation of atrial fibrillation by ectopic beats originating from the pulmonary veins: electrophysiological characteristics, pharmacological responses, and effects of radiofrequency ablation. Circulation. 1999;100(18):1879–86.
11. Boutilier JK, et al. Gene expression networks in the murine pulmonary myocardium provide insight into the pathobiology of atrial fibrillation. G3 (Bethesda). 2017;7(9):2999–3017.
12. Basson CT, et al. Mutations in human TBX5 [corrected] cause limb and cardiac malformation in Holt-Oram syndrome. Nat Genet. 1997;15(1):30–5.
13. Li QY, et al. Holt-Oram syndrome is caused by mutations in TBX5, a member of the Brachyury (T) gene family. Nat Genet. 1997;15(1):21–9.
14. McDermott DA, et al. TBX5 genetic testing validates strict clinical criteria for Holt-Oram syndrome. Pediatr Res. 2005;58(5):981–6.
15. Elek C, Vitez M, Czeizel E. Holt-Oram syndrome. Orv Hetil. 1991;132(2):73–4.. 77-78
16. Barisic I, et al. Holt Oram syndrome: a registry-based study in Europe. Orphanet J Rare Dis. 2014;9:156.
17. Holt M, Oram S. Familial heart disease with skeletal malformations. Br Heart J. 1960;22:236–42.
18. Basson CT, et al. The clinical and genetic spectrum of the Holt-Oram syndrome (heart-hand syndrome). N Engl J Med. 1994;330(13):885–91.
19. Newbury-Ecob RA, Leanage R, Raeburn JA, Young ID. Holt-Oram syndrome: a clinical genetic study. J Med Genet. 1996;33(4):300–7.
20. Huang T, et al. Causes of clinical diversity in human TBX5 mutations. Cold Spring Harb Symp Quant Biol. 2002;67:115–20.
21. Bohm J, et al. Functional analysis of the novel TBX5 c.1333delC mutation resulting in an extended TBX5 protein. BMC Med Genet. 2008;9:88.
22. Boogerd CJ, et al. Functional analysis of novel TBX5 T-box mutations associated with Holt-Oram syndrome. Cardiovasc Res. 2010;88(1):130–9.
23. Bruneau BG, et al. A murine model of Holt-Oram syndrome defines roles of the T-box transcription factor Tbx5 in cardiogenesis and disease. Cell. 2001;106(6):709–21.
24. Steimle JD, et al. Evolutionarily conserved Tbx5-Wnt2/2b pathway orchestrates cardiopulmonary development. Proc Natl Acad Sci U S A. 2018;115(45):E10615–24.
25. Peng T, et al. Coordination of heart and lung co-development by a multipotent cardiopulmonary progenitor. Nature. 2013;500(7464):589–92.
26. Nadadur RD, et al. Pitx2 modulates a Tbx5-dependent gene regulatory network to maintain atrial rhythm. In: Sci Transl Med 8(354):354ra115; 2016.
27. Tripathi S, et al. Meta- and orthogonal integration of influenza "OMICs" data defines a role for UBR4 in virus budding. Cell Host Microbe. 2015;18(6):723–35.
28. Bapat A, Anderson CD, Ellinor PT, Lubitz SA. Genomic basis of atrial fibrillation. Heart. 2018;104(3):201–6.
29. van Setten J, et al. PR interval genome-wide association meta-analysis identifies 50 loci associated with atrial and atrioventricular electrical activity. Nat Commun. 2018;9(1):2904.
30. Kramer A, Green J, Pollard J Jr, Tugendreich S. Causal analysis approaches in Ingenuity Pathway Analysis. Bioinformatics. 2014;30(4):523–30.
31. Goette A, et al. Increased expression of extracellular signal-regulated kinase and angiotensin-converting enzyme in human atria during atrial fibrillation. J Am Coll Cardiol. 2000;35(6):1669–77.
32. Brundel BJ, et al. Alterations in potassium channel gene expression in atria of patients with persistent and paroxysmal atrial fibrillation: differential regulation of protein and mRNA levels for K+ channels. J Am Coll Cardiol. 2001;37(3):926–32.
33. Barth AS, et al. Reprogramming of the human atrial transcriptome in permanent atrial fibrillation: expression of a ventricular-like genomic signature. Circ Res. 2005;96(9):1022–9.
34. Lamirault G, et al. Gene expression profile associated with chronic atrial fibrillation and underlying valvular heart disease in man. J Mol Cell Cardiol. 2006;40(1):173–84.

35. Cardin S, et al. Contrasting gene expression profiles in two canine models of atrial fibrillation. Circ Res. 2007;100(3):425–33.
36. De Souza AI, et al. Proteomic and metabolomic analysis of atrial profibrillatory remodelling in congestive heart failure. J Mol Cell Cardiol. 2010;49(5):851–63.
37. Riley G, Syeda F, Kirchhof P, Fabritz L. An introduction to murine models of atrial fibrillation. Front Physiol. 2012;3:296.
38. Deshmukh A, et al. Left atrial transcriptional changes associated with atrial fibrillation susceptibility and persistence. Circ Arrhythm Electrophysiol. 2015;8(1):32–41.
39. Mahida S. Transcription factors and atrial fibrillation. Cardiovasc Res. 2014;101(2):194–202.
40. Gudbjartsson DF, et al. Variants conferring risk of atrial fibrillation on chromosome 4q25. Nature. 2007;448(7151):353–7.
41. Chinchilla A, et al. PITX2 insufficiency leads to atrial electrical and structural remodeling linked to arrhythmogenesis. Circ Cardiovasc Genet. 2011;4(3):269–79.
42. Kirchhof P, et al. PITX2c is expressed in the adult left atrium, and reducing Pitx2c expression promotes atrial fibrillation inducibility and complex changes in gene expression. Circ Cardiovasc Genet. 2011;4(2):123–33.
43. Wang J, et al. Pitx2 prevents susceptibility to atrial arrhythmias by inhibiting left-sided pacemaker specification. Proc Natl Acad Sci U S A. 2010;107(21):9753–8.
44. Tao Y, et al. Pitx2, an atrial fibrillation predisposition gene, directly regulates ion transport and intercalated disc genes. Circ Cardiovasc Genet. 2014;7(1):23–32.
45. Mommersteeg MT, et al. Pitx2c and Nkx2-5 are required for the formation and identity of the pulmonary myocardium. Circ Res. 2007;101(9):902–9.
46. Soufan AT, et al. Reconstruction of the patterns of gene expression in the developing mouse heart reveals an architectural arrangement that facilitates the understanding of atrial malformations and arrhythmias. Circ Res. 2004;95(12):1207–15.
47. Huang RT, Xue S, Xu YJ, Zhou M, Yang YQ. A novel NKX2.5 loss-of-function mutation responsible for familial atrial fibrillation. Int J Mol Med. 2013;31(5):1119–26.
48. Xie WH, et al. Prevalence and spectrum of Nkx2.5 mutations associated with idiopathic atrial fibrillation. Clinics (Sao Paulo). 2013;68(6):777–84.
49. Qiu XB, et al. PITX2C loss-of-function mutations responsible for idiopathic atrial fibrillation. Clinics (Sao Paulo). 2014;69(1):15–22.
50. Wang J, et al. Pitx2-microRNA pathway that delimits sinoatrial node development and inhibits predisposition to atrial fibrillation. Proc Natl Acad Sci U S A. 2014;111(25):9181–6.
51. Christoffels VM, et al. Formation of the venous pole of the heart from an Nkx2-5-negative precursor population requires Tbx18. Circ Res. 2006;98(12):1555–63.
52. Xie L, et al. Tbx5-hedgehog molecular networks are essential in the second heart field for atrial septation. Dev Cell. 2012;23(2):280–91.
53. Ye W, et al. A common Shox2-Nkx2-5 antagonistic mechanism primes the pacemaker cell fate in the pulmonary vein myocardium and sinoatrial node. Development. 2015;142(14):2521–32.
54. Ventura A, et al. Restoration of p53 function leads to tumour regression in vivo. Nature. 2007;445(7128):661–5.
55. Kim D, et al. TopHat2: accurate alignment of transcriptomes in the presence of insertions, deletions and gene fusions. Genome Biol. 2013;14(4):R36.
56. Trapnell C, Pachter L, Salzberg SL. TopHat: discovering splice junctions with RNA-Seq. Bioinformatics. 2009;25(9):1105–11.
57. Barnett DW, Garrison EK, Quinlan AR, Stromberg MP, Marth GT. BamTools: a C++ API and toolkit for analyzing and managing BAM files. Bioinformatics. 2011;27(12):1691–2.
58. Pertea M, Kim D, Pertea GM, Leek JT, Salzberg SL. Transcript-level expression analysis of RNA-seq experiments with HISAT, StringTie and Ballgown. Nat Protoc. 2016;11(9):1650–67.
59. Pertea M, et al. StringTie enables improved reconstruction of a transcriptome from RNA-seq reads. Nat Biotechnol. 2015;33(3):290–5.
60. R Core Team. R: A language and environment for statistical computing. R Foundation for Statistical Computing. 2017.

61. Robinson MD, McCarthy DJ, Smyth GK. edgeR: a Bioconductor package for differential expression analysis of digital gene expression data. Bioinformatics. 2010;26(1):139–40.
62. Ritchie ME, et al. limma powers differential expression analyses for RNA-sequencing and microarray studies. Nucleic Acids Res. 2015;43(7):e47.
63. Wickham H. ggplot2: Elegant graphics for data analysis. New York: Springer; 2009.
64. Wickham H. Scales: Scale Functions for Visualization. R package version 0.5.0. 2017.
65. Nowak KJ, et al. Mutations in the skeletal muscle alpha-actin gene in patients with actin myopathy and nemaline myopathy. Nat Genet. 1999;23(2):208–12.
66. Perera D, et al. Bub1 maintains centromeric cohesion by activation of the spindle checkpoint. Dev Cell. 2007;13(4):566–79.
67. Christodoulou A, Lederer CW, Surrey T, Vernos I, Santama N. Motor protein KIFC5A interacts with Nubp1 and Nubp2, and is implicated in the regulation of centrosome duplication. J Cell Sci. 2006;119(Pt 10):2035–47.
68. Chan GK, Jablonski SA, Starr DA, Goldberg ML, Yen TJ. Human Zw10 and ROD are mitotic checkpoint proteins that bind to kinetochores. Nat Cell Biol. 2000;2(12):944–7.
69. Barton PJ, et al. The myosin alkali light chains of mouse ventricular and slow skeletal muscle are indistinguishable and are encoded by the same gene. J Biol Chem. 1985;260(14):8578–84.
70. Moldovan GL, et al. Inhibition of homologous recombination by the PCNA-interacting protein PARI. Mol Cell. 2012;45(1):75–86.
71. Lu X, et al. The cytokine-driven regulation of secretoglobins in normal human upper airway and their expression, particularly that of uteroglobin-related protein 1, in chronic rhinosinusitis. Respir Res. 2011;12:28.
72. Kitamura T, Takagi S, Naganuma T, Kihara A. Mouse aldehyde dehydrogenase ALDH3B2 is localized to lipid droplets via two C-terminal tryptophan residues and lipid modification. Biochem J. 2015;465(1):79–87.
73. Tomsig JL, Creutz CE. Copines: a ubiquitous family of Ca(2+)-dependent phospholipid-binding proteins. Cell Mol Life Sci. 2002;59(9):1467–77.
74. Fagerberg L, et al. Analysis of the human tissue-specific expression by genome-wide integration of transcriptomics and antibody-based proteomics. Mol Cell Proteomics. 2014;13(2):397–406.
75. Yue F, et al. A comparative encyclopedia of DNA elements in the mouse genome. Nature. 2014;515(7527):355–64.
76. Yoshida H, et al. KIAA1199, a deafness gene of unknown function, is a new hyaluronan binding protein involved in hyaluronan depolymerization. Proc Natl Acad Sci U S A. 2013;110(14):5612–7.
77. Eyre D. Collagen of articular cartilage. Arthritis Res. 2002;4(1):30–5.
78. Erle DJ, Ruegg C, Sheppard D, Pytela R. Complete amino acid sequence of an integrin beta subunit (beta 7) identified in leukocytes. J Biol Chem. 1991;266(17):11009–16.
79. Pang YL, Poruri K, Martinis SA. tRNA synthetase: tRNA aminoacylation and beyond. Wiley Interdiscip Rev RNA. 2014;5(4):461–80.
80. Smith CL, et al. Mouse Genome Database (MGD)-2018: knowledgebase for the laboratory mouse. Nucleic Acids Res. 2018;46(D1):D836–42.
81. Lopez Jimenez N, et al. Examination of FGFRL1 as a candidate gene for diaphragmatic defects at chromosome 4p16.3 shows that Fgfrl1 null mice have reduced expression of Tpm3, sarcomere genes and Lrtm1 in the diaphragm. Hum Genet. 2010;127(3):325–36.
82. Jisaka M, Kim RB, Boeglin WE, Nanney LB, Brash AR. Molecular cloning and functional expression of a phorbol ester-inducible 8S-lipoxygenase from mouse skin. J Biol Chem. 1997;272(39):24410–6.
83. Lu Z, et al. Molecular Architecture of Contactin-associated Protein-like 2 (CNTNAP2) and Its Interaction with Contactin 2 (CNTN2). J Biol Chem. 2016;291(46):24133–47.
84. Stevens DR, et al. Hyperpolarization-activated channels HCN1 and HCN4 mediate responses to sour stimuli. Nature. 2001;413(6856):631–5.
85. Darzacq X, et al. Cajal body-specific small nuclear RNAs: a novel class of 2′-O-methylation and pseudouridylation guide RNAs. EMBO J. 2002;21(11):2746–56.

86. Burgoyne RD. Neuronal calcium sensor proteins: generating diversity in neuronal Ca^{2+} signalling. Nat Rev Neurosci. 2007;8(3):182–93.
87. DeChiara TM, Efstratiadis A, Robertson EJ. A growth-deficiency phenotype in heterozygous mice carrying an insulin-like growth factor II gene disrupted by targeting. Nature. 1990;345(6270):78–80.
88. Schluter OM, Schmitz F, Jahn R, Rosenmund C, Sudhof TC. A complete genetic analysis of neuronal Rab3 function. J Neurosci. 2004;24(29):6629–37.
89. Steinberg SJ, Wang SJ, McGuinness MC, Watkins PA. Human liver-specific very-long-chain acyl-coenzyme A synthetase: cDNA cloning and characterization of a second enzymatically active protein. Mol Genet Metab. 1999;68(1):32–42.
90. Huang W, et al. The long non-coding RNA SNHG3 functions as a competing endogenous RNA to promote malignant development of colorectal cancer. Oncol Rep. 2017;38(3):1402–10.

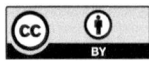

The Endocardium as a Master Regulator of Ventricular Trabeculation

52

Xianghu Qu and H. Scott Baldwin

Abstract

Ventricular chamber morphogenesis, characterized by trabeculae formation, is crucial for cardiac function and embryonic viability and depends on cellular interactions between the endocardium and myocardium. The ang1-Tie2 pathway is required for normal heart chamber development, but its molecular effectors are not well defined. Here we show that loss of Tie2 in endocardial cells (EC) results in mid-gestation lethality due to heart defects including hyperplastic myocardium trabeculation (fewer but thicker trabeculae), thinner compact myocardium and simplified endocardial network. The thicker trabeculae phenotype results from enhanced proliferation of trabecular cardiomyocytes. Meanwhile, endocardial loss of Tie2 reduces proliferation and production of ECs and impairs endocardial sprouting, which provides necessary support for trabecular assembly and extension, thus resulting in a dramatically simplified trabecular meshwork. These findings reveal two seemingly apposing functions of Tie2 in myocardium trabeculation: ensuring normal trabeculation by supporting EC proliferation and sprouting while preventing hypertrabeculation by inhibiting trabecular cardiomyocyte proliferation.

X. Qu (✉)
Department of Pediatrics (Cardiology), Vanderbilt University Medical Center, Nashville, TN, USA
e-mail: Xianghu.qu@vumc.org

H. S. Baldwin
Department of Pediatrics (Cardiology), Vanderbilt University Medical Center, Nashville, TN, USA

Department of Cell and Development Biology, Vanderbilt University Medical Center, Nashville, TN, USA
e-mail: scott.baldwin@vumc.org

331

T. Nakanishi et al. (eds.), *Molecular Mechanism of Congenital Heart Disease and Pulmonary Hypertension*, https://doi.org/10.1007/978-981-15-1185-1_52

Keywords
Tie2 · Endocardium · Myocardium trabeculation · RA signaling · Conditional knockout

52.1   Introduction

Congenital heart diseases are some of the most common human birth defects. In many congenital heart diseases, genetic defects lead to impaired embryonic heart development or growth. A key development process in cardiac ontogeny is ventricular chamber formation. One of the first signs of chamber development is the formation of trabeculae [1]. Lack of trabeculation frequently causes embryonic lethality in mice and excess trabeculation causes cardiomyopathy and heart failure in humans [2]. A number of signaling molecules from myocardium, endocardium and cardiac extracellular matrix (ECM) have been implicated in trabeculation and an intimate communication between endocardium and myocardium promotes cardiomyocyte (CM) proliferation and differentiation leading to trabeculae formation [2]. The Notch signaling pathway has been the most intensely investigated in this process with Bmp10, Nrg1 and EphrinB2 identified as downstream targets of Notch signaling during trabeculation [3]. However, the molecular and cellular mechanisms controlling trabeculation are still poorly understood.

The Tie (tyrosine kinase with immunoglobulin-like and EGF homology) receptors, Tie1 and Tek/Tie2, are type 1 transmembrane protein receptor tyrosine kinases (RTKs) [4]. Along with the vascular endothelial growth factor (VEGF) receptors, these are the only known endothelial cell (EC)-specific RTKs. Although deficiency in Tie1 results in cardiovascular demise in utero [5–7], Tie1 is dispensable for cardiac trabeculation. Mutations in Tie2 have been described to cause ventricular septal defects and cutaneomucosal venous malformations in humans [8, 9]. Previous reports have suggested a role for Tie2 signaling in trabeculation because Tie2-null embryos have no trabeculae [5, 10] and deficiency *of Ang1*; the primary agonist for Tie2 results in a marked reduction in cardiac trabeculation [11, 12]. However, the molecular basis for these phenotypes has remained elusive. In addition, *Tie2*-deficient mouse embryos with abnormal trabeculation also had lethal vascular defects raising the question of whether the cardiac defects observed were primary or secondary to more global vascular compromise. Here, we show that loss of endocardial Tie2 results in embryonic heart failure that is characterized by impaired endocardial growth and hyperplastic trabeculation.

52.2   Mouse Models for Endocardial Specific Gene Deletion

In order to allow temporal and tissue-specific gene inactivation, we have developed a conditional allele of the mouse *Tie2* gene by introducing Cre recombinase recognition sites (*loxP*) into the *Tie2* locus. This strategy involved introducing a *loxP* site

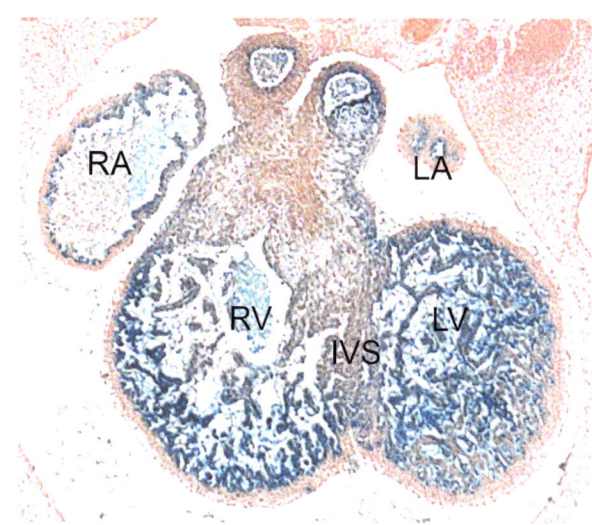

Fig. 52.1 *Nfatc1^{Cre}* mediates *loxP* excision exclusively in the endocardium. X-gal staining of *R26^{fslz};Nfatc1^{Cre}* heart sections at E12.5 shows that *Nfatc1^{Cre}*-mediated recombination is restricted to the embryonic atrial and ventricular endocardium but not in the endothelial cells (ECs) of the peripheral vasculature. *RA* right atrium, *RV* right ventricle, *LA* left atrium, *LV* left ventricle, *IVS*, interventricular septum

within the first intron, and another *loxP* site just upstream of the minimal promoter region. To specifically determine the role of Tie2 in cardiac trabeculation, we utilized this floxed *Tie2* allele and an endocardial specific Cre transgenic line previously generated in our lab (*Nfatc1^{Cre}*) [13]. We first analyzed Cre activity by X-gal staining of *R26^{fslz};Nfatc1^{Cre}* heart sections showing that Cre expression was restricted to the endocardium from E9.0 but not in the ECs of the peripheral vasculature (Fig. 52.1).

52.3   Tie2 Is Essential for Ventricular Chamber Development

Mice with a floxed *Tie2* allele were crossed with the *Nfatc1^{Cre}* line. We refer to *Nfatc1$^{Cre/+}$;Tie2$^{f/f}$* mice as *Tie2* conditional knockout (*Tie2-cko*). Similar to the global deletion of *Tie2*, no endocardial *Tie2-cko* animals survived to birth. *Tie2-cko* embryos were grossly indistinguishable from their littermates until E12.5 at which point most began to show dorsal edema that increased until demise at E13.0–E13.5. Histological analysis of their hearts confirmed abnormal trabeculation, thin compact myocardium and ventricular septal defects compared with littermate controls (*Tie2$^{+/f}$* and *Tie2$^{f/f}$*). Dual-fluorescence staining of heart sections with antibodies for troponin T (myocardial marker) and endomucin (which identifies ECs) (Fig. 52.2) revealed fewer but thicker trabeculae in *Tie2-cko* hearts. In addition, the endomucin-positive endocardial network and sproutings were abnormal.

To determine if the thicker trabeculae in *Tie2-cko* hearts were due to enhanced proliferation rate in myocardium, we assessed MCs proliferation rate by BrdU pulse labeling. There is no significant difference in the percentage of BrdU-positive cardiomyocytes in the compact zone between the control and *Tie2-cko* hearts at E11.5 and E12.5. However, in the trabecular zone the percentage of BrdU-positive MCs in

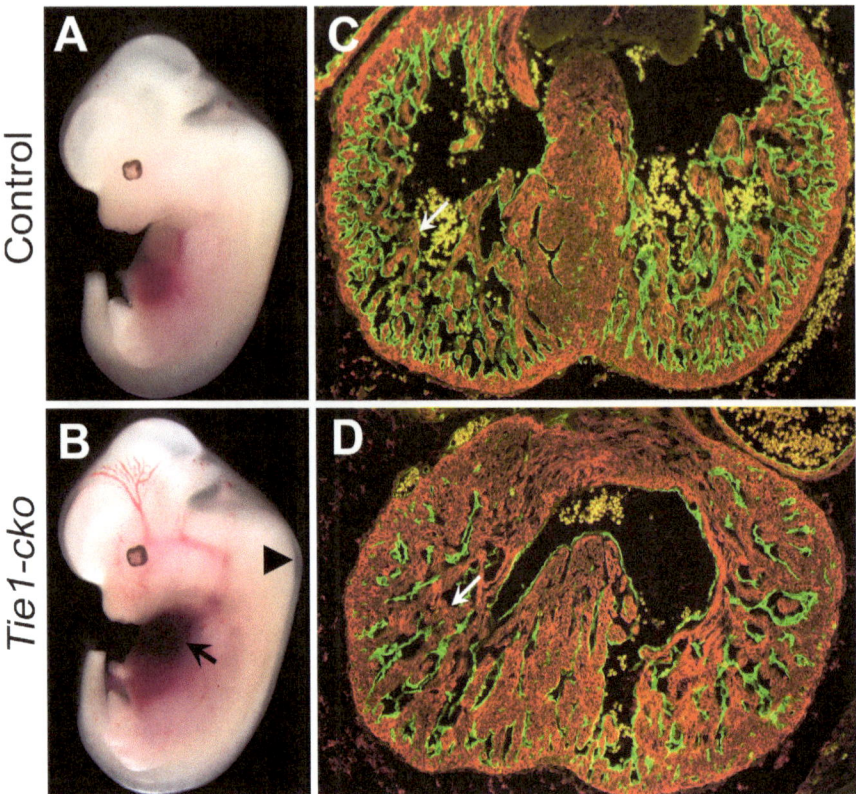

Fig. 52.2 Endocardial specific deletion of Tie2 results in abnormal trabeculation. (**a, b**) Gross images of control (**a**) and *Tie2-cko* (**b**) embryos at E12.5 showing pericardial effusions (arrow) and edema (arrowhead) in the mutant embryos. (**c, d**) Control and *Tie2-cko* ventricular sections at E12.5 were stained with troponin T (myocardial marker, red) and endomucin (endocadial marker, green) antibodies. Compared to the control, the mutant heart had fewer but thicker trabeculae (arrows), thinner compact myocardium and simplified endocardial network

the *Tie2-cko* was significantly higher than that in the control, 36.6% vs. 24.6% at E11.5 and 32.4 vs. 11.8% at E12.5. Co-immunostaining for endomucin and Erg (EC-specific ETS transcription factor) revealed that the reduced endocardial sprout-ings in *Tie2-cko* mice was accompanied by a decreased number of ECs; the total endocardial EC number was determined by counting cells positive for Erg (Fig. 52.3). BrdU analysis also revealed that EC proliferation in the *Tie2-cko* endo-cardium was reduced by nearly 50% compared with control mice at E10.5 and E11.5. Thus, endocardial attenuation of *Tie2* leads to impaired endocardial growth and hyperplastic trabeculation.

In summary, we propose a model of trabeculation regulation by Endocardial Tie2 (Fig. 52.4). In wild-type mice, at E9.0, the first stage or initiation of trabeculation is characterized by endocardial sprout formation and touchdown coincident with

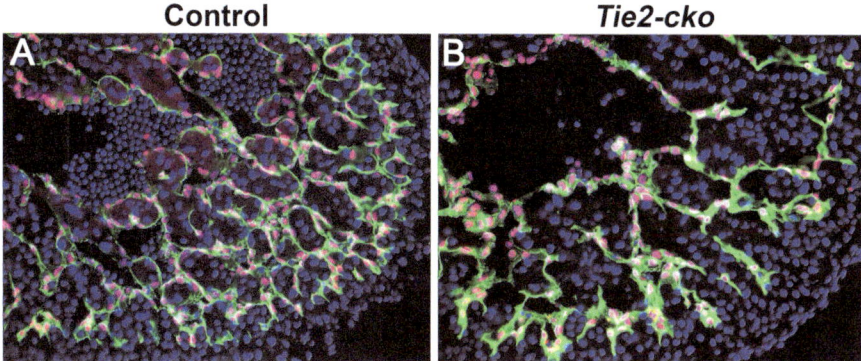

Fig. 52.3 Endocardial attenuation of Tie2 results in decreased EC number and simplified endocardial network. Dual immunostaining of control and *Tie2-cko* heart sections (left ventricle) for Erg (red) and endomucin (green) at E11.5 reveals a significant decrease in Erg-positive endocardial cell number in the mutant ventricles (**b**) compared to control ventricles (**a**) following endocardial loss of Tie2. DAPI, blue

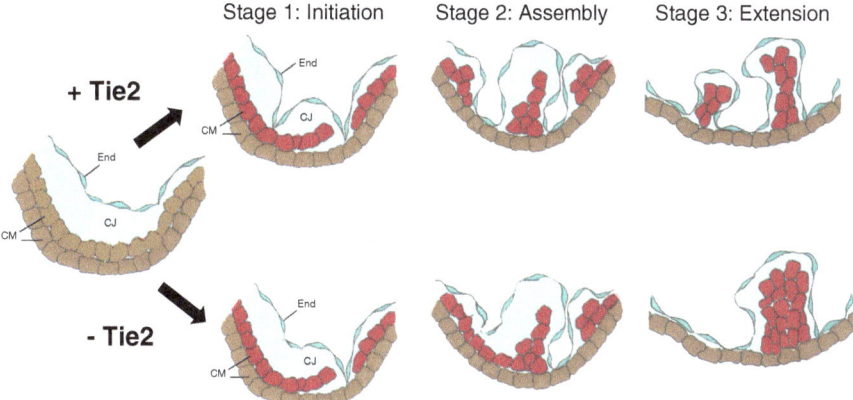

Fig. 52.4 Proposed model of trabeculation regulation by endocardial Tie2. In wild-type mice, myocardial trabeculation develops as a three-step model: stage 1 at E9.0, initiation of trabeculation, stage 2 at E9.25, trabecular assembly and stage 3 at E9.5, trabecular extension. In *Tie2-cko* mice, only limited endocardial sproutings reached the outer layer myocardium. Although the myocardial wall in mutant ventricles was able to thicken to a multicellular layer and form sheet-like protrusions (myocardial lamina), assembly and extension of trabeculae were impaired, thus leading to thicker but reduced trabeculae. *CJ* cardiac jelly, *CM* cardiomyocytes, *End*, endocardium

myocardial delamination. Next endocardial sproutings progress laterally beneath the myocardial lamina resulting in isolated clusters of myocardial cells within a "bubble" of cardiac ECM, covered by endocardium. By E9.25 the endocardial sprouting-enveloped myocardial lamina assemble to isolated short trabecular clusters (stage 2: assembly), which is followed by trabecular extension (stage 3) at E9.5, leading to finger-like long trabecular structures. In *Tie2-cko* mice, only limited endocardial sproutings reached the outer myocardial layer. Although the myocardial wall in mutant ventricles was able to thicken and form multicellular sheet-like protrusions (myocardial lamina), assembly and extension of trabeculae were impaired, thus leading to thicker but reduced trabeculae.

52.4   Future Directions and Clinical Implications

Despite the absolute requirement for functional Tie2 signaling in normal cardiovascular development as well as its essential role in the progression of adult heart and vascular diseases, there is a paucity of information delineating the mechanism(s) of Tie2 activation or the subsequent signaling events that modulate heart ontogeny. This work reveals a critical role for the endocardium in the orchestration of ventricular trabeculation which is dependent on endocardial RTK Tie2 signaling. Tie2 not only plays a primary autocrine function in support of EC proliferation and angiogenic sprouting and touchdown but also is instrumental in the generation of paracrine signaling that results in inhibition of trabecular CM proliferation that prevents hypertrabeculation. Further investigation on this project will focus on delineating downstream targets of Tie2 activation in both endocardium (cell autonomous effect) and myocardium (paracrine effect) during ventricular trabeculation. These new insights will be important in further defining mechanisms of disease pathology related to ventricular chamber morphogenesis and function and will ultimately be critical in elucidating the etiology of congenital heart diseases.

Acknowledgments This work was supported by grants from NHLB/NIH: RL1HL0952551 (H.S.B.).

References

1. Sedmera D, Pexieder T, Vuillemin M, Thompson RP, Anderson RH. Developmental patterning of the myocardium. Anat Rec. 2000;258(4):319–37.
2. Zhang W, Chen H, Qu X, Chang CP, Shou W. Molecular mechanism of ventricular trabeculation/compaction and the pathogenesis of the left ventricular noncompaction cardiomyopathy (LVNC). Am J Med Genet C Semin Med Genet. 2013;163C(3):144–56.
3. Captur G, et al. Morphogenesis of myocardial trabeculae in the mouse embryo. J Anat. 2016;229(2):314–25.
4. Augustin HG, et al. Control of vascular morphogenesis and homeostasis through the angiopoietin-Tie system. Nat Rev Mol Cell Biol. 2009;10(3):165–77.
5. Sato TN, et al. Distinct roles of the receptor tyrosine kinases Tie-1 and Tie-2 in blood vessel formation. Nature. 1995;376(6535):70–4.
6. Puri MC, et al. The receptor tyrosine kinase TIE is required for integrity and survival of vascular endothelial cells. EMBO J. 1995;14(23):5884–91.
7. Qu X, Tompkins K, Batts LE, Puri M, Baldwin S. Abnormal embryonic lymphatic vessel development in Tie1 hypomorphic mice. Development. 2010;137(8):1285–95.
8. Szot JO, Cuny H, Blue GM, Humphreys DT, Ip E, Harrison K, Sholler GF, Giannoulatou E, Leo P, Duncan EL, Sparrow DB, Ho JWK, Graham RM, Pachter N, Chapman G, Winlaw DS,

Dunwoodie SL. A screening approach to identify clinically actionable variants causing congenital heart disease in exome data. Circ Genom Precis Med. 2018;11(3):e001978.

9. Wouters V, Limaye N, Uebelhoer M, Irrthum A, Boon LM, Mulliken JB, et al. Hereditary cutaneomucosal venous malformations are caused by TIE2 mutations with widely variable hyper-phosphorylating effects. Eur J Hum Genet. 2010;18:414–20.

10. Dumont DJ, et al. Dominant-negative and targeted null mutations in the endothelial receptor tyrosine kinase, tek, reveal a critical role in vasculogenesis of the embryo. Genes Dev. 1994;8(16):1897–909.

11. Suri C, et al. Requisite role of angiopoietin-1, a ligand for the TIE2 receptor, during embryonic angiogenesis. Cell. 1996;87(7):1171–80.

12. Jeansson M, et al. Angiopoietin-1 is essential in mouse vasculature during development and in response to injury. J Clin Invest. 2011;121(6):2278–89.

13. Wu B, et al. Endocardial cells form the coronary arteries by angiogenesis through myocardial-endocardial VEGF signaling. Cell. 2012;151(5):1083–96.

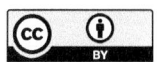

The Role of Alternative mRNA Splicing in Heart Development

53

Douglas C. Bittel, Nataliya Kibiryeva, Naoya Kenmochi, Prakash Patil, Tamayo Uechi, Brenda Rongish, Mike Filla, Jennifer Marshall, Michael Artman, Rajasingh Johnson, and James E. O'Brien Jr

Abstract

Research in the last 10 years has led to improved understanding of the genetic regulation of vertebrate heart development, but despite this effort, approximately 70% of all congenital heart defects (CHDs) still have an unknown etiology. Alternative splicing of mRNA has been documented to play roles in normal and abnormal development. Dysregulated splicing of mRNA has been shown to cause heart defects in mice, however a link between mRNA splicing and CHDs has not yet been shown in humans. We reported that more than 50% of genes associated with heart development were alternatively spliced in the right ventricle (RV) of infants with tetralogy of Fallot (TOF) relative to the RV of normally developing infants. Moreover, there was a significant decrease in the level of 12 scaRNAs

D. C. Bittel (✉)
Ward Family Heart Center, Children's Mercy Hospital,
University of Missouri–Kansas City School of Medicine, Kansas City, MO, USA

Department of Pediatrics, Children's Mercy Hospital,
University of Missouri–Kansas City School of Medicine, Kansas City, MO, USA

The Kansas City University of Medicine and Bioscience, Kansas City, MO, USA
e-mail: dbittel@kcumb.edu

N. Kibiryeva · J. Marshall · J. E. O'Brien Jr
Ward Family Heart Center, Children's Mercy Hospital,
University of Missouri–Kansas City School of Medicine, Kansas City, MO, USA

N. Kenmochi · P. Patil · T. Uechi
Frontier Science Research Center, University of Miyazaki, Miyazaki, Japan

B. Rongish · M. Filla · R. Johnson
University of Kansas Medical Center, Kansas City, KS, USA

M. Artman
Department of Pediatrics, Children's Mercy Hospital,
University of Missouri–Kansas City School of Medicine, Kansas City, MO, USA

© The Editor(s) (if applicable) and The Author(s) 2020
T. Nakanishi et al. (eds.), *Molecular Mechanism of Congenital Heart Disease and Pulmonary Hypertension*, https://doi.org/10.1007/978-981-15-1185-1_53

339

(small cajal body associated RNAs) in the RV from infants with TOF. These small noncoding RNAs guide the biochemical modification of specific nucleotides in spliceosomal RNAs that are critical for spliceosomal function. We used primary cells derived from the RV of infants with TOF to show a direct link between scaRNA levels and alteration in mRNA splicing of several genes that regulate heart development. We modified the expression of sets of scaRNAs and consequentially documented distinctive mRNA splicing, accompanied by corresponding protein isoform changes suggesting a unique contribution by each scaRNA. Furthermore, we knocked down two homologous scaRNAs in zebrafish and saw a disruption of heart development with an accompanying alteration in splice isoforms of cardiac regulatory genes. These combined results provide compelling evidence that scaR-NAs contribute to the regulation of cardiac development by fine-tuning the fidelity of the spliceosome that adjusts exon retention as cell differentiation occurs. Importantly, our findings are consistent with the concept that disruption of mRNA splicing patterns during early embryonic development disturbs normal signaling pathways, resulting in conotruncal misalignment and TOF.

Keywords
Congenital heart defects · snoRNA · scaRNA · Alternative mRNA splicing · Spliceosome

53.1   Introduction

Congenital heart defects (CHDs) are the most common birth defects and represent a substantial health care burden even in countries with advanced health care systems [1]. Approximately 70% of all CHD cases are idiopathic and a significant effort has been made in the last 10 years to identify the genetic basis of CHDs. However, there remains a significant gap in our understanding of the genetic heritability of CHDs. Splicing in the vertebrate heart has been shown to be dynamic and carefully regulated [2–5]. However, no direct link between alternative splicing and CHDs has been established. In the developing embryo, precise spatial and temporal signaling is required between the first heart field from which the left ventricle is derived and the second heart field (SHF) from which the right ventricle and the conotruncal outflow tract are derived [3, 6–11]. The regulatory networks that control heart morphogenesis are mediated by multiple master regulatory genes (e.g. *NKX2.5*, *GATA4*, *MBNL1*) that control key pathways, including the WNT and NOTCH pathways, all of which have alternatively spliced messages.

Nearly all protein-coding genes in eukaryotic genomes contain introns (94% in humans) which must be removed to produce a mature messenger RNA [12]. Additionally, recent estimates of alternative splicing suggest as many as 90% of human genes have alternative transcript isoforms [13, 14]. There is growing appreciation for the role that alternative splicing plays in normal development and pathogenesis [2, 15–19]. The spliceosome facilitates pre-mRNA processing (splicing) of almost all primary transcripts in eukaryotic genomes. The primary spliceosome, termed the U2 spliceosome, is a multi-megadalton ribonucleoprotein complex composed of numerous proteins and five small nuclear RNAs (snRNAs or spliceosomal RNAs, U1, U2, U4, U5 and U6). The conformation and composition of the spliceosome are highly dynamic and conserved between yeast and humans [20]. Elaborate RNA–RNA–protein interactions align the reactive subgroups and repeatedly rearrange as each intron is identified, intron-exon boundaries are located, and catalysis proceeds to remove each intron in every pre-mRNA.

Some exons are constitutive, that is, they are present in every mature message; however, there are a surprising number of alternatively spliced transcripts that dramatically increase the complexity of the transcriptome and thus the proteome. The significance of alternative splicing for vertebrate evolution was highlighted by two companion papers in the December 21, 2012, issue of *Science* [21, 22]. Alternative splicing is temporally and spatially controlled resulting in unique splice variants in different tissues and at different time points in the same tissue. Recently, the transition from a fetal to postnatal pattern of a conserved set of alternatively spliced isoforms was shown to regulate mouse heart development [23]. Clearly, mRNA splicing plays a significant role in mammalian cardiac development, but the potential contribution to human heart pathology remains unknown.

Only about 2% of the human genome is translated into protein, but it is now evident that as much as 80% of the genome is transcribed [24]. The importance of noncoding RNA (ncRNA) for heart development has recently been shown by the requirement for correct spatiotemporal expression of specific microRNAs to ensure proper heart development [25]. In addition, there are clear spatial and temporal transcript splicing transitions that are conserved in the vertebrate heart during fetal and postnatal development [23, 26]. It is likely that there are multiple checkpoints to ensure proper transcriptome content for correct heart development. If these checkpoints fail, it is likely that cardiac development will also fail. It is possible that some of the checkpoints may be encoded in ncRNA families yet to be investigated.

A significant class of evolutionarily conserved ncRNA is the small nucleolar RNAs (snoRNAs) with homologs in all eukaryotes. The snoRNAs primarily guide biochemical modifications of specific nucleotides (e.g., methylation and pseudouridylation) of ribosomal RNAs and small nuclear RNAs (snRNAs, also referred to as spliceosomal RNAs). Those snoRNAs that target spliceosomal RNAs are associated with Cajal bodies in the nucleus and are known as scaRNAs (small Cajal-body-specific RNAs). In most vertebrate species, snoRNAs reside in the introns of other genes and require splicing to initiate snoRNA maturation [27]. Interestingly, intron-encoded snoRNAs may have special promoters to drive transcription, suggesting tissue specificity [28]. While the biochemical targets of snoRNAs have been clearly elucidated over the last 20 years, there is a surprising paucity of information regarding the developmental significance of this abundant class of ncRNA.

Our initial studies focused on analyzing the transcriptome of cardiac tissues discarded after surgical correction of tetralogy of Fallot (TOF), a congenital heart disease which is phenotypically representative of disruption of normal conotruncal development. Our preliminary data demonstrated that scaRNAs and their target spliceosomal RNAs are reduced in TOF myocardium [29]. It is therefore possible that reduced levels of scaRNAs may impact stability or fidelity of the spliceosome, causing alterations in mRNA maturation that contributes to TOF. The accumulation of moderate reductions in scaRNA level may cause alterations in spliceosomal function, thus contributing noise to the communication between the first and second heart fields, and resulting in conotruncal misalignment. We hypothesize that tissue-specific control of the pattern of scaRNA expression could provide temporal and spatial specificity to the spliceosome, thus providing a ubiquitous mechanism for regulating splicing in the developing embryo.

While the epigenetic role that scaRNAs play in maintaining spliceosomal integrity and precision is currently unexplored in terms of human health, we have collected substantial evidence that scaRNAs and splicing patterns are tissue-specific and indeed play a critical role in vertebrate cardiac development. We have examined the impact on spliceosome function made by dysregulated scaRNAs using human primary cells derived from the right ventricle of infants with TOF and from normally developing infant heart tissue. In addition, using the well-established zebrafish model, we characterized the nature of scaRNA interaction and its impact on vertebrate heart development. These experiments allowed us to confirm that these epigenetic elements affect vertebrate heart development, which represents a paradigm shift in our understanding of human heart development.

scaRNAs direct the posttranslational biochemical modification of spliceosomal RNAs. Without this modification the spliceosome will fail to function properly [30]. Recent studies show that without site-specific modification the RNA–RNA interactions of the spliceosomal RNAs, U2 and U6 do not achieve the correct conformation [31]. We previously identified 12 scaRNAs that were moderately but significantly reduced in TOF myocardium [29], similar to fetal levels of expression of the scaRNAs (Fig. 53.1). Interestingly, the majority of these scaRNAs target nucleotides that

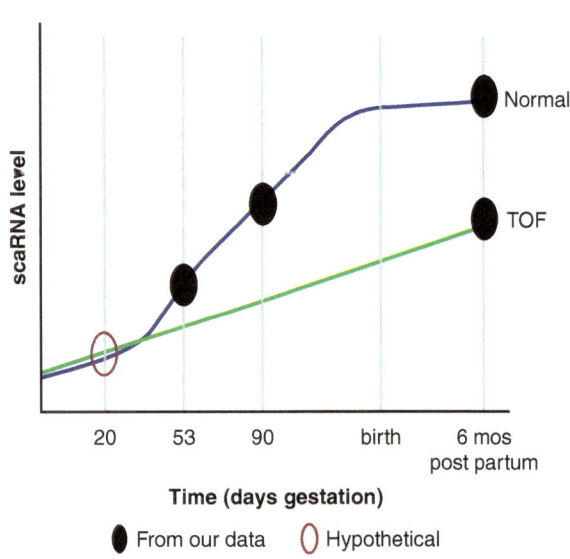

Fig. 53.1 ScaRNAs have reduced expression in fetal and TOF myocardium compared to normal myocardium

are important for conformational integrity of the U2–U6 complex [31]. Reduced levels of scaRNAs in TOF myocardium suggest a failure of adequate regulation of the scaRNA level early in gestation resulting in inadequate spliceosomal function. In the proposed investigation, we will carefully characterize the synergy between scaRNAs and assess the impact on spliceosome function (i.e., splicing) and vertebrate heart development. It is our contention that scaRNA function may serve as a checkpoint in transcriptional processing, regulating many aspects of development, including heart formation.

53.2 Subjects

Our subjects were children less than 1 year of age with CHDs: TOF; tranposition of the great arteries (TGA); or pulmonary atresia with intact ventricular septum (PA/IVS) requiring surgical reconstruction. Informed consent was obtained from a parent or legal guardian after reviewing the consent document and having their questions answered (IRB #11120627). Our original observations were based on analysis of tissue from 16 infants with idiopathic TOF (nonsyndromic, without 22q11.2 deletions, 11 males, 5 females), comparison tissues from eight normally developing infants (3 males, 5 females). In addition, we have now characterized scaRNA, spliceosomal RNAs and the splicing pattern of 6 key transcription factors from an additional 21 infants with idiopathic TOF. Our acquisition and characterization of control human infant heart tissues and human fetal heart tissue have been previously described [29, 32]. The fetal hearts were dissected by Dr. James O'Brien, a pediatric cardiac surgeon and co-investigator, who performed the reconstruction of the conotruncal defects to ensure the tissue analyzed was from a similar location as the tissues removed during surgery.

53.3 Results and Discussion

53.3.1 scaRNAs Target U2 and U6 snRNAs and Both snRNAs Are Significantly Reduced in TOF

We used the scaRNABase database (http://www-scarna.biotoul.fr/index.php) to identify the nucleotides targeted for modification by the 12 scaRNAs that are reduced in TOF. Only two snRNAs were predicted to be targeted: U2 and U6 snRNAs. Six of the scaRNAs targeted 10 nucleotides (of 23 nucleotides that are known to be modified by scaRNAs) in U2 and 6 scaRNAs targeted 5 nucleotides (of 8 total modified nucleotides) in U6. Interestingly, U2 and U6 had significantly reduced expression in our 16 TOF samples compared to the 8 controls (U2 was reduced 1.8-fold in TOF RV, $p = 0.04$, and U6 was reduced 3.2-fold in TOF RV $p < 0.0001$). This is consistent with reduced stability of U2 and U6 as a consequence of inefficient scaRNA biochemical modification.

53.3.2 Cardiac Regulatory Networks Are Enriched for Alternative Splice Isoforms in TOF

Coordinated control of alternative splicing modifies the transcriptome and hence the proteome, while participating in most developmental processes [33, 34]. Studies of animal models have shown the importance of appropriate splicing for proper heart development [3, 5, 23, 35]. Still, knowledge of the sequence of events leading to tissue-specific alternative splicing is limited. More importantly with respect to the current proposal, nothing is known about the significance of scaRNA-guided nucleotide modification in spliceosomal RNAs and the potential impact on transcript splicing. Intriguingly, our analyses of splicing variants in TOF myocardium revealed a substantial increase of alternative transcript isoforms which were enriched in gene networks known to be critical for regulating heart development, including the WNT and NOTCH pathways. More importantly, ~50% of these alternative isoforms are present in normal fetal RV, suggesting regulation of splicing did not proceed properly during heart development in the infants with TOF (Alternative splicing of mRNA is dynamic in human fetal heart development, in prep). Figure 53.2 shows representative examples of alternative splicing, *DICER* and *DAAM1*, which have a similar pattern of splicing in fetal and TOF tissues (blue and green lines) compared to the control tissue (red line). *Dicer* was shown to be important in mouse heart development playing a role in splicing regulation [3], and splice variants of *Daam1*, a member of the WNT pathway, were recently shown to impact angiogenesis and endothelial cell migration and tube formation [36].

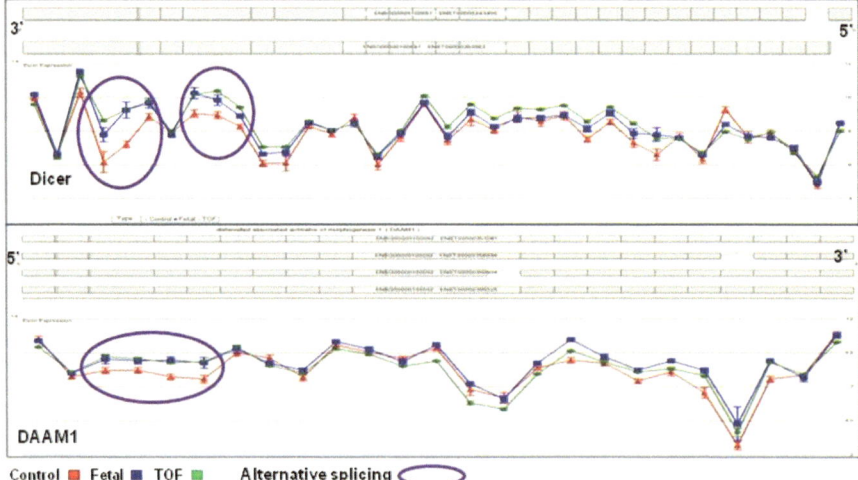

Fig. 53.2 Alternative splicing (e.g., DICER and DAAM1) is similar in TOF and fetal myocardium

53.3.3 Reduced scaRNA Expression and Alternative Splicing Are Not a Consequence of Hypertrophy

Hypertrophy is known to reactivate the expression of some fetal genes. Thus we wanted to determine if the fetal expression patterns we observed could be a consequence of hypertrophy. As a comparison to TOF, we analyzed right ventricular samples from infants with TGA and PA/IVS. The embryological origins of TOF and TGA likely share some common features involving miscommunication between the first and second heart fields. However, PA/IVS is distinct and probably less complex in terms of origin of the regulatory defect. Nevertheless, TOF, TGA and PA/IVS share a common attribute: right ventricular hypertrophy. We observed only ten snoRNAs with differential expression in PA/IVS right ventricular tissue compared to control tissue. The ten snoRNAs that were reduced in PA/IVS were in common with TOF, and all target the 28S rRNA. In addition, U2 and U6 levels were not reduced in PA/IVS relative to the control tissue, and splice isoforms were essentially unchanged relative to the controls. On the other hand, RV from children with TGA bore a striking resemblance to the TOF pattern of scaRNA, spliceosomal RNA expression and fetal type splice isoforms. Therefore, the fetal type pattern of scaRNA and spliceosomal RNA expression, as well as fetal splice isoforms, does not appear to be simply a consequence of hypertrophy since they were not present in PA/IVS RV samples. These findings support our postulation that scaRNAs are of key importance in regulating heart development and not simply a consequence of hypertrophy.

53.3.4 Primary Cell Lines Derived from TOF Myocardium Retain the Same Relative Expression Patterns as the Tissue

We have derived primary cell lines from right ventricular myocardium obtained from 15 infants with TOF (TOF primary cells—TOFpc). These cells are most likely fibroblasts. The cell type is somewhat inconsequential since what we wish to examine is spliceosome response to changing levels of scaRNAs. We compared scaRNA levels, U2 and U6 levels, and splice isoform patterns between TOFpcs and primary myocytes derived from normally developing infant heart tissue. TOFpcs retained the same fetal type pattern of scaRNA, spliceosomal RNA expression and splicing isoforms of index genes relative to cells derived from normally developing neonatal cardiac tissue (data not shown). Splicing patterns also retained a TOF pattern in the TOFpcs relative to the normal cells. These changes were consistent through at least four passages of the cell lines.

53.3.5 Overexpression of ACA26 and SCARNA1 (ACA35) in TOF Primary Cells Was Associated with an Increase in U2 Levels and a Decrease in Fetal Splice Isoforms

The scaRNAs were cloned into an intron sequence between hemoglobin exons 3 and 4 so that they would be correctly processed in vivo and expression was

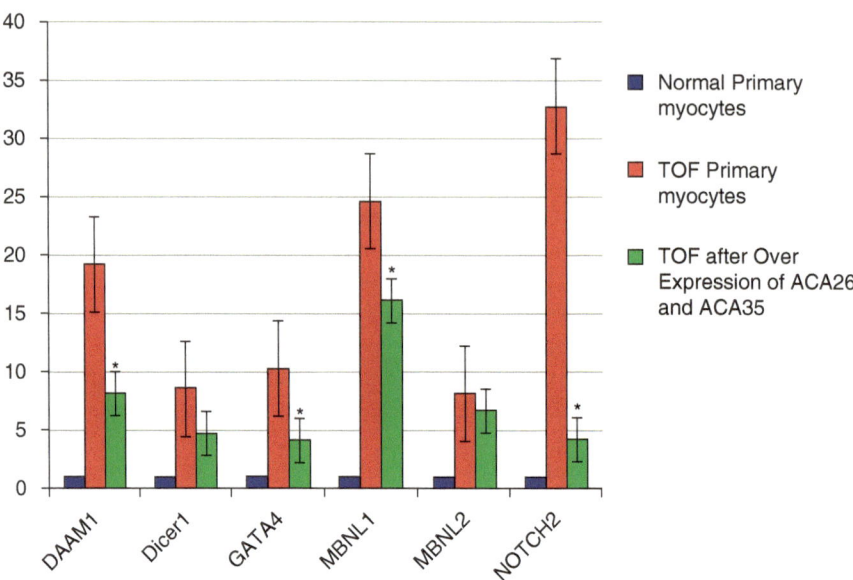

Fig. 53.3 Levels of fetal splice isoforms are reduced after overexpression of scaRNAs. Data are fold change, averaged from three different TOF primary cell lines (genotypes). *Significantly different from levels in sham transfected TOF primary cells

driven with the CMV promoter [37]. When either plasmid was transfected alone, there was an increase in the scaRNA but no change in U2 level or in splicing (data not shown). However, when we simultaneously transfected plasmids pCGL-ACA26 and pCGL-SCARNA1 into TOF primary myocytes, there was modest (~50%) but significant upregulation in U2 level. This is consistent with the idea that the scaRNA-directed modification of snRNAs is necessary for snRNA stability. More importantly, there was a reduction in the level of the fetal type splice form (Fig. 53.3). These data were repeated in TOFpcs from three different infants (genotypes). This is an exciting discovery which squarely supports our hypothesis that the scaRNAs are playing a role in spliceosomal function. These novel new findings support the critical role that scaRNAs play in mammalian heart development. This connection has not been investigated previously.

53.3.6 Knockdown of scaRNAs (scaRNA1 Targeting U2, or snord94 Targeting U6) Causes Heart Defects in Zebrafish

Studies of snoRNA-directed modification of ncRNA in archaea and lower eukaryotes have shown that nucleotide modifications are crucial for ncRNA functions [38, 39]. However, similar studies in vertebrates have not been described until the recent report of the developmental significance of snoRNAs in zebrafish by Kenmochi and colleagues [40]. In summary, they suppressed the expression of several snoRNAs, including U26, in zebrafish (U26 was one of the snoRNAs that we identified as being down regulated in myocardium from infants with TOF). Using a unique highly sensitive mass spec analysis that they developed, they found that decreased U26 snoRNA expression reduced the snoRNA-guided methylation of the target nucleotides. Impaired rRNA modification, even at a single site, led to severe morphological defects and embryonic lethality in zebrafish. Thus, nucleotide modifications in rRNA play an essential role in vertebrate development. Additionally, as a preliminary study this past summer, in collaboration with Kenmochi and colleagues we have suppressed the expression of two scaRNAs, scarna1 and snord94 (both are homologous to scaRNAs identified by our screens of TOF myocardium) in zebrafish embryos. The knockdown of the scaRNAs resulted in developmental abnormalities, including heart malformations (Fig. 53.4) and altered splicing of genes that regulate heart development. This is an exciting finding and taken together with our observations that scaRNA levels impact splicing in TOF primary cardiomyocytes, suggesting that scaRNAs play a critical and, as yet, unrecognized role in vertebrate heart development. Furthermore, it appears that these particular scaRNAs primarily affect heart developmental processes. Collectively, these data provide firm support of our overarching hypothesis.

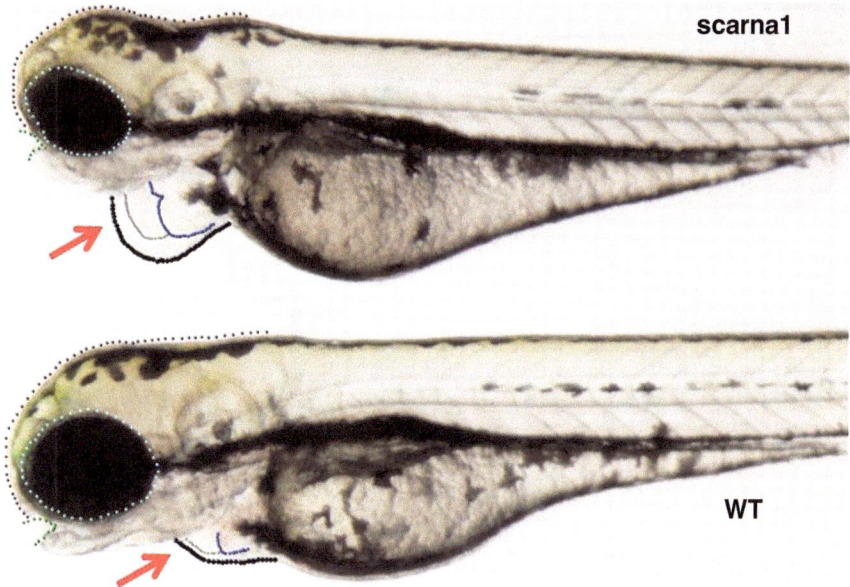

Fig. 53.4 Representative example of zebrafish morphant at 72 hpf (hours post fertilization, knockdown targeted at scarna1). Arrows indicate the heart, blue and grey outlines indicate enlargement of both the atria and ventricle, respectively. Eye and head size are slightly changed but other organs, brain, notochord, otic vesicles, and fins appear essentially normal at this stage

53.3.7 Splice Isoforms Change During Development in Zebrafish and After Targeted Knockdown of scaRNAs

We downloaded RNA-Seq data from the Gene Expression Omnibus derived from developing zebrafish at 0.75 h, 6 h, 1 day, 2 days, 3 days and 5 days postfertilization (GEO#: GSE30603) and analyzed for alternative splicing. We found clear changes in ratios of splice isoforms of a large proportion of genes, including genes important for heart development (e.g., *Gata4, Mbnl1, Notch1, Dicer*, data not shown). We performed RNA-Seq on RNA extracted from 24hpf zebrafish embryos treated with antisense morpholinos directed at scaRNA1 or snord94 and WT untreated embryos and embryos treated with mismatch morpholinos. Paired-end sequencing runs were performed with 101 base reads on the Illumina HiSeq 1500. RNA-Seq data were analyzed using the "Tuxedo suite." There were no appreciable differences between mismatch morpholino and WT-type embryos. snord94 was reduced by 40%, and scaRNA1 was not detectable in their respective knockdown morphants compared to WT or mismatch treated embryos. We saw a clear shift in the predominant isoforms of our index genes after treatment with the antisense morpholino (Fig. 53.5 shows results of validation of the WNT pathway gene splicing variants in zebrafish morphants). These analyses clearly demonstrate that, as in mammals, splicing in developing zebrafish is dynamic.

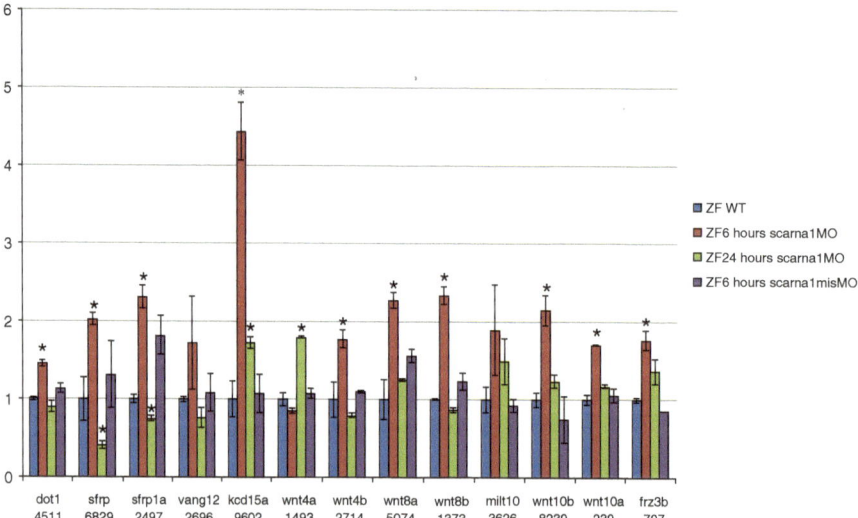

Fig. 53.5 Splicing of WNT pathway genes is altered in zebrafish morphants. Treating zebrafish embryos with anti-scarna1 morpholino causes changes in exon retention of cardiac regulatory genes. Eleven of 39 members of the WNT family have changes in exon retention after treatment with antisense morpholino (assessed by RNA-Seq and qRT-PCR; values shown are from qRT-PCR data). The mismatch morpholino has no significant effect on splicing

Furthermore, the knockdown experiments strongly support our hypothesis that scaR-NAs are important for regulating splice variants and heart development. Furthermore, snord94 and scaRNA1 appear to be important for heart development.

53.4 Conclusions

We examined the noncoding transcriptome in myocardial tissue from children with tetralogy of Fallot (TOF) and observed changes in mRNA splice isoforms of genes that are critical for regulating heart development [29]. In parallel, we found a modest but significant reduction in the levels of 12 small Cajal body-specific RNAs (scaRNAs are a subset of snoRNAs and direct the biochemical processing of spliceosomal RNA) [29]. These patterns of scaRNA expression and splicing are similar to patterns we saw in the fetal myocardium. To explore the potential relevance of these findings, we manipulated the expression of two of these scaRNAs in cell cultures and zebrafish. We saw clear changes in splicing patterns and, importantly, developmental deficiencies including heart defects in zebrafish. Our findings support a direct role for scaRNAs in fine tuning the fidelity of the spliceosome in a manner that is critical to support splicing transitions that are essential for correct heart development. Our observations open the door on a new paradigm in developmental regulation and potentially may explain a substantial portion of the missing genetic heritability of CHDs. Importantly, by accurately characterizing the role of scaRNAs in disrupting genetic signaling, it is possible that this could lead to the identification of "targets" that may be amenable to change through intervention as is the case with microRNAs.

References

1. American Heart Association: https://www.heart.org/en/health-topics/congenital-heart-defects (2011).
2. Kalsotra A, Cooper TA. Functional consequences of developmentally regulated alternative splicing. Nat Rev Genet. 2011;12:715–29.
3. Kalsotra A, Wang K, Li PF, Cooper TA. MicroRNAs coordinate an alternative splicing network during mouse postnatal heart development. Genes Dev. 2010;24:653–8.
4. Bland CS, et al. Global regulation of alternative splicing during myogenic differentiation. Nucleic Acids Res. 2010;38:7651.
5. Salomonis N, et al. Alternative splicing in the differentiation of human embryonic stem cells into cardiac precursors. PLoS Comput Biol. 2009;5:e1000553.
6. Bentham J, Bhattacharya S. Genetic mechanisms controlling cardiovascular development. Ann N Y Acad Sci. 2008;1123:10–9.
7. Bruneau BG. The developmental genetics of congenital heart disease. Nature. 2008;451:943–8.
8. Buckingham M, Meilhac S, Zaffran S. Building the mammalian heart from two sources of myocardial cells. Nat Rev Genet. 2005;6:826–35.
9. Huang JB, et al. Molecular mechanisms of congenital heart disease. Cardiovasc Pathol. 2009;19:e183–93.
10. Thum T, Catalucci D, Bauersachs J. MicroRNAs: novel regulators in cardiac development and disease. Cardiovasc Res. 2008;79:562–70.

11. Wessels MW, Willems PJ. Genetic factors in non-syndromic congenital heart malformations. Clin Genet. 2010;78:103–23.
12. Ward AJ, Cooper TA. The pathobiology of splicing. J Pathol. 2010;220:152–63.
13. Wang ET, et al. Alternative isoform regulation in human tissue transcriptomes. Nature. 2008;456:470.
14. Pan Q, Shai O, Lee LJ, Frey BJ, Blencowe BJ. Deep surveying of alternative splicing complexity in the human transcriptome by high-throughput sequencing. Nat Genet. 2008;40:1413–5.
15. Singh RK, Cooper TA. Pre-mRNA splicing in disease and therapeutics. Trends Mol Med. 2012;18:472.
16. Kaida D, Schneider-Poetsch T, Yoshida M. Splicing in oncogenesis and tumor suppression. Cancer Sci. 2012;103:1611–6.
17. Tanackovic G, et al. PRPF mutations are associated with generalized defects in spliceosome formation and pre-mRNA splicing in patients with retinitis pigmentosa. Hum Mol Genet. 2011;20:2116–30.
18. Mannoor K, Liao J, Jiang F. Small nucleolar RNAs in cancer. Biochim Biophys Acta. 2012;1826:121–8.
19. Williams GT, Farzaneh F. Are snoRNAs and snoRNA host genes new players in cancer? Nat Rev Cancer. 2012;12:84–8.
20. Will CL, Luhrmann R. Spliceosome structure and function. Cold Spring Harb Perspect Biol. 2011;3 https://doi.org/10.1101/cshperspect.a003707.
21. Merkin J, Russell C, Chen P, Burge CB. Evolutionary dynamics of gene and isoform regulation in Mammalian tissues. Science. 2012;338:1593–9.
22. Barbosa-Morais NL, et al. The evolutionary landscape of alternative splicing in vertebrate species. Science. 2012;338:1587–93.
23. Kalsotra A, et al. A postnatal switch of CELF and MBNL proteins reprograms alternative splicing in the developing heart. Proc Natl Acad Sci U S A. 2008;105:20333–8.
24. Cheng J, et al. Transcriptional maps of 10 human chromosomes at 5-nucleotide resolution. Science. 2005;308:1149–54.
25. Liu N, Olson EN. MicroRNA regulatory networks in cardiovascular development. Dev Cell. 2010;18:510–25.
26. Castle JC, et al. Expression of 24,426 human alternative splicing events and predicted cis regulation in 48 tissues and cell lines. Nat Genet. 2008;40:1416–25.
27. Kiss T, Filipowicz W. Exonucleolytic processing of small nucleolar RNAs from pre-mRNA introns. Genes Dev. 1995;9:1411–24.
28. Deng W, et al. Organization of the Caenorhabditis elegans small non-coding transcriptome: genomic features, biogenesis, and expression. Genome Res. 2006;16:20–9.
29. O'Brien JE Jr, et al. Noncoding RNA expression in myocardium from infants with tetralogy of Fallot. Circ Cardiovasc Genet. 2012;5:279–86.
30. Karijolich J, Yu YT. Spliceosomal snRNA modifications and their function. RNA Biol. 2010;7:192–204.
31. Karunatilaka KS, Rueda D. Post-transcriptional modifications modulate conformational dynamics in human U2-U6 snRNA complex. RNA. 2013;20:16–23.
32. Bittel DC, et al. Gene expression in cardiac tissues from infants with idiopathic conotruncal defects. BMC Med Genomics. 2011;4:1.
33. Johnson JM, et al. Genome-wide survey of human alternative pre-mRNA splicing with exon junction microarrays. Science. 2003;302:2141–4.
34. Wang GS, Cooper TA. Splicing in disease: disruption of the splicing code and the decoding machinery. Nat Rev Genet. 2007;8:749–61.
35. Stennard FA, et al. Cardiac T-box factor Tbx20 directly interacts with Nkx2-5, GATA4, and GATA5 in regulation of gene expression in the developing heart. Dev Biol. 2003;262:206–24.
36. Ju R, et al. Activation of the planar cell polarity formin DAAM1 leads to inhibition of endothelial cell proliferation, migration, and angiogenesis. Proc Natl Acad Sci U S A. 2010;107:6906–11.
37. Darzacq X, et al. Cajal body-specific small nuclear RNAs: a novel class of 2'-O-methylation and pseudouridylation guide RNAs. EMBO J. 2002;21:2746–56.

38. Matera AG, Terns RM, Terns MP. Non-coding RNAs: lessons from the small nuclear and small nucleolar RNAs. Nat Rev Mol Cell Biol. 2007;8:209–20.
39. Liang B, et al. Structure of a functional ribonucleoprotein pseudouridine synthase bound to a substrate RNA. Nat Struct Mol Biol. 2009;16:740–6.
40. Higa-Nakamine S, et al. Loss of ribosomal RNA modification causes developmental defects in zebrafish. Nucleic Acids Res. 2012;40:391–8.

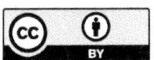

Progress in the Generation of Multiple Lineage Human-iPSC-Derived 3D-Engineered Cardiac Tissues for Cardiac Repair

54

Fei Ye, Shuji Setozaki, William J. Kowalski, Marc Dwenger, Fangping Yuan, Joseph P. Tinney, Takeichiro Nakane, Hidetoshi Masumoto, and Bradley B. Keller

Abstract

Despite improvements over the past 30 years, 10-year pediatric heart transplantation survival rates remain low and mechanical support is both expensive and relatively unavailable. In contrast to isolated cell therapies,

F. Ye · W. J. Kowalski · M. Dwenger · F. Yuan · J. P. Tinney · B. B. Keller (✉)
Kosair Charities Pediatric Heart Research Program and Department of Pediatrics,
University of Louisville, Louisville, KY, USA
e-mail: brad.keller@louisville.edu

S. Setozaki
Kosair Charities Pediatric Heart Research Program and Department of Pediatrics,
University of Louisville, Louisville, KY, USA

Department of CV Surgery, Okamura Memorial Hospital, Shizuoka, Japan

T. Nakane
Kosair Charities Pediatric Heart Research Program and Department of Pediatrics,
University of Louisville, Louisville, KY, USA

Department of Cell Growth and Differentiation, Center for iPS Cell Research
and Application, Kyoto University, Kyoto, Japan

Department of CV Surgery, Kyoto University Graduate School of Medicine, Kyoto, Japan

H. Masumoto
Kosair Charities Pediatric Heart Research Program and Department of Pediatrics,
University of Louisville, Louisville, KY, USA·

Department of Cell Growth and Differentiation, Center for iPS Cell Research
and Application, Kyoto University, Kyoto, Japan

Department of CV Surgery, Kyoto University Graduate School of Medicine, Kyoto, Japan

Clinical Translational Research Program, RIKEN Center for Biosystems Dynamics Research,
Kobe, Japan

353

T. Nakanishi et al. (eds.), *Molecular Mechanism of Congenital Heart Disease
and Pulmonary Hypertension*, https://doi.org/10.1007/978-981-15-1185-1_54

implantable engineered cardiac tissues (ECTs) recover myocardial mass and function, creating the opportunity for cardiac recovery rather than replacement. Our ECT research has progressed from using embryonic avian and rodent cell compositions to human induced pluripotent stem cell (h-iPSC)-derived, multiple cell lineage formulations with the goal of clinical translation. We generate ECTs from h-iPSC-derived cardiomyocytes (CM), endothelial cells (EC), and vascular mural cells (MC) in both linear (15 × 1 mm) and large format (LF, 20 × 20 mm) geometries using rodent-derived and human-compatible reagents. H-iPSC ECTs undergo rapid gel compaction and begin intrinsic beating by day 3. CM fraction at ECT formation is approximately 60%. The ECT maximum capture rates increased during in vitro culture up to 28 days and in response to optogenetic pacing (OP) using AAV-ChIEF from day 7 to 14. ECT relaxation times decreased, force-frequency relations became more neutral, and beat-to-beat hysteresis decreased with prolonged culture or OP. H-iPSC-derived ECTs generated using human collagen I and human compatible MaxGel have comparable structural and functional features to rodent-derived ECTs. Linear and LF-ECTs implanted onto xenotolerant infarcted rat hearts survived, engrafted, improved ejection fraction, normalized regional echo strain, and reduced scar area at 4 weeks. Thus, these h-iPSC ECT compositions show promise as a strategy for pediatric myocardial recovery.

Keywords

Cardiomyocytes · Cardiac repair and regeneration · Engineered cardiac tissues · Induced pluripotent stem cells

54.1   Introduction

Despite dramatic progress in the surgical management and survival of infants with complex congenital heart defects, myocardial injury following cardiac surgery and progressive cardiac dysfunction results in significant morbidity and mortality. There are currently many cardiac "cellular therapies" undergoing pre-clinical and clinical trials in adults. There have been small, encouraging clinical trials using stem cells in infants with hypoplastic left heart syndrome in Japan [1–3] that have led to similar trials in the United States [4–6]. It is clear that injected or implanted cells do not survive and that functional improvement occurs via paracrine mechanisms that impact angiogenesis and/or remodeling. Rapid advances in tissue engineering over the past two decades have resulted in the generation of functional, multicellular, 3D cardiac tissues with the potential for translation to human cardiac repair and regeneration [7–14]. This chapter provides a concise overview of some of the key issues in the generation, maturation, and translation of these engineered cardiac tissues (ECTs) and related work in our laboratory.

54.2 Continued Expansion of Engineered Cardiac Tissues (ECTs)

Following the initial description of 3D-reconstituted heart tissue using embryonic chick CM [7], CM species used to generate ECTs include chicken, mouse, and rat embryonic and post-natal CM, and a range of embryonic stem cells and induced pluripotent stem cells from rodents and human cell lines [8–16]. While initial formulations used a combination of cells, matrix factors, and collagen, additional compositions have utilized fibrin rather than collagen to reduce the effect of matrix stimulated inflammation [17] and tunable matrix compositions [18]. ECTs became increasingly popular as in vitro platforms for drug toxicology models [19] as well as for in vitro models for cardiac genetic disease modeling and repair [20].

54.3 Human Induced Pluripotent Stem Cell (H-iPSC) Linear ECTs

While cells from multiple vertebrate species have been used to investigate ECT structural and functional maturation and to model cardiomyopathies, it is clear that human cells are required for clinical trials and future therapies. H-iPSCs can be differentiated to cardiac lineages and produced in the quantities required for pre-clinical and future clinical trials. Multiple studies have validated the ability of h-iPSC-derived CM to mature and form implantable cell sheets [21]. To advance this paradigm, we developed and validated methods to generate linear (15 mm length × 1 mm diameter) ECTs from human iPSCs-derived CV lineages (h-iPSC-ECTs) [11]. We found that the coexistence of EC and MC vascular lineages with CMs within the 3D ECT compositions promoted tissue maturation (Fig. 54.1). Furthermore, we demonstrated the therapeutic potential of h-iPSC ECTs in an immune-tolerant rat myocardial infarction (MI) model showing the improvement of cardiac function with regenerated myocardium and enhanced angiogenesis [11].

54.4 Generation and Characterization of Large Format H-iPSC ECTs

Larger-format ECTs have been described using pre-vascularization, stacking cell sheets, scalable scaffolds, and bioprinting [12, 22]. Building on our success with linear h-iPSC ECTs and guided by initial works from the Bursac lab using polydimethylsiloxane (PDMS) molds, we fabricated a range of mold geometries from 0.5 mm thick PDMS sheets to generate a novel large-format hiPSC-ECT (LF-ECT, Fig. 54.2). As with our linear h-iPSC ECTs, these h-iPSC LF-ECTs undergo gel compaction, spontaneously and then synchronously beat, develop CM alignment along the internal bundle long axis, and survive in vivo implantation to recover myocardial function in an immune-tolerant rodent MI model [12]. Though unpublished, we have scaled this LF-ECT geometry to 30 × 30 mm, suitable for large animal pre-clinical studies.

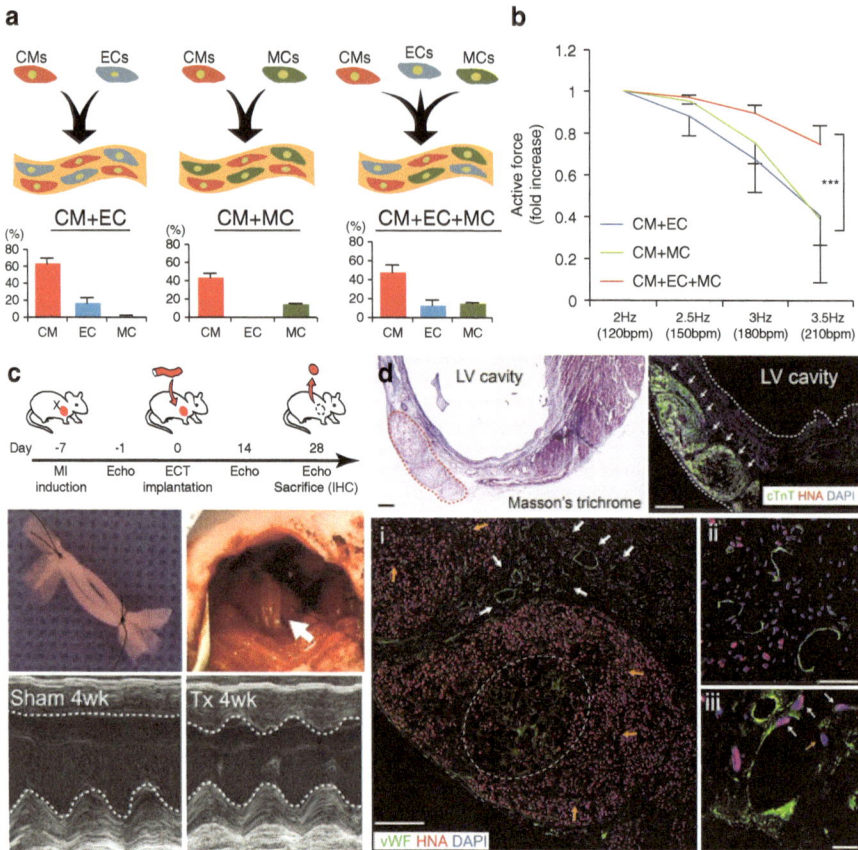

Fig. 54.1 H-iPSC linear ECTs generate functional cardiac tissues that recover cardiac structure and function following injury. (**A**) Schematic diagrams for three ECT compositions (upper) containing cardiomyocytes (CM), endothelial cells (EC), and/or mural cells (MC) and the proportions of each cell type used to generate ECTs (lower). (**B**) CM + EC + MC composition best preserved active force at increasing pacing rates. (**C**) Schematic timeline of rat MI surgery and ECT implantation (upper panel), three hiPSC-ECTs bundled for implantation (middle panel), and representative M-mode images for sham-operated (left) and ECT-implanted (right) rats 4 weeks after surgery (lower panel). (**D**) (a–c) Left ventricular (LV) histology 4 weeks after implantation of h-iPSC ECTs with Masson's trichrome staining (upper left panel, 500 μm scale bar), double immunostaining for cTnT and HNA (human cell marker) with arrows indicating engrafted myocardium (upper right panel, 500 μm scale bar): (i) lower magnification with white arrows indicating capillary formation around grafted tissue; orange arrows indicate penetrating vasculature and white dotted line indicates vasculature within the ECT graft (200 μm) with higher magnification in (ii) 50 μm scale bar and (iii) 20 μm scale bar. (Adapted from [11])

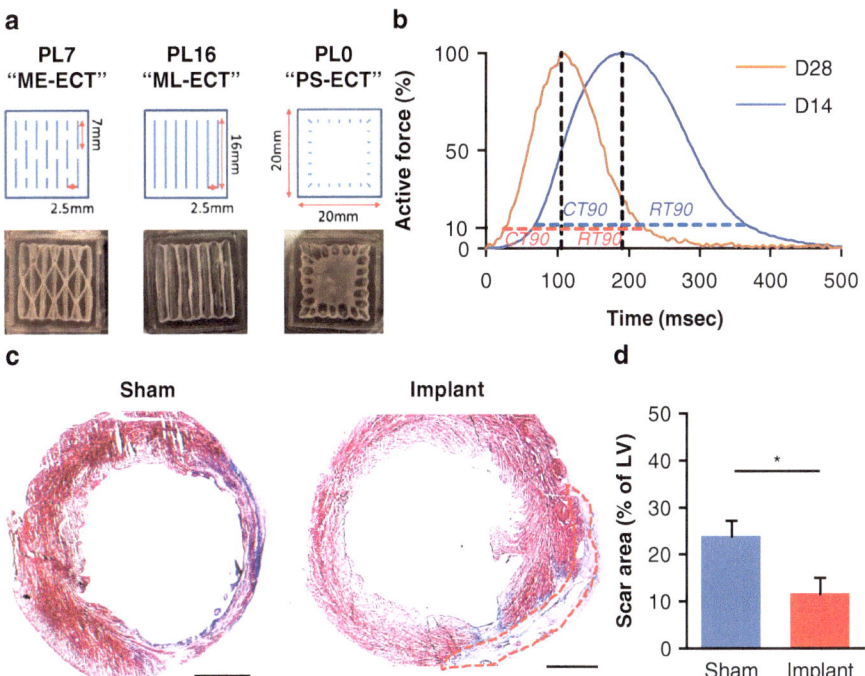

Fig. 54.2 H-iPSC large format LF-ECTs generate functional cardiac tissues that can recover cardiac structure and function following injury. (**a**) Schematic diagrams for three ECT compositions of LF-ECTs: ME-ECT with 7 mm posts in a pattern to generate a mesh, ML-ECT with 16 mm posts to generate multiple linear bundles, and PS-ECT to generate a central cell sheet (upper) and representative images after 14 days in vitro. (**b**) Prolonging in vitro culture from 14 days (blue) to 28 days (red) increased the rate of force generation and relaxation. Dashed lines highlight 90% contraction time (CT) and relaxation time (RT). (**c**) Representative Masson's trichrome staining of SHAM and ME-ECT h-iPSC LF-ECT IMPLANT rat hearts 4 weeks post-implant. Red dotted line indicates engrafted area. Scale bar: 2 mm. (**d**) ME-ECT implantation reduced scar area (% of LV). (Adapted from [12])

54.5   Optogenetic Pacing of H-iPSC ECTs

One of the barriers to h-iPSC-derived ECT clinical translation is the relative electrophysiologic and contractile immaturity of h-iPSC-derived CMs. Strategies to mature CM within tissue-engineered structures include cyclic mechanical loading and electric field stimulation. As a novel approach, we designed proof-of-principle experiments to transfect h-iPSC-derived ECTs with a desensitization-resistant, chimeric channel rhodopsin, ChR (ChIEF) protein and then optically pace (OP) ECTs to accelerate maturation. We transfected h-iPSC ECTs using an AAV-packaged ChIEF and then verified OP by whole-cell patch clamp. ECTs were then chronically OP (C-OP) above their intrinsic beat rates in vitro from day 7 to 14. C-OP resulted in improved ECT electrophysiological properties and subtle changes in the expression

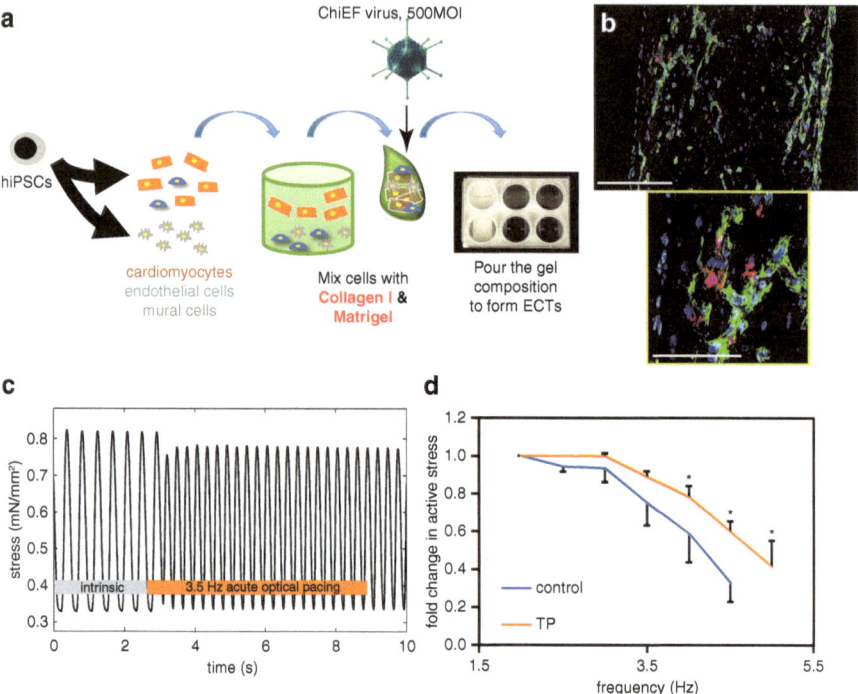

Fig. 54.3 Optogenetic pacing (OP) of h-iPSC linear ECTs results in functional maturation. (**a**) Schematic for the generation of h-iPSC linear ECTs with CHiEF virus. (**b**) D14 chronic C-OP ECT showing 52% CM and 13% ChIEF-transfected cells. Nuclei (DAPI-blue), CM (cTnT-green), ChIEF-transfected cells with tdTomato (red). CM were predominantly located at the outer surface and the majority of transfected cells were CM. Inset in (**b**) shows higher magnification of double-positive cTnT and tdTomato cells. (**c**) Force measurement during intrinsic beating and during OP via 470 nm LED at 3.5 Hz. (**d**) Stress-frequency curves showed a less negative relationship after chronic (C-OP) or prolonged culture to D28 (unpublished data)

of some cardiac relevant genes though active force generation and histology were unchanged (Fig. 54.3). These results validate the feasibility of a novel C-OP paradigm for non-invasive and scalable OP-induced ECT maturation strategies.

54.6 Incorporating Human Compatible Biomaterials into H-iPSC ECTs

An additional barrier to the clinical translation of h-iPSC-derived ECTs is the qualification of all reagents for human use as required by the FDA. Therefore, we revised our h-iPSC ECT formulation to replace rodent-derived Matrigel with human-derived and clinically acceptable MaxGel and replaced rodent type with human type I collagen. These experiments required multiple variations in composition but ultimately resulted in a human compatible h-iPSC-derived linear ECT with structural

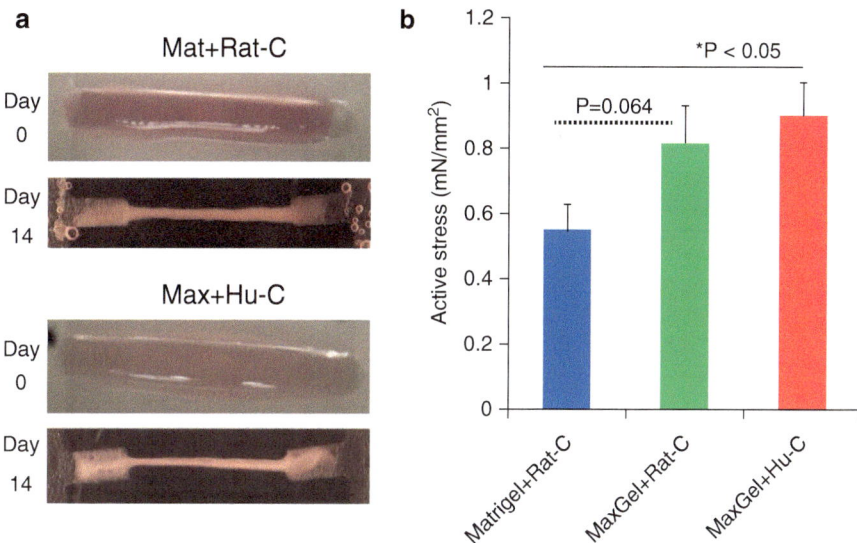

Fig. 54.4 Comparison of rodent-derived and human component-derived h-iPSC linear ECTs. (**a**) Representative images of rodent-derived (Matrigel and rat collagen I) and human compatible component (MaxGel and human collagen I) h-iPSC linear ECTs immediately after pouring on day 0 and after 14 days of in vitro culture. (**b**) Comparison of active stress on day 14 between 3 ECT compositions: Matrigel and rat collagen I, MaxGel and rat collagen I, and MaxGel and human collagen I. Active stress was greatest in human component ECTs (unpublished data)

and functional features equivalent or better than ECTs formulated with rodent-derived matrix reagents (Fig. 54.4). While higher cost, these experiments provide additional insights for the formulations required for h-iPSC translation to humans.

54.7   Future Directions and Clinical Implications

Clearly, biological repair and replacement of lost myocardium using h-iPSCs that can form myocardium (versus skeletal muscle) are feasible, and clinical trials to determine safety and feasibility in adult heart failure patients should occur in the near future. It is important to note that many adult stem cell trials have shown statistically and clinically significant improvements in heart failure patients, and studies using stem cells have shown encouraging results for children with congenital heart disease [1–4]. The use of isolated cells, or the exosomes extracted from cells, may represent a much simpler therapeutic product to manufacture, verify, and distribute for future clinical therapy compared to the complexities of generating engineered tissues (multi-layer cell sheets and ECTs). Translation of these more complex formulations will require the engagement of biotechnology and biopharma companies with expertise in semi-automated manufacturing techniques and complex biologic quality controls not available in academic environments. Fortunately, every innovation in CV care for infants and children has been shown to also be valuable for the treatment of the much larger adult market. Therefore, the opportunities to translate h-iPSC ECTs towards infants and children with significant myocardial injury and heart failure remain encouraging.

Acknowledgments This research was funded by the Kosair Charities Pediatric Heart Research Endowment Fund. All h-iPSCs used for this research were provided under a materials transfer agreement between the University of Louisville Research Foundation and the Center for iPS Cell Research and Application, Kyoto University. The authors acknowledge the collaborative support of Dr. Jun K. Yamashita, Principal Investigator, Department of Cell Growth and Differentiation, Center for iPS Cell Research and Application, Kyoto University.

References

1. Tsilimigras DI, Oikonomou EK, Moris D, et al. Stem cell therapy for congenital heart disease: a systematic review. Circulation. 2017;136(24):2373–85.
2. Sano T, Ousaka D, Goto T, et al. Impact of cardiac progenitor cells on heart failure and survival in single ventricle congenital heart disease. Circ Res. 2018;122:994. https://doi.org/10.1161/CIRCRESAHA.117.312311.
3. ClinicalTrials.gov. NCT01829750: Cardiac Progenitor Cell Infusion to Treat Univentricular Heart Disease (PERSEUS). Phase I study to investigate the efficacy of intracoronary infusion of cardiac progenitor cells in patients with univentricular heart disease. Dr. Hidemasa Oh, PI.
4. Kaushal S, Wehman B, Pietris N, et al. Study design and rationale for ELPIS: a phase I/IIb randomized pilot study of allogeneic human mesenchymal stem cell injection in patients with hypoplastic left heart syndrome. Am Heart J. 2017;192:48–56.
5. ClinicalTrials.gov. NCT01883076: Autologous Umbilical Cord Blood Cells for HLHS. Phase I study to determine the safety and feasibility of injections of autologous umbilical cord blood (UCB) cells into the right ventricle of Hypoplastic Left Heart Syndrome (HLHS) children undergoing a scheduled Glenn surgical procedure. Dr. Tim Nelson, PI.
6. ClinicalTrials.gov. NCT02781922: Cardiac Stem/Progenitor Cell Infusion in Univentricular Physiology (APOLLON Trial). The purpose of this study is to evaluate the efficacy and safety of intracoronary injection of autologous cardiac stem cells (JRM-001) after reconstructive surgery in pediatric patients with functional single ventricle Japan Regenerative Medicine Co., Ltd, PI.
7. Eschenhagen T, Fink C, Remmers U, et al. Three-dimensional reconstitution of embryonic cardiomyocytes in a collagen matrix: a new heart muscle model system. FASEB J. 1997;11(8):683–94.
8. Tobita K, Liu LJ, Janczewski AM, et al. Engineered early embryonic cardiac tissue retains proliferative and contractile properties of developing embryonic myocardium. Am J Physiol Heart Circ Physiol. 2006;291(4):H1829–37.
9. Fujimoto KL, Clause KC, Liu LJ, et al. Engineered fetal cardiac graft preserves its cardiomyocyte proliferation within post-infarcted myocardium and sustains cardiac function. Tissue Eng Part A. 2011;17(5–6):585–96.
10. Tulloch NL, Muskheli V, Razumova MV, et al. Growth of engineered human myocardium with mechanical loading and vascular coculture. Circ Res. 2011;109:47–59.
11. Masumoto H, Nakane T, Tinney JP et al 2016 The potential of three-dimensional engineered cardiac tissues composed of multiple human iPS cell-derived cardiovascular cell lineages for cardiac regeneration. Sci Rep 6:29933. YouTube: https://www.youtube.com/watch?v=dDUtxP-zcP0.

12. Nakane T, Masumoto H, Tinney JP, et al. Development of a large-format engineered cardiac tissue from human induced pluripotent stem cells-derived multiple lineage cardiac cells. Sci Rep. 2017;7:45641.
13. Kowalski WJ, Yuan FP, Nakane T, et al. Quantification of cardiomyocyte alignment from 3D confocal microscopy of engineered tissue. Microsc Microanal. 2017;23:826–42.
14. Fujita B, Zimmermann WH. Myocardial tissue engineering for regenerative applications. Curr Cardiol Rep. 2017;19(9):78. Review.
15. Tiburcy M, Hudson JE, Balfanz P, et al. Defined engineered human myocardium with advanced maturation for applications in heart failure modeling and repair. Circulation. 2017;135(19):1832–47.
16. Li RA, Keung W, Cashman TJ, et al. Bioengineering an electro-mechanically functional miniature ventricular heart chamber from human pluripotent stem cells. Biomaterials. 2018;163:116–27.
17. Conradi L, Schmidt S, Neofytou E, et al. Immunobiology of fibrin-based engineered heart tissue. Stem Cells Transl Med. 2015;4(6):625–31.
18. Williams C, Budina E, Stoppel WL, et al. 3rd Cardiac extracellular matrix-fibrin hybrid scaffolds with tunable properties for cardiovascular tissue engineering. Acta Biomater. 2015;14:84–95.
19. Feric NT, Radisic M. Towards adult-like human engineered cardiac tissue: maturing human pluripotent stem cell-derived cardiomyocytes in human engineered cardiac tissues. Adv Drug Deliv Rev. 2016;96:110–34.
20. Long C, Li H, Tiburcy M, Rodriguez-Caycedo C, et al. Correction of diverse muscular dystrophy mutations in human engineered heart muscle by single-site genome editing. Sci Adv. 2018;4(1):eaap9004.
21. Masumoto H, Ikuno T, Takeda M, et al. Human iPS cell-engineered cardiac tissue sheets with cardiomyocytes and vascular cells for cardiac regeneration. Sci Rep. 2014;4:6716. https://doi.org/10.1038/srep06716.
22. Miyagawa S, Domae K, Yoshikawa Y, et al. Phase I clinical trial of autologous stem cell-sheet transplantation therapy for treating cardiomyopathy. J Am Heart Assoc. 2017;6(4). pii: e003918) https://doi.org/10.1161/JAHA.116.003918.

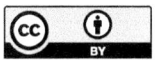

Quantification of Contractility in Stem Cell-Derived Cardiomyocytes

55

Konrad Brockmeier, Moritz Haustein, Markus Khalil, and Tobias Hannes

Abstract

Murine embryonic stem cell derived cardiomyocytes (mESC-CMs) and murine induced pluripotent stem cell derived cardiomyocytes (miPS-CMs) were differentiated and co-cultured with irreversibly injured myocardial tissue slices. When beating clusters had integrated morphologically into the damaged tissue, isometric force measurements were performed. Effects of Ca(2+), nifedipine, and beta-adrenergic modulation were studied during loaded contractions and compared with the contractile behavior of native murine myocardial slices. Both CM variants conferred force to the myocardial tissue. Contraction increased with higher concentrations of Ca(2+) and Isoproterenol, and decreased with nifedipine in all slice variants. Differences between mESC-CMs and miPS-CMs were non-significant, however, significantly different ($P < 0.05$), when compared to native myocardial slices.

Keywords

Stem cells · iPS · Force measurements · Damaged myocardium

K. Brockmeier (✉) · M. Haustein · T. Hannes
Pediatric Cardiology, University of Cologne, Cologne, Germany
e-mail: konrad.brockmeier@uk-koeln.de

M. Khalil
Pediatric Cardiology, University of Giessen, Giessen, Germany

55.1   Introduction

Therapy for heart failure is a challenge also in the setting of congenital heart disease. Up to now, there is no true solution of a repair of damaged myocytes. Stem cell-derived cardiomyocytes are believed to offer possible solutions in the future. The possibility to potentially replace failing myocardium with stem cell-derived cardiomyocytes will depend to a major part on the contractile properties of these cells.

In order to quantify the contractility of stem cell-derived cardiomyocytes, we present an in vitro model using slices of murine ventricles.

The aim of our work was to compare the contractile properties of (1) murine embryonic stem cell-derived cardiomyocytes (mESC-CMs), (2) murine induced pluripotent stem cell-derived cardiomyocytes (miPS-CMs) and (3) contractile properties of native murine ventricular myocardium at a comparable age of differentiation.

As assumed in a prior work, it is almost impossible to assign myocardial contractile properties of transplanted cells in vivo; we therefore developed a tissue culture model mimicking the situation in vivo [1].

55.2   Materials and Methods

Experiments were carried out according to the Principles of Laboratory Animal care.

We prepared avital tissue slices from neonatal murine ventricles, which were used as a non-contractile matrix as described elsewhere [2]. In summary, neonatal murine ventricles were embedded in 4% low-melting agarose and cut into 300-μm-thick slices along the short axis with a microtome (Leica Microsystems, Wetzlar, Germany), kept in cold (4 °C) Ca^{2+}-free Tyrode's solution, continuously aerated with pure oxygen and supplemented with $CaCl^2$ if needed. Finally, the ventricular tissue slices were exposed to irreversible myocardial injury by severe and long-standing deprivation of oxygen and glucose.

MESC-CMs and miPS-CMs were generated as described previously [3]. Beating clusters of miPS-CMs and mESC-CMs were microdissected 11 days after initiation of in vitro differentiation and co-cultured for 5–7 days on top of the oxygen- and glucose-deprived ventricular slices, placing the non-vital slices into a funnel-shaped cavity and adding CM clusters in a very cautious way using a score to estimate attachment and "integration" under microscopic control. For the experiments of contractility measurements, those two types of co-culture preparations and native embryonic heart slices were mounted onto two steel needles connected to an isometric force transducer in a customized dish within Tyrode's solution. All three types of slices were conditioned stepwise by extending their length until maximal force resulted during continuous pacing at 2–4 Hz. Signals from the force measurement transducer and electrical pacing were A/D converted, amplified and recorded on a digital medium using DASYLab software (National Instruments) with a sampling rate of 1 kHz, high and low pass filtered (0.05–15 Hz) and signal averaged. Isometric force was measured in Tyrode's solution after 5 min of spontaneous beating at constant resting conditions. The amplitudes of 20 contractions before and after stimulation were normalized and analyzed.

Effects of Ca^{2+} were analyzed in Ca^{2+}-free Tyrode's solution by increasing concentrations of Ca^{2+} (0.5, 2.5, 4.5, 6.5 and 8.5 mM, 10 min for each concentration). In addition, the effects of the Ca^{2+}-blocker nifedipine (0.01–10 M) and ß-adrenergic isoproterenol (10.9–10.6 M) were analyzed.

Means and standard deviations, and ranges were calculated. Paired and unpaired t tests or one-way analysis of variance (ANOVA) was performed. $P < 0.05$ was considered statistically significant.

55.3   Results

Native embryonic heart tissue as well as co-cultured preparations with mESC-CMs or miPS-CMs showed spontaneous contractions. During spontaneous contractions no difference between the beating frequency of preparations with mESC-CMs [2.9 ± 0.4(1.3–4.3) Hz, $n = 11$] and miPS-CMs [2.2 ± 0.2(1.5–4.0) Hz, $n = 12$] was found. There was significant slower contraction rate in native embryonic heart slices [0.8 ± 0.1(0.1–1.4) Hz, $n = 8$, $P < 0.05$]. In Ca^{2+}-free Tyrode's solution no contraction occurred. Contraction increased with increasing concentration of Ca^{2+} in mESC-CMs, miPS-CMs and native embryonic heart slices. Native embryonic heart slices showed significantly stronger contractility ($P < 0.05$ vs. both miPS-CMs and mESC-CMs). Comparison was achieved after data normalization using the force values at Ca^{2+} = 2.5 mM of individual experiments. 3/4 miPS-CMs preparations and 2/4 mESC-CMs preparations showed decreasing contraction at a concentration of 1 µmol and stopped contraction at concentrations of 10 µmol nifedipine. Native embryonic heart slices continued contractions also at high nifedipine doses. Dose-dependent negative inotropy of nifedipine was seen in all three groups (Fig. 55.1).

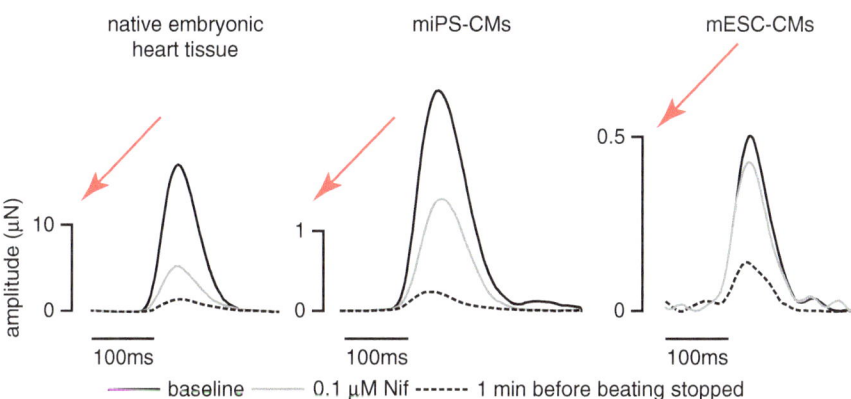

Fig. 55.1   The effect of nifedipin(NIF) is shown in the three preparations: native embryonic heart tissue, murine induced pluripotent cell derived cardiomyocytes (miPS-CMs) and murine embryologic stem cell derived cardiomyocytes (mESC-CMs). Note the similar behavior of all three preparations. Important the different scales of amplitudes (micro Newton)—chosen for relative comparison

A positive inotropic effect of isoproterenol was seen in all three groups. The inotropic effect of isoproterenol was significantly stronger in native embryonic heart tissue. Differences between mESC-CMs and miPS-CMs were non-significant.

55.4   Discussion

The results demonstrate that our ventricular slice model for analysis and comparison of contractility of co-cultured preparations with mESC-CMs, miPS-CMs and native embryonic heart tissue works sufficiently. The primary finding from this study is that stem cell-derived cardiomyocytes, both mESC-CMs and miPS-CMs attached to avital myocardial slices, showed quantifiable force/contractility after co-culture under defined conditions. There were only minor differences between such mESC-CM and miPS-CM preparations. However, significant differences in contraction behavior were found when compared to native embryonic heart slices of comparable age. Calcium dependency was demonstrated in all three preparations in a relative similar fashion, however, in a much lesser amplitude level seen in the pluripotent stem cell-derived cardiomyocyte preparations. MESC-CM and miPS-CM slice preparations exhibited contractile behavior of possibly immature sarcoplasmic reticulum. The Ca^{2+}-channel antagonist nifedipine induced a dose-dependent negative inotropy on the force of contraction of all three preparations underlining the importance of L-type calcium channels for contractility regulation. The stem cell-derived cardiomyocytes showed significantly diminished ß-adrenergic response compared to native embryonic heart slices.

So far there is no data that convincingly support the hypothesis that pluripotent stem cell-derived cardiomyocytes are capable of developing into a cardiomyocyte phenotype that is identical to mature ventricular cardiomyocytes in vitro [4]. The potential development of mature sarcoplasmatic reticulum in stem cell-derived cardiomyocytes is still an issue, and the understanding of factors involved in differentiation toward a functional and a mature cardiac phenotype is still incomplete [5].

References

1. Pillekamp F, Reppel M, Dinkelacker V, Duan Y, Jazmati N, Bloch W, Brockmeier K, Hescheler J, Fleischmann BK, Koehling R. Force measurements of human embryonic stem cell-derived cardiomyocytes in an in vitro transplantation model. Cell Physiol Biochem. 2007;16:127–32.
2. Pillekamp F, Reppel M, Rubenchyk O, Pfannkuche K, Matzkies M, Bloch W, Sreeram N, Brockmeier K, Hescheler J. Force measurements of human embryonic stem cell-derived cardiomyocytes in an in vitro transplantation model. Stem Cells. 2007;25:174–80.
3. Kolossov E, Bostani T, Roell W, Breitbach M, Pillekamp F, Nygren JM, Sasse P, Rubenchik O, Fries JW, Wenzel D, Geisen C, Xia Y, Lu Z, Duan Y, Kettenhofen R, Jovinge S, Bloch W, Bohlen H, Welz A, Hescheler J, Jacobsen SE, Fleischmann BK. Engraftment of engineered ES cell-derived cardiomyocytes but not BM cells restores contractile function to the infarcted myocardium. J Exp Med. 2006;203:2315–27.
4. Dolnikov K, Shilkrut M, Zeevi-Levin N, Gerecht-Nir S, Amit M, Danon A, Itskovitz-Eldor J, Binah O. Functional properties of human embryonic stem cell-derived cardiomyocytes:

intracellular Ca2 handling and the role of sarcoplasmic reticulum in the contraction. Stem Cells. 2006;24:236–45.

5. Xi J, Khalil M, Shishechian N, Hannes T, Pfannkuche K, Liang H, Fatima A, Haustein M, Suhr F, Bloch W, Reppel M, Sarie T, Wernig M, J rnigi R, Brockmeier K, Hescheler J, Pillekamp F. Comparison of contractile behavior of native murine ventricular tissue and cardiomyocytes derived from embryonic or induced pluripotent stem cells. FASEB J. 2010;24:2739–51.

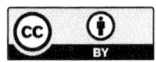

A Neurotrophic Factor Receptor GFRA2, a Specific Surface Antigen for Cardiac Progenitor Cells, Regulates the Process of Myocardial Compaction

56

Hidekazu Ishida, Shigeru Miyagawa, Keiichi Ozono, Ken Suzuki, Yoshiki Sawa, and Kenta Yashiro

Keywords

GFRA2 · Surface antigen · Cardiac progenitor cells · Non-compaction cardiomyopathy

A surface marker specific for cardiac progenitors (CPs) allows the robust isolation of CPs, effectively circumventing the necessity of genetic modification. Recently, we have reported that glial cell line–derived neurotrophic factor receptor alpha 2 (*Gfra2*), which is anchored to the plasma membrane via Glycosylphosphatidylinositol, specifically marks CPs of both the first and second heart fields within the early mouse embryo [1], identified by single-cell expression profiling on mouse embryonic CPs (Fig. 56.1) [2, 3].

H. Ishida · K. Ozono
Department of Paediatrics, Graduate School of Medicine, Osaka University, Suita, Osaka, Japan

S. Miyagawa · Y. Sawa
Department of Cardiovascular Surgery, Graduate School of Medicine, Osaka University, Suita, Osaka, Japan

K. Suzuki
Centre for Microvascular Research, William Harvey Research Institute, Barts and The London School of Medicine and Dentistry, Queen Mary University of London, London, UK

K. Yashiro (✉)
Department of Cardiac Regeneration and Therapeutics, Graduate School of Medicine, Osaka University, Suita, Osaka, Japan

Centre for Endocrinology, William Harvey Research Institute, Barts and The London School of Medicine and Dentistry, Queen Mary University of London, London, UK

Department of Anatomy, Division of Anatomy and Developmental Biology, Kyoto Prefectural University of Medicine, Kyoto, Japan
e-mail: kyashiro@kotp.kpu-m.ac.jp

Mouse developement

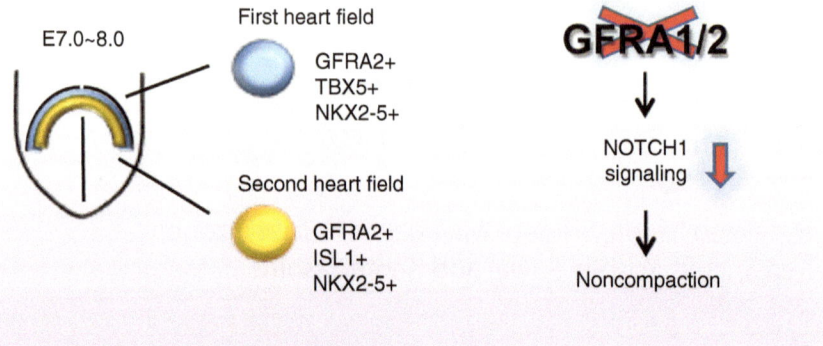

Pluripotent stem cell differention

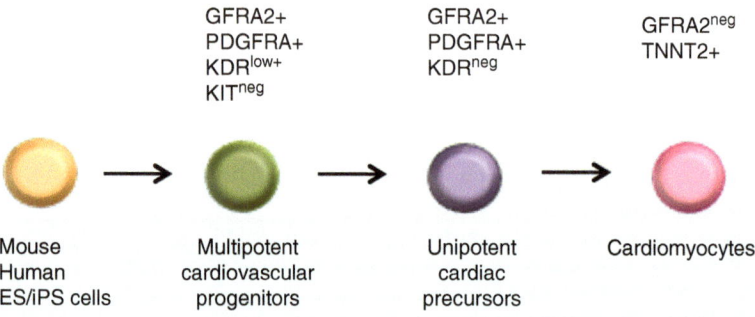

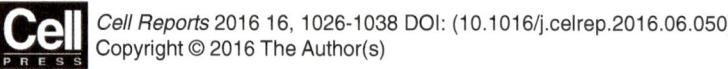

Cell
PRESS
Cell Reports 2016 16, 1026-1038 DOI: (10.1016/j.celrep.2016.06.050)
Copyright © 2016 The Author(s)

Fig. 56.1 GFRA2 is a specific marker for CPs which governs myocardial compaction. *Upper case*: A signal transduction via GFRA1/2 is upstream of NOTCH signal that is indispensable for the myocardial compaction process. *Lower case*: GFRA2 is a specific surface antigen to identify CPs from differentiating pluripotent stem cells in mice and humans. This illustration is cited from Ishida, H et al. Cell Rep. 2016 Jul 26;16(4):1026–38, and is licensed under the Creative Commons Attribution 4.0 International License. To view a copy of this license, visit http://creativecommons. org/licenses/by/4.0/ or send a letter to Creative Commons, PO Box 1866, Mountain View, CA 94042, USA

- GFRA2 facilitates the isolation of CPs by fluorescence-activated cell sorting from differentiating mouse and human pluripotent stem cells. If utilizing pan-mesoderm marker PDGFRA and hemangioblastic marker KDR in conjunction with GFRA2, multipotent CPs giving rise to cardiomyocytes, smooth muscle cells and endothelial cells are identified as GFRA2$^+$/PDGFRA$^+$/KDR$^+$ whereas CPs already committed only to cardiomyocytes are identified as GFRA2$^+$/PDGFRA$^+$/KDR^{neg}.

- In loss-of-function of *Gfra2*, the functional redundancy of GFRA1 compensated for the cardiac GFRA2 signal in the mutant mouse embryos. Compound mutant of *Gfra1/2* showed non-compaction cardiomyopathy due to the down-regulation of NOTCH signal in the developing heart. Cardiac GFRA2 signal is distinct from the canonical pathway that depends on the RET tyrosine kinase and its established ligands.

Collectively our findings establish a platform for investigating the biology of CPs as a foundation for the future development of CP transplantation therapies for treating heart failure.

Acknowledgments   This work was supported by MRC New Investigator Research Grant G0900105 and MRC Research Grant MR/J007625/1 to K.Y., Japan Heart Foundation/Bayer Yakuhin Research Grant Abroad and JSPS (Japan Society for the Promotion of Science) Postdoctoral Fellowship for Research Abroad to H.I. We thank Ruchaya PJ at Kings College London for the support in writing.

References

1. Ishida H, Saba R, Kokkinopoulos I, et al. GFRA2 identifies cardiac progenitors and mediates cardiomyocyte differentiation in a RET-independent signaling pathway. Cell Rep. 2016;16(4):1026–38.
2. Brouilette S, Kuersten S, Mein C, et al. A simple and novel method for RNA-seq library preparation of single cell cDNA analysis by hyperactive Tn5 transposase. Dev Dyn. 2012;241(10):1584–90.
3. Kokkinopoulos I, Ishida H, Saba R, et al. Single-cell expression profiling reveals a dynamic state of cardiac precursor cells in the early mouse embryo. PLoS One. 2015;10(10):e0140831.

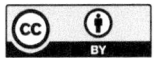

Cardiac Cell Specification by Defined Factors

57

Yuika Morita and Jun Takeuchi

Our previous study has shown that Tbx5-Gata4-Baf60c-induced functional cardio-myocytes via the ectopic expression of *Nkx2-5/Islet1* in the mesodermal cells, but not in the endodermal/ectodermal cells [1, 2] (Fig. 57.1). Mesp1 is one of the major transcriptional regulators specifying the mesodermal lineage, but it also induces skeletal muscle, hematopoietic and vascular cells as well as cardiac cells [3–5]. Eomesodermin (Eomes), an upstream player of Mesp1, regulates mesodermal cell lineages, but it does not have a potential for specification of cardiac cell fate from cardiovascular lineages either [6]. Therefore, the study of cardiac cell fate specification from the embryonic stem cells by the defined factors still remains at least two major questions.

1. How the cardiac lineage is committed from the mesoderm via repressing skeletal muscle, hematopoietic and vascular cell fates?
2. Are there any factors specifying the cardiac lineage directly from the undifferentiated stem cells?

Y. Morita
MRI, Tokyo Medical and Dental University, Tokyo, Japan

Department of Cardiology, Keio University, Tokyo, Japan

J. Takeuchi (✉)
MRI, Tokyo Medical and Dental University, Tokyo, Japan

© The Editor(s) (if applicable) and The Author(s) 2020
T. Nakanishi et al. (eds.), *Molecular Mechanism of Congenital Heart Disease and Pulmonary Hypertension*, https://doi.org/10.1007/978-981-15-1185-1_57

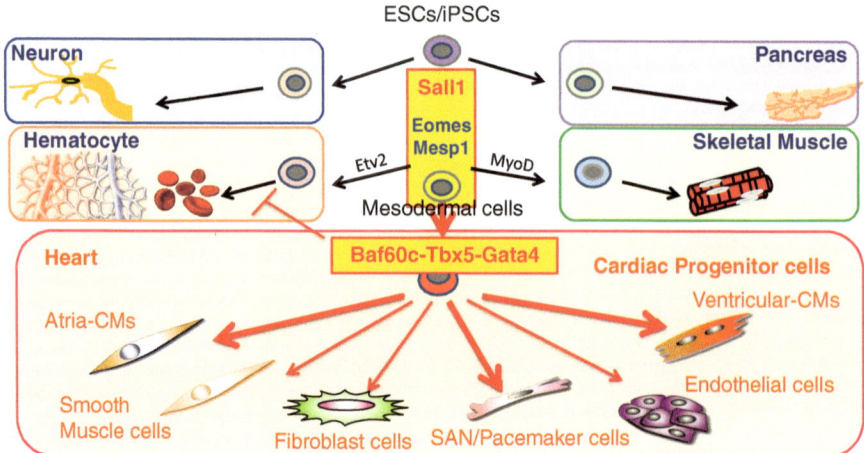

Fig. 57.1 The defined factors for cardiogenesis

To disclose these questions, we performed RNA sequencing from the anterior field at the early cardiac crescent stage, and we identified Sall1 gene as a suitable key regulator for the cardiac cell lineage [7]. Overexpression of Sall1 in mouse ES accelerated cardiogenesis and also promoted cardiac cell fate in human iPS cells with upregulation of several cardiac transcriptional genes (*ISLET1/NKX2-5/MEF2C*) and sarcomeric genes (*TNNT2/MYL7/MYH6/MYH7*). Sall1 also acts as a modulator to recruit the histone-modification/the chromatin remodeling factors and the other transcriptional factors to commit the cardiac cell fate. Interestingly, permanent expression of Sall1 in differentiating human iPS cells increased the number of cardiac progenitor cells [7] (Fig. 57.2). These data suggest that Sall1 acts as a key factor to promote and maintain the cardiac progenitor cell phase from undifferentiating stem cells, and down-regulation of Sall1 expression after induction of cardiac progenitor cells is necessary to shift the cell fate to cardio-myocyte differentiation.

Our data just show that a novel gene, Sall1, programs cardiac cell fate and accelerates cardiogenesis, but this factor may act as a defined player for the cardiac cell fate with and the other transcriptional factors to define. Thus, the study for isolation of in vivo Sall1 partners and establishment of its regulation will give us the next window for the program/reprogram research (Fig. 57.1).

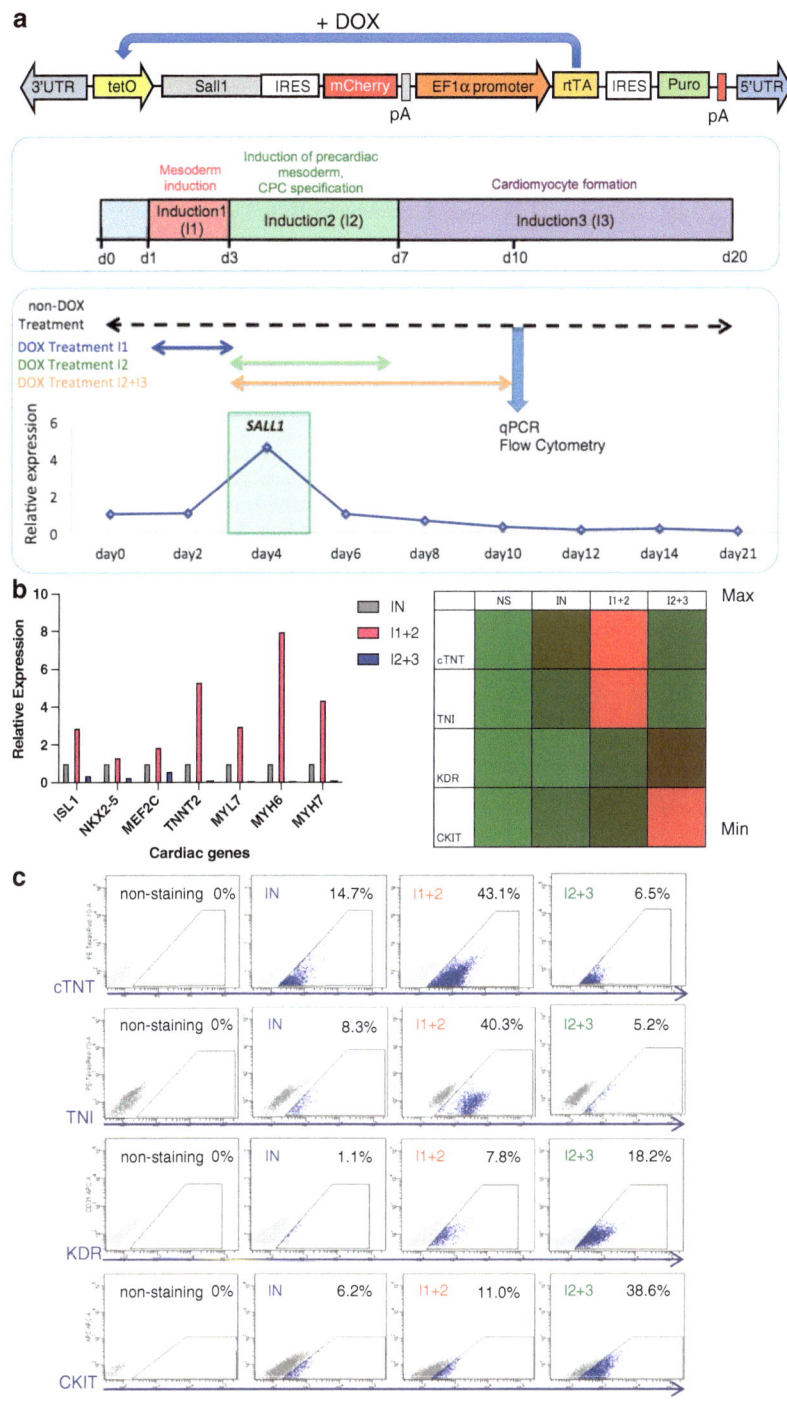

Fig. 57.2 The critical expression of Sall1 for promoting cardiogenesis

References

1. Takeuchi JK, Bruneau BG. Direct transdifferentiation of mouse mesoderm to heart tissue by defined factors. Nature. 2009;459:708–11.
2. van Weerd JH, Koshiba-Takeuchi K, Kwon C, Takeuchi JK. Epigenetic factors and cardiac development. Cardiovasc Res. 2011;91:203–11.
3. Bondue A, Lapouge G, Paulissen C, Semeraro C, Iacovino M, Kyba M, Blanpain C. Mesp1 acts as a master regulator of multipotent cardiovascular progenitor specification. Cell Stem Cell. 2008;3:69–84.
4. Chan S, Shi X, Toyama A, Arpke RW, Dandapat A, Iacovino M, Kang J, Le G, Hagen HR, Garry DJ, Kyba M. Mesp1 patterns mesoderm into cardiac, hematopoietic, or skeletal myogenic progenitors in a context-dependent manner. Cell Stem Cell. 2013;12:587–601.
5. Lescroat F, Wang X, Lin X, Swedlund B, Gargouri S, Sanchez-Danes A, Moignard V, Dubois C, Paulissen C, Kinston S, Gottgens B, Blanpain C. Defining the earliest step of cardiovascular lineage segregation by single-cell RNA-seq. Science. 2018;359(6380):1177–81.
6. Van den Ameele J, Tiberi L, Bondue A, Paulissen C, Herpoel A, Lacovino M, Kyba M, Blanpain C, Vanderhaeghen P. Eomesodermin inducesMesp1 expression and cardiac differentiation from embryonic stem cells in the absence of Activin. EMBO Rep. 2012;13(4):355–62.
7. Morita Y, Andersen P, Hotta A, Tsukahara Y, Sasagawa N, Hayashida N, Koga C, Nishikawa M, Saga Y, Evans SM, Koshiba-Takeuchi K, Nishinakamura R, Yoshida Y, Kwon C, Takeuchi JK. Sall1 transiently marks undifferentiated heart precursors and regulates their fate. J Mol Cell Cardiol. 2016;92:158–62.

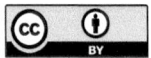

A Temporo-Spatial Regulation of Sema3c Is Essential for Interaction of Progenitor Cells during Cardiac Outflow Tract Development

58

Kazuki Kodo, Shinsuke Shibata, Sachiko Miyagawa-Tomita, Sang-Ging Ong, Hiroshi Takahashi, Tsutomu Kume, Hideyuki Okano, Rumiko Matsuoka, and Hiroyuki Yamagishi

K. Kodo · H. Yamagishi (✉)
Division of Pediatric Cardiology, Department of Pediatrics, Keio University School of Medicine, Tokyo, Japan
e-mail: hyamag@keio.jp

S. Shibata · H. Okano
Department of Physiology, Keio University School of Medicine, Tokyo, Japan

S. Miyagawa-Tomita
Department of Pediatric Cardiology, Tokyo Women's Medical University, Tokyo, Japan

Department of Physiological Chemistry and Metabolism, Graduate School of Medicine, The University of Tokyo, Bunkyo City, Tokyo, Japan

Department of Veterinary Technology, Yamazaki Gakuen University, Hachioji, Tokyo, Japan

S.-G. Ong
Department of Pharmacology, University of Illinois at Chicago, Chicago, IL, USA

H. Takahashi
Department of Neurology, National Hospital Organization, Tottori Medical Center, Tottori, Japan

T. Kume
Feinberg Cardiovascular Research Institute, Feinberg School of Medicine, Northwestern University, Chicago, IL, USA

R. Matsuoka
Department of Pediatric Cardiology, TWMU, Tokyo, Japan

© The Editor(s) (if applicable) and The Author(s) 2020
T. Nakanishi et al. (eds.), *Molecular Mechanism of Congenital Heart Disease and Pulmonary Hypertension*, https://doi.org/10.1007/978-981-15-1185-1_58

Keywords
Cardiac neural crest cell · Second heart field · TBX1 · Congenital heart disease

The two cardiac progenitor cell lineages, cardiac neural crest cells (cNCCs) and the second heart field (SHF), play key roles in the development of the cardiac outflow tract (OFT). Both cardiac progenitor cells interact with each other and contribute to OFT formation cooperatively. The neurovascular guiding molecule, semaphorin 3c (Sema3c), is thought to serve as a key attractant for the migration of cNCCs. A previous study reported that Tbx1 null mice showed a significant reduction in Sema3c expression in the OFT region [1]. However, the regulatory effect of Tbx1 on Sema3c was unclear. Here, we show that Sema3c plays key roles in cNCCs-SHF interactions through the regulation by Tbx1 and other molecules during OFT development [2].

By generating reporter transgenic mice harboring *Sema3c* enhancer fragments and lacZ transgene, we found that Foxc1/c2 directly regulated Sema3c expression in the OFT via direct binding to the Fox-site on the 5′ flanking sequence of *Sema3c* where Tbx1 synergistically enhanced the Foxc1/c2 function. In comparison, Tbx1 in the SHF inhibited ectopic Sema3c expression in cNCCs within the pharyngeal arch region via Fgf8-ERK signaling. Consistently, the ectopic expression of Sema3c in the cNCCs of *Tbx1* hypomorphic mouse embryos caused abnormal migration and/or aggregation, and the overexpression of Sema3c in cultured cNCCs inhibited their migration, resulting in their aggregation. These results suggest that Tbx1-Fgf8-ERK signaling negatively regulates Sema3c expression in cNCCs for the proper guidance of their migration from the dorsal pharyngeal region to the OFT.

In conclusion, a proper temporo-spatial expression of Sema3c, which is tightly regulated positively by Foxc1/c2 and negatively by the Tbx1-Fgf8 cascade, is essential for the correct navigation of cNCCs towards the OFT (Fig. 58.1). This report is the first evidence of a detailed signal transduction mechanism for the interaction between cNCCs and SHF progenitor cells through Sema3c, providing a new molecular basis for a potential therapeutic strategy for congenital heart diseases involving OFT defects.

This work was supported by MEXT KAKENHI, Grant-in-Aid for Scientific Research (B) and Grant-in-Aid for Young Scientists (B), Keio University Academic Development Funds and Brain/MINDS project from AMED, Japan.

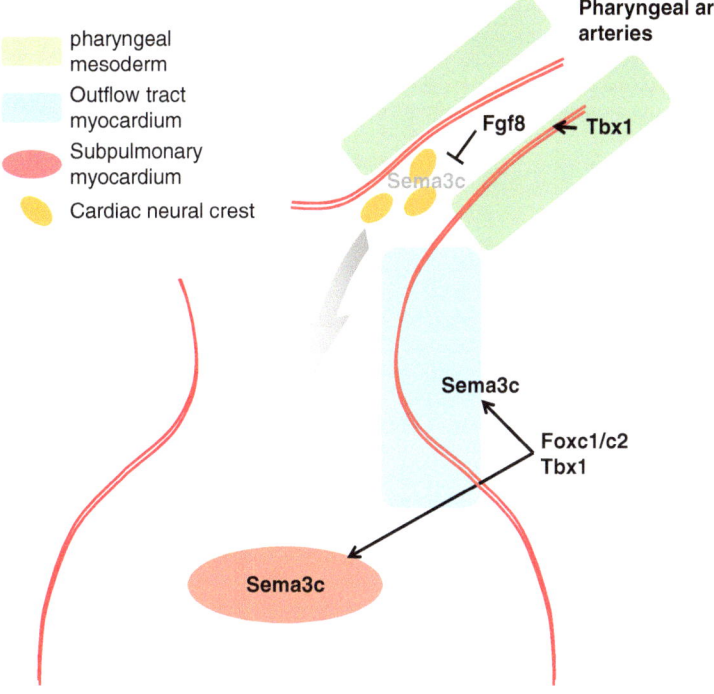

Fig. 58.1 Temporo-spatial regulation of Sema3c by Foxc1/c2 and Tbx1-Fgf8 cascade from the second heart field for proper navigation of cardiac neural crest cells towards the developing outflow tract

References

1. Kodo K, Shibata S, Miyagawa-Tomita S, et al. Regulation of Sema3c and the interaction between cardiac neural crest and second heart field during outflow tract development. Sci Rep. 2017;7:6771.
2. Théveniau-Ruissy M, Dandonneau M, Mesbah K, et al. The del22q11.2 candidate gene Tbx1 controls regional outflow tract identity and coronary artery patterning. Circ Res. 2008;103:142–8.

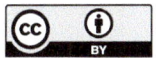

Spatiotemporally Restricted Developmental Alterations in the Anterior and Secondary Heart Fields Cause Distinct Conotruncal Heart Defects

59

Mayu Narematsu and Yuji Nakajima

Abstract

During the early heart development, heart outflow tract elongates by the addition of cardiomyocytes from the anterior heart field (AHF)/secondary heart field (SHF). Dye-marking experiments in early chick embryos clarified that each AHF/SHF migrates to distinct conotruncal regions. Local administration of retinoic acid to the AHF/SHF causes distinct conotruncal heart defects in a region and stage dependent manner. For example, impaired development of AHF at HH stage 12 (corresponding to Carnegie stages 10–11 in human embryos) causes dextroposed aorta including transposition of the great arteries (TGA), while SHF at HH stage 12 persistent truncus arteriosus (PTA). Our results indicated that the abnormal development of certain AHF/SHF at certain stages causes specific spectrum of conotruncal heart defects.

Keywords

Second heart field · Heart outflow tract · Transposition of great arteries · Congenital heart defects · Retinoic acid

Developmental alterations of the heart outflow tract (OFT) cause conotruncal heart defects (CTHDs), which are often diagnosed in infants with congenital heart defects. During the early heart development, the OFT elongates by the addition of

M. Narematsu · Y. Nakajima (✉)
Department of Anatomy and Cell Biology, Graduate School of Medicine, Osaka City University, Osaka, Japan
e-mail: narematsu@med.osaka-cu.ac.jp; yuji@med.osaka-cu.ac.jp

Table 59.1 Conotruncal heart defects produced by local administration of RA to the AHF or SHF at early looped-heart stage in chick embryonic hearts

RA addition	At stage 12[a]	At stage 14[b]
To AHF	TGA, DORV	PTA
To SHF	PTA	PTA, DORV

[a]Corresponding to embryonic day (ED) 8.5 in mouse and Carnegie stage 10 in human
[b]ED 9.0 in mouse and Carnegie stage 11 in human

cardiomyocytes from the second lineage of heart-forming regions, which reside in the first and second pharyngeal arches (anterior heart field [AHF]) as well as in the splanchnic mesoderm of the pericardial coelom in the posterior pharyngeal arches (secondary heart field [SHF]) [1]. As the arterial pole moves in the anterior-to-posterior (cranial-to-caudal) direction, the AHF is first added to the OFT followed by the SHF. Therefore, abnormal development of certain parts of the AHF or SHF at certain stages may cause specific CTHDs.

Dye-marking experiments in chick embryos at the early looped-heart stage showed that the right and left AHFs migrate ipsilaterally to form the proximal OFT, whereas SHFs migrate rotationally to form the distal OFT beneath the semilunar valves [2]. The results indicated that each AHF/SHF migrates to generate distinct conotruncal regions.

Retinoic acid (RA) is a potent teratogen to induce CTHDs. Local administration of RA to the AHF in chick embryos at early looped-heart stage (stage 12) caused a truncated OFT, thereby resulting in transposition of the great arteries (TGA) and double outlet right ventricle (DORV) (Table 59.1) [3]. The left AHF was more sensitive to RA in the development of TGA. Accordingly, the proximal OFT, especially the subpulmonic region, may play a role in conotruncal rotation to establish the left ventricle-to-aortic connection [4]. Persistent truncus arteriosus (PTA) occurred when RA was added to the SHF at stage 12 as well as to the AHF/SHF at stage 14 (Table 59.1). Accordingly, normal development of the distal OFT is necessary for conotruncal septation involving the aortico-pulmonary septum, a derivative of the cardiac neural crest. In conclusion, AHF at the early looped-heart stage, corresponding to Carnegie Stages 10–11 in human embryos, is the region responsible, and impediment of which causes a dextroposed aorta including TGA.

References

1. Nakajima Y. Second lineage of heart forming region provides new understanding of conotruncal heart defects. Congenit Anom (Kyoto). 2010;50:8–14.
2. Takahashi M, Terasako Y, Yanagawa N, et al. Myocardial progenitors in the pharyngeal regions migrate to distinct conotruncal regions. Dev Dyn. 2012;241:284–93.
3. Narematsu M, Kamimura T, Yamagishi T, et al. Impaired development of left anterior heart field by ectopic retinoic acid causes transposition of the great arteries. J Am Heart Assoc. 2015;4 https://doi.org/10.1161/JAHA.115.001889.
4. Nakajima Y. Mechanism responsible for D-transposition of the great arteries: is this part of the spectrum of right isomerism? Congenit Anom (Kyoto). 2016;56:196–202.

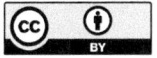

Significance of Transcription Factors in the Mechanisms of Great Artery Malformations

60

Yusuke Watanabe and Osamu Nakagawa

Keywords

Congenital cardiovascular disease · Great arteries · Notch signaling

Members of the Hey transcriptional factor family are Notch target genes [1], and they have unique and redundant functions in cardiovascular development. Among them, we recently reported that Hey1 had an indispensable role for the great artery formation (Fig. 60.1) [2].

Dysfunction of several transcription factors is correlated with anomalies of the great arteries. Human *TBX1* is the gene responsible for 22q11.2 deletion syndrome, and mutant mice for *Tbx1* recapitulate the phenotypes such as interruption of aortic arch type B and right-sided aortic arch. These defects are originated from the impaired development of the fourth pharyngeal arch arteries (PAAs) at early embryonic stages, and migration, proliferation and survival of the neural crest cells are affected in *Tbx1* mutant mice [3]. Similarly, the deficiency of upstream and downstream transcription factors of Tbx1, such as Foxc2, Gbx2 and Hes1, results in abnormal great arteries.

The malformation of great arteries in *Hey1* knockout mice is also associated with the fourth PAA defect although the expression of Tbx1 and target genes as well as the behavior of neural crest cells are normal [2]. Interestingly, the tubular endothelial structure is disturbed, and the expression of a Notch ligand, Jagged1, in endothelial cells is markedly reduced in the defective fourth PAAs of *Hey1* knockout embryos (Fig. 60.1) [2], suggesting that Hey1 is necessary for the endothelial organization of the fourth PAA. Elucidating the mechanism of Hey actions, especially

Y. Watanabe (✉) · O. Nakagawa
Department of Molecular Physiology, National Cerebral and Cardiovascular Center Research Institute, Suita, Osaka, Japan
e-mail: ywatanabe@ncvc.go.jp; osamu.nakagawa@ncvc.go.jp

385

T. Nakanishi et al. (eds.), *Molecular Mechanism of Congenital Heart Disease and Pulmonary Hypertension*, https://doi.org/10.1007/978-981-15-1185-1_60

Fig. 60.1 Defects of great artery morphogenesis and pharyngeal arch artery development in Hey1 knockout mice

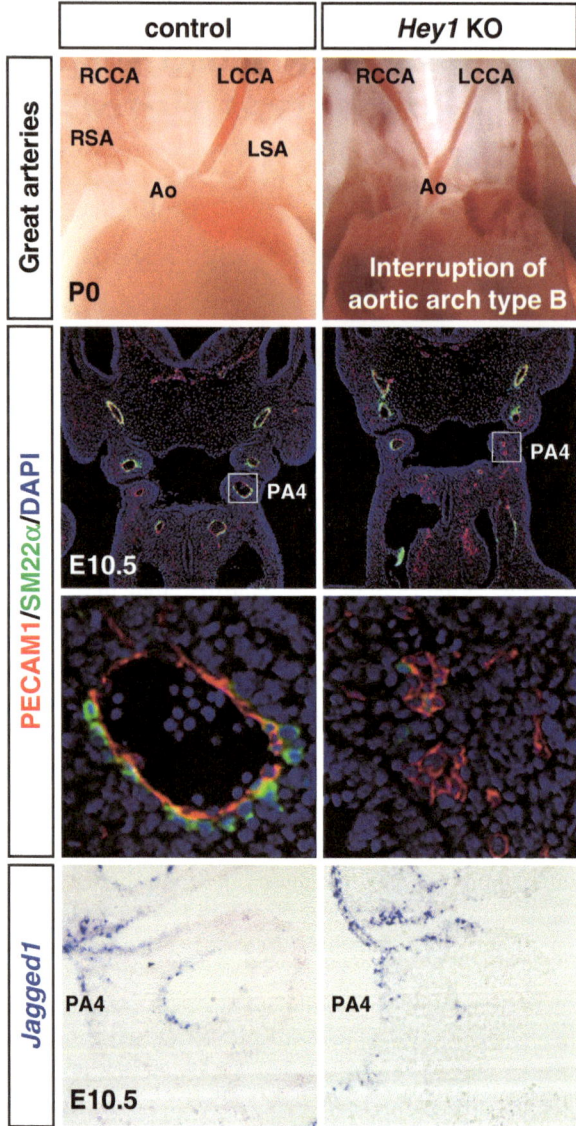

tissue specificity and direct target genes, and relationship with Tbx1 pathway will provide further understanding of the fourth PAA development and related human congenital cardiovascular diseases.

References

1. Nakagawa O, McFadden DG, Nakagawa M, Yanagisawa H, Hu T, Srivastava D, Olson EN. Members of the HRT family of basic helix-loop-helix proteins act as transcriptional repressors downstream of Notch signaling. Proc Natl Acad Sci U S A. 2000;97(25):13655–60.
2. Fujita M, Sakabe M, Ioka T, Watanabe Y, Kinugasa-Katayama Y, Tsuchihashi T, Utset MF, Yamagishi H, Nakagawa O. Pharyngeal arch artery defects and lethal malformations of the aortic arch and its branches in mice deficient for the Hrt1/Hey1 transcription factor. Mech Dev. 2016;139:65–73.
3. Lindsay EA, Vitelli F, Su H, Morishima M, Huynh T, Pramparo T, Jurecic V, Ogunrinu G, Sutherland HF, Scambler PJ, et al. Tbx1 haploinsufficiency in the DiGeorge syndrome region causes aortic arch defects in mice. Nature. 2001;410(6824):97–101.

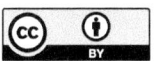

The Different c-kit Expression in Human Induced Pluripotent Stem (iPS) Cells Between With Feeder Cells and Without Feeder Cells

61

Nanako Kawaguchi, Emiko Hayama, Yoshiyuki Furutani, and Toshio Nakanishi

Keywords

c-kit · Induced pluripotent stem cell · iPS · Cardiomyocyte differentiation · Gene expression

c-kit is a stem cell factor (SCF) receptor and is known to be expressed in hematopoietic stem cells, prostate stem cells, mast cells, and melanocytes. Since c-kit was reportedly expressed in cardiac stem cells, which are believed to have the ability to become cardiac myocytes or to support cardiac myocyte survival [1, 2], this protein has been used as a marker for cardiac regeneration [3].

iPS cells have been established and used for cardiac regenerative medicine and for developing disease models [4]. However, c-kit expression during cardiomyocyte differentiation using human iPS cells has not yet been studied. Therefore, we characterized the gene expression levels in cultured iPS cells and the change in expression levels during cardiomyocyte differentiation by reverse transcription quantitative polymerase chain reaction (RT-qPCR).

c-kit expression was positive, and its level was much higher in iPS cells cultured with feeder cells than in iPS cells cultured without feeder cells. The RNA from feeder cells was extremely low, and the primer for c-kit expression did not contain the murine-specific sequence, suggesting that c-kit expression in the iPS cells cultured with feeder cells was from the iPS cells. c-kit expression was not detected or was detected at extremely low levels in the feeder-free iPS cells. In both cell conditions (with or without feeder), c-kit expression was detected in the early phase of

N. Kawaguchi · E. Hayama · Y. Furutani · T. Nakanishi (✉)
Department of Pediatric Cardiology, Tokyo Women's Medical University, Tokyo, Japan
e-mail: nakanishi.toshio@twmu.ac.jp

cardiomyocyte differentiation (1–3 days after iPS cells were treated with differentiation medium) before Brachyury was expressed. Brachyury is the transcription factor that is essential for mesoderm formation. c-kit was not expressed thereafter. We examined the SCF expression level in iPS cells cultured with or without feeder cells, but SCF was not detected in either condition.

These results suggest that SCF is independent of c-kit expression, and c-kit might affect the early stage of cardiac differentiation.

References

1. Miyamoto S, Kawaguchi N, Ellison GM, Matsuoka R, Shin'oka T, Kurosawa H. Characterization of long-term cultured cardiac stem cells (CSCs) derived from adult rat hearts. Stem Cells Dev. 2010;19(1):105–16.
2. Kawaguchi N, Smith A, Waring C, Hasan K, Miyamoto S, Matsuoka R, Ellison GM. Gata4high CSCs foster cardiac myocyte survival. PLoS One. 2010;5(12):e14297.
3. Kawaguchi N, Nakanishi T. Cardiomyocyte regeneration using stem cells. Cells. 2013;2(1):6782. https://doi.org/10.3390/cells2010067.
4. Kawaguchi N, Hayama E, Furutani Y, Nakanishi T. Prospect of in vitro heart disease model. Stem Cell Int. 2012:e439219.

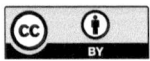

Establishment of Induced Pluripotent Stem Cells from Immortalized B Cell Lines and Their Differentiation into Cardiomyocytes

62

Emiko Hayama, Yoshiyuki Furutani, Nanako Kawaguchi,
Eiko Oomichi, Mitsuyo Shimada, Kei Inai,
and Toshio Nakanishi

Collection of peripheral blood from many patients over a long period of time has resulted in the establishment of a library composed of more than 4400 immortalized B cell lines, which have been used to identify mutated genes responsible for congenital heart defects (CHD). Because of the current progress in induced pluripotent stem cell (iPSC) technology and the ability of these iPSC lines to differentiate into cardiomyocytes, we started a project to establish an *in vitro* cardiac disease model using patient specific-iPSC-derived cardiomyocytes. As part of this project, we have established more than 20 iPSC lines from patients with CHD and from normal controls. All generated iPSC lines expressing pluripotent stem cell marker genes and proteins were alkaline phosphatase-positive. After reprogramming, the mutated genes were not altered and normal karyotypes were observed; Epstein–Barr viral genes were also not expressed. Most iPSC lines were confirmed to be able to differentiate into ectoderm, mesoderm and endoderm *in vivo*, indicating that we had successfully established iPSC lines. These iPSC lines were then induced to differentiate into cardiomyocytes. Most of these iPSC lines were observed to differentiate into beating cardiomyocytes, with some diversity in cardiomyocyte differentiation among the cell lines. In this study, we examined the effect of serial dilutions of agents on early stages of cardiomyocyte differentiation. In a floating culture system, varying concentrations of Activin A (0–10 ng/mL) and BMP4 (0–10 ng/mL) with FGF-2 (5 ng/mL) in StemPro 34 (ThermoFisher Scientific, Waltham, MA) medium

E. Hayama (✉) · Y. Furutani · N. Kawaguchi · E. Oomichi · M. Shimada · K. Inai
T. Nakanishi
Department of Pediatric Cardiology, Tokyo Women's Medical University, Tokyo, Japan
e-mail: emiko-ha@twmu.ac.jp; nakanishi.toshio@twmu.ac.jp

T. Nakanishi et al. (eds.), *Molecular Mechanism of Congenital Heart Disease and Pulmonary Hypertension*, https://doi.org/10.1007/978-981-15-1185-1_62

were used to induce mesoderm formation. The optimum concentrations of the agents for cardiomyocyte induction in iPSC lines were varied; 0–5 ng/mL Activin A and 1.25–10 ng/mL BMP4 were generally effective. We further investigated some additives for enhancement of embryoid body (EB) formation, and hyaluronate and Matrigel (BD Biosciences, San Jose, CA) addition relatively improved EB formation. Induction of functioning cardiomyocytes was associated with the ability to form appropriately sized EB in floating culture. Thus, further studies are required to improve the cell differentiation ability in some iPSC lines for establishment of stable disease models using patient-specific iPSC-derived cardiomyocytes.

Acknowledgment This work was supported in part by grants from the Japan Research Promotion Society for Cardiovascular Diseases.

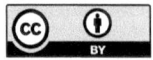

Establishment of an In Vitro LQT3 model Using Induced Pluripotent Stem Cells from LQT3 Patient-Derived Cardiomyocytes

63

Yoshiyuki Furutani, Emiko Hayama, Nanako Kawaguchi, Yasuhiro Katsube, Eiko Oomichi, Mitsuyo Shimada, Kei Inai, and Toshio Nakanishi

Cardiomyocytes derived from induced pluripotent stem cells (iPSC) are used to evaluate the function and risk factors of genetic variations linked to congenital and adult heart diseases in human beings. Our purpose in this study was to establish an in vitro cardiac disease model from an immortalized B-cell line stock using patient-specific iPSC-derived cardiomyocytes. Long QT syndrome (LQTS) 3 is caused by a gain-of-function mutation in the SCN5A gene, resulting in a prolonged QT interval as well as the development of early after-depolarizations (EADs). We generated LQT3-iPSC lines from immortalized B-cell lines transformed from peripheral blood obtained from a 24-day-old male (patient #1) and an 11-year-old female (patient #2), both diagnosed with type-3 LQTS due to SCN5A missense mutation (patient #1: exon 28, G4868A, R1623Q; patient #2: exon 20, G3578A, R1193Q). Several control iPSC lines were also created from samples collected from healthy candidates (26–36-year-old male and female). In both the generated patient iPSC lines, mutated genes were not altered after reprogramming, and normal karyotypes were observed. The pluripotency of all these iPSC lines was proven by in vivo teratoma formation and the expression of pluripotent stem cell marker genes and proteins. To evaluate the electrophysiological properties at the multicellular level, we studied the iPSC-derived cardiac cell layers with a microelectrode array mapping system (MED 64, Alpha MED Scientific Inc.). The recorded extracellular

Y. Furutani (✉) · E. Hayama · N. Kawaguchi · E. Oomichi · M. Shimada · K. Inai
T. Nakanishi
Department of Pediatric Cardiology, Tokyo Women's Medical University, Tokyo, Japan
e-mail: yfurutani@twmu.ac.jp; nakanishi.toshio@twmu.ac.jp

Y. Katsube
Department of Pediatrics, Nippon Medical School, Tokyo, Japan

393

T. Nakanishi et al. (eds.), *Molecular Mechanism of Congenital Heart Disease and Pulmonary Hypertension*, https://doi.org/10.1007/978-981-15-1185-1_63

electrograms were analyzed to measure the field-potential duration (FPD), which was normalized to account for variations in beating frequency, using Fridericia's correction (FPDcF, analogous to the QTc interval in the electrocardiogram). FPDcF was observed to be longer in LQT3 patient-derived specimens when compared to that in healthy control specimens (patient #1: $P < 0.05$, $N = 17$ and patient #2: $P < 0.0001$, $N = 19$ when compared to healthy control $N = 39$). Moreover, EADs were observed in both LQT3 patient specimens after 15–30 nM of E-4031 was added exclusively to patient samples. The results indicated that LQT3 patient iPSC-derived cardiac cells expressed prolonged QT duration (a common pathophysiological feature of LQTS) and EAD development with marked arrhythmogenicity in our in vitro disease model system.

Further Reading

Navarrete EG, Liang P, Lan F, Sanchez-Freire V, Simmons C, Gong T, Sharma A, Burridge PW, Patlolla B, Lee AS, Wu H, Beygui RE, Wu SM, Robbins RC, Bers DM, Wu JC. Screening drug-induced arrhythmia using human induced pluripotent stem cell-derived cardiomyocytes and low-impedance microelectrode arrays. Circulation. 2013;128:S3–13.

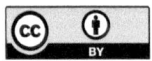

Genetic Assessments for Clinical Courses of Left Ventricle Noncompaction

64

Yoshitsugu Nogimori, Akio Kato, Kazuhisa Sato, Yosuke Kitagawa, Takuya Wakamiya, Shin Ono, Ki-Sung Kim, Sadamitsu Yanagi, and Hideaki Ueda

Keywords

Left ventricle noncompaction · *TBX 20* · *GATA 4*

Left ventricle noncompaction (LVNC) is a clinically heterogeneous disorder. Although several genetic mutations have been reported, only a little is known about its genotype–phenotype correlation. We report two cases of LVNC with different mutations and different clinical courses for each. Case 1 was a 15-year-old boy with atrial septum defect and pulmonary valve stenosis. He was diagnosed as LVNC when he was 3 years old, but his cardiac function was maintained and no medication was necessary. A 432 kb deletion in chromosome 8p 23.1, including *GATA4*, was found. Case 2 was a boy who was referred to our hospital at the age 6 for apparent right ventricle hypertrophy in electrocardiogram carried out for screening. We recognized severe pulmonary hypertension (PH) and LVNC with attenuated cardiac diastolic function and fair systolic function. In spite of medications for both heart failure and PH, the response was poor. A genetic investigation revealed a point mutation at exon 6 of *TBX20*, c.655-2A>G.

Both *GATA4* and *TBX20* have been reported to cause LVNC, but their clinical courses are not well known. Blinder et al. reported a case with *GATA4* mutation [1], presenting a normal cardiac function. While Wang et al. reported genetic pathogenic variants to be independent risk factors for adverse events [2], there may be some relatively favorable mutations as our case1 and the report by Blinder et al. *GATA4* is known as one of the earliest-expressed transcriptional factors in cardiac progenitor

Y. Nogimori (✉) · A. Kato · K. Sato · Y. Kitagawa · T. Wakamiya · S. Ono · K.-S. Kim
S. Yanagi · H. Ueda
Department of Cardiology, Kanagawa Children's Medical Center,
Yokohama, Kanagawa, Japan
e-mail: nogimori-tky@umin.ac.jp

T. Nakanishi et al. (eds.), *Molecular Mechanism of Congenital Heart Disease
and Pulmonary Hypertension*, https://doi.org/10.1007/978-981-15-1185-1_64

cells, and the expression continues throughout life in cardiomyocytes. It concerns to differentiation of myocardium together with TBX5, but how and when it affects myocardium compaction is unknown. In case 2, the severe PH could not be explained only by passive etiology, and pulmonary arterial hypertension also existed. *TBX20* is related to various cardiac disorders including cardiomyopathy, intracardiac septal defects and abnormal valvulogenesis. Although the relation between the *TBX20* mutation and PH was not clear in our case, it is interesting that Edwin et al. reported a familial case of dilated cardiomyopathy (DCM) with *TBX20* mutation with primary PH [3]. Provided that both DCM and LVNC fall in a spectrum of cardiomyopathy, association of PH might be a key to find the function of *TBX20* in these similar cases.

In summary, we report two cases of LVNC, one with *GATA4* deletion and slight symptoms and the other with *TBX20* mutation with severe PH and diastolic dysfunction, which were resistant to treatments.

References

1. Blinder JJ, et al. Noncompaction of the left ventricular myocardium in a boy with a novel chromosome 8p 23.1 deletion. Am J Med Genet. 2011;155A(9):2215–20.
2. Wang C, et al. A wide and specific spectrum of genetic variants and genotype-phenotype correlations revealed by next-generation sequencing in patients with left ventricular noncompaction. J Am Heart Assoc. 2017;6(9):e006210.
3. Edwin PK, et al. Mutations in cardiac T-Box factor gene *TBX20* are associated with diverse cardiac pathologies, including defects of septation and valvulogenesis and cardiomyopathy. Am J Hum Genet. 2007;81(2):280–91.

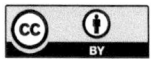

Elucidating the Pathogenesis of Congenital Heart Disease in the Era of Next-Generation Sequencing

65

Yu Nakagama and Ryo Inuzuka

Keywords

Next-generation sequencing · Whole-exome sequencing · Variant · Mutation · Congenital heart disease

Over the last decade, genetic screening has become increasingly available for patients with congenital heart disease (CHD). Chromosomal microarray has proved to be promising, particularly in the diagnosis of syndromic CHDs, and is now considered first-tier cytogenetic testing [1]. Whole-exome sequencing (WES) is another approach for genetic screening aimed towards identifying single-gene mutations [2]. Trio- and pedigree-based WES facilitate the identification of de novo and compound heterozygous variants throughout the entire coding region. Filtering of variants based on allele frequency, in silico predictions and segregation status, effectively narrows down the putative mutation. Thus, application of next-generation sequencing (NGS) has the potential of enhancing gene discovery in CHD pathogenesis.

Despite all the progress, underlying causes for the vast majority of CHDs remain unknown. The present study revealed ~1 de novo coding variant per trio by WES of a heterotaxy cohort. In a familial case of CHD, WES identified compound heterozygous, loss-of-function variants cosegregating with the phenotype [3]. Now, the major challenge lies in interpreting so-called "private" mutations that are specific to each pedigree. Distinguishing a truly causal mutation from benign variants requires well-designed functional studies. Future investigations must focus on establishing vertebrate models that recapitulate human CHD pathogenesis, based on the accumulating mutational data on CHD patients.

Y. Nakagama · R. Inuzuka (✉)

Department of Pediatrics, Graduate School of Medicine, The University of Tokyo, Tokyo, Japan

e-mail: inuzukar-tky@umin.ac.jp

T. Nakanishi et al. (eds.), *Molecular Mechanism of Congenital Heart Disease and Pulmonary Hypertension*, https://doi.org/10.1007/978-981-15-1185-1_65

Acknowledgements All work was supported by JSPS KAKENHI Grant JP16K10059. Grateful acknowledgement is rendered to Professor Seishi Ogawa, Department of Pathology and Tumor Biology, Graduate School of Medicine, Kyoto University, for support of NGS. The authors also acknowledge the Human Genome Center, Institute of Medical Science, The University of Tokyo, for providing computing resources (https://genomon-project.github.io/GenomonPagesR/).

References

1. Nakagama Y, Inuzuka R et al. Chromosomal microarray analysis for the diagnosis of Mowat-Wilson syndrome in two patients with syndromic congenital heart disease. Paper presented at the 52nd annual meeting of the Japanese Society of Pediatric Cardiology and Cardiac Surgery, Tokyo Dome Hotel, Tokyo, 6–8 July 2016.
2. Nakagama Y, Inuzuka R et al. TGA as a heterotaxy-spectrum heart defect: lessons learned from two primary ciliary dyskinesia cases with AV- or VA-discordant hearts. Paper presented at the 53rd annual meeting of the Japanese Society of Pediatric Cardiology and Cardiac Surgery, Act City Hamamatsu, Shizuoka, 7–9 July 2017.
3. Nakagama Y, Inuzuka R et al. The role of next-generation sequencing in elucidating the pathogenesis of congenital heart disease. Paper presented at the 8th TAKAO international symposium, Kunibiki Messe, Shimane, 6–8 October 2017.

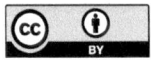

Index

© The Editor(s) (if applicable) and The Author(s) 2020
T. Nakanishi et al. (eds.), *Molecular Mechanism of Congenital Heart Disease and Pulmonary Hypertension*, https://doi.org/10.1007/978-981-15-1185-1